# ANTIGEN AND ANTIBODY MOLECULAR ENGINEERING IN BREAST CANCER DIAGNOSIS AND TREATMENT

# ADVANCES IN EXPERIMENTAL MEDICINE AND BIOLOGY

A Continuation Order Plan is available for this series. A continuation order will bring delivery of each new volume immediately upon publication. Volumes are billed only upon actual shipment. For further information please contact the publisher.

# ANTIGEN AND ANTIBODY MOLECULAR ENGINEERING IN BREAST CANCER DIAGNOSIS AND TREATMENT

Edited by

## Roberto L. Ceriani
Cancer Research Fund of Contra Costa
Walnut Creek, California

SPRINGER SCIENCE+BUSINESS MEDIA, LLC

Library of Congress Cataloging-in-Publication Data

International Workshop on Breast Cancer Research (5th : 1992 : San
  Francisco, Calif.)
    Antigen and antibody molecular engineering in breast cancer
  diagnosis and treatment / edited by Roberto L. Ceriani.
        p.    cm. -- (Advances in experimental medicine and biology ; v.
  353)
    "Proceedings of the Fifth International Workshop on Breast Cancer
  Research, held November 16-17, 1992, in San Francisco, California"-
  -T.p. verso.
    Includes bibliographical references and index.
    ISBN 978-0-306-44720-4    ISBN 978-1-4615-2443-4 (eBook)
    DOI 10.1007/978-1-4615-2443-4
    1. Breast--Cancer--Immunotherapy--Congresses. 2. Breast--Cancer-
  -Immunodiagnosis--Congresses. 3. Breast--Cancer--Molecular aspects-
  -Congresses.    I. Ceriani, Roberto L.    II. Title.    III. Series.
  RC280.B8I573    1992
  616.99'449061--dc20                                            94-7977
                                                                    CIP

Proceedings of the Fifth International Workshop on Breast Cancer Research, held
November 16–17, 1992, in San Francisco, California


ISBN 978-0-306-44720-4

© 1994 Springer Science+Business Media New York
Originally published by Plenum Press, New York in 1994

5th INTERNATIONAL WORKSHOP ON BREAST CANCER
RESEARCH AND IMMUNOLOGY

San Francisco, California
November 16-17, 1992

Organized by Cancer Research Fund of Contra Costa, with the cooperation of the
International Association for Breast Cancer Research

WORKSHOP CHAIRPERSON

Dr. Roberto L. Ceriani
Cancer Research Fund of Contra Costa

ORGANIZING COMMITTEE

| Chairperson: | Dr. Roberto L. Ceriani |
| --- | --- |
| Members: | Dr. Jerry A. Peterson |
| | Dr. Ricardo Mesa-Tejada |
| | Ms. Laura Majauskas |
| | Mr. John Weaver |

# PREFACE

Today, advances in the area of immunology and breast cancer are made at an increasing rate, yielding an amount of information that can become unwieldy. The opportunity for scientists in this area of research to gather together to exchange results and working hypotheses represents, in my belief, a very attractive proposition. With this in mind, these workshops have been convened with two year intervals for the last ten years. In each of them, selected topics have been highlighted.

The present workshop underscores the large advancements made in the molecular biology of both breast cancer associated antigens and their corresponding antibodies. Understanding the genetic information for the expression of these antigens has been recently advanced leading to preparation of molecularly engineered reagents for use in vaccination, serum assays, and immunizations for novel antibody production. In the anti-breast cancer antibody field the availability of molecular engineering approaches to humanize murine antibodies has induced intense interest in the creation of less immunogenic antibody forms that are now available for clinical testing. Clinical studies using anti-breast murine antibody continue to be carried out and are presented at this meeting establishing a base line for safety and efficaciousness in imaging and immunotherapy that it is hoped will be superseded by the humanized forms.

Basic immunology and immunochemistry studies in breast cancer are also included in this workshop that demonstrate the fast pace at which this research is advancing in many laboratories worldwide. These seminal immunological studies are now being translated into new approaches for diagnosis, prognosis and immunotherapy in breast cancer also included in this workshop.

The international character of this workshop has to be emphasized. Also, it must be mentioned the clearing house function for studies in breast cancer immunology that this and former meetings of this series have had. Original observations of the early eighties have now developed into entire systems that represent the scope of the work of individual laboratories. Overall, the introduction of elaborate molecular engineering technology to this field of study has helped validate early research postulates and achieve goals considered before to be insurmountable. The excitement generated by the opportunities now available to us, I am sure, will help maintain the present day high level of achievement and induce us to consider our ultimate research goal achievable, the management and eventual cure of breast cancer.

R.L. Ceriani

ACKNOWLEDGEMENTS

The Organizing Committee for the 5th International Workshop on Breast Cancer Research and Immunology, together with the Cancer Research Fund of Contra Costa, gratefully acknowledge the support of the following in making the Workshop possible:

SPONSORS

COULTER Immunology
CIBA-GEIGY
BRISTOL-MYERS SQUIBB
Lily Research Laboratories
DuPont
Burroughs Wellcome Company
Abbott Laboratories
Mt. Diablo Medical Center
American Speedy Printing
Toys 2 Go (Discovery Toys) - Judy Corley

# CONTENTS

## SESSION III

# BREAST MUCIN AND ASSOCIATED ANTIGENS IN DIAGNOSIS AND THERAPY

Jerry A. Peterson and Roberto L. Ceriani

Cancer Research Fund of Contra Costa
2055 North Broadway
Walnut Creek, CA 94596

## INTRODUCTION

The human milk fat globule (HMFG) membrane has been the source of antigens for the production of polyclonal and monoclonal antibodies against normal and malignant breast epithelial cells that have found important applications in diagnosis and therapy of breast cancer (Ceriani et al., 1977). Monoclonal antibodies (MoAbs) prepared against the HMFG membrane, for the first time, identified a highly glycosylated, large molecular weight glycoprotein (breast mucin) as a major component of the surface membrane of breast epithelial cells (Ceriani et al., 1983). In addition, MoAbs against smaller glycoproteins of the HMFG have identified new and potentially important components of breast epithelial cell membranes, namely two glycoproteins of 70 kDa and a 46 kDa, respectively (Ceriani et al., 1983; Peterson et al., 1990). The 70 kDa glycoprotein (BA70) has been shown to be associated with the breast mucin by disulfide linkages, suggesting it to be a putative linker protein (Duwe et al., 1989) for the breast mucin. The 46 kDa glycoprotein (BA46) appears to be a member of a family of proteins having a domain with homology with the C1C2 domain of human coagulation factors V and VIII (Larocca et al., 1991). In this paper we will summarize the characteristics of the breast mucin and the 46 kDa antigen, present evidence on their epitopic heterogeneity, and suggest possible molecular strategy for selecting the most appropriate MoAbs for use in breast cancer diagnosis and therapy.

## THE BREAST MUCIN AND EPITOPIC HETEROGENEITY OF THE TANDEM REPEAT

The breast mucin appears to be a highly immunogenic surface antigen on breast epithelial cell membranes, since it is the antigen recognized by the vast majority of MoAbs developed against both breast carcinoma cells and HMFG. Moreover, nearly all the MoAbs that recognize the polypeptide core of this highly glycosylated mucin

*Antigen and Antibody Molecular Engineering in Breast Cancer Diagnosis*
*and Treatment*, Edited by R.L. Ceriani, Plenum Press, New York, 1994

1

have been found to be against an immunodominant region of 20 amino acid tandem repeat domain (Burchell et al., 1989). The entire cDNA for the breast mucin has been sequenced and found to code for a polypeptide containing a long central domain of a variable number of these 20 amino acid tandem repeats (20-80), a N-terminal region containing a signal peptide sequence, and a C-terminal region containing a putative transmembrane domain (Gendler et al., 1990; Wreschner et al., 1990; Ligtenberg et al., 1990). Cloning of the cDNA for the pancreatic mucin has revealed a virtually identical core protein (Lan et al., 1990). The tandem repeat domain is rich in serine and threonine and contains multiple O-linked glycosylation sites that is typical of mucins. The difference between the breast mucin and the pancreatic mucin appears to be in the type and degree of glycosylation, since the breast mucin is approximately 50% carbohydrate and the pancreatic mucin is 80% carbohydrate. MoAbs against the pancreatic mucin usually identify carbohydrate epitopes, while many MoAbs against the breast mucin, especially those against the core protein, do not react with pancreas. Secretory epithelial cells from other tissues, such as ovary, lung, salivary gland, and sebaceous gland, also appear to contain this cell-associated mucin coded by the gene MUC-1 (Peat et al., 1992), and also appear to exhibit tissue specific glycosylation patterns.

It has also become evident that breast carcinomas differ considerably from normal breast in their glycosylation patterns, usually being less glycosylated than in the normal gland. This has resulted in the development of MoAbs with a certain degree of tumor specificity when they recognize polypeptide epitopes that are masked on the fully glycosylated mucin. A similar situation must also exist in other tissues, such as in the case of ovary where many MoAbs against the breast mucin core protein that bind strongly with normal breast epithelial cells and breast carcinomas do not react with normal ovary but do react with ovarian carcinomas (Peterson et al., 1990).

This breast mucin is also secreted by breast carcinomas and has provided the basis for serum assays in breast cancer patients (Nicolini et al., 1991; Ceriani et al., 1992). The mechanism by which the breast mucin is released into circulation has not yet been clearly resolved; however, there is evidence that it may be due to variation in mRNA splicing that results in two different mRNAs, one of which codes for a membrane-associated mucin that contains the transmembrane region, and a secreted mucin lacking the transmembrane region (Hareuveni et al., 1991). An alternative mechanism has also been proposed that involves the cellular release of the mucin as the result of proteolytic cleavage (Hilkens et al., 1988). The role of these two mechanisms in the appearance of circulating antigen has not yet been clearly resolved.

In this paper we present evidence that there are important differences between the secreted and cell-associated breast mucin, and that MoAbs recognizing different epitope structures on the tandem repeat can have significantly different potentials for detecting circulating antigen, and for tumor localization and therapy. A large number of MoAbs against the breast mucin have been shown to bind to overlapping amino acid sequences in the most hydrophilic region of the tandem repeat (Table 1). Their epitopes comprise various combinations of an 8 amino acid sequence (Table 1). In spite of this, they exhibit considerable difference in their binding in immunohistochemistry among both normal and tumor tissue (Peterson et al., 1990), and exhibit cell heterogeneity of expression among and within breast tumors (Ceriani et al., 1984). This epitope heterogeneity is apparently due to alterations in glycosylation that occurs in breast carcinomas. In order to investigate this we have analysed the epitopes of two MoAbs (Mc5 and BrE3), that differ considerably in their effectiveness in breast cancer therapy (radioimmunotherapy) and diagnosis (serum assays). Epitope mapping of the polypeptide epitopes of Mc5 and BrE3 on the tandem repeat region of the breast mucin reveals that they have overlapping linear amino acid sequences of DTRPAP and TRP in their epitopes (Table 1) (Peterson et al., 1991). In spite of this, the binding affinity of Mc5 is significantly affected by the degree of glycosylation of the breast mucin, in that, the affinity on the fully glycosylated, mature breast mucin isolated from HMFG is significantly higher (disassociation constant; $3.63 \times 10^{-9}$) than on the deglycosylated mucin (hydrogen floride method) ($1.62 \times 10^{-8}$) or on the nonglycosylated core protein produce in bacteria as a fusion protein ($1.0 \times 10^{-7}$) (Larocca et al., 1992). This indicates that oligosaccharide structures on the mature mucin are either part of the Mc5 epitope or glycosylation alters the polypeptide configuration to yield the highest affinity epitope on the breast mucin. In contrast, the affinity constant for BrE3 is not affected by the degree of glycosylation; being $1.66 \times 10^{-8}$ for the mature mucin, $1.56 \times 10^{-8}$ for the deglycosylated mucin, and $1.15 \times 10^{-8}$ for the fusion protein. MoAb Mc5 binds strongly to both normal breast (though only apical staining) and breast carcinomas (membrane and cytoplasmic staining), while BrE3 binds strongly to breast carcinomas (both surface and cytoplasmic, preferentially the latter), but only weakly to normal breast epithelial cells.

**Table 1.** MoAbs that react with the breast mucin core polypeptide and have defined epitopes on the tandem repeat.

| MoAb | Antigen for Immunization | Epitope TSAPDTRPAPGST |
|---|---|---|
| Mc5 | HMFG | TRPAP |
| M15 | Mucin peptide | TRPA |
| BrE2 | HMFG | TRP |
| BrE3 | HMFG | TRP |
| DF3 | Breast Ca | TRP |
| RINA 1/8 | T47D | DTRPA |
| 139H2 | HMFG | PDTRPA |
| B27.29 | Milk mucin | DTRPAP |
| HMFG-1 | HMFG | PDTRP |
| EMA | Br Ca | PDTRP |
| BrE1 | HMFG | DTRP |
| Mc1 (HMFG2) | HMFG-milk cells | DTR |
| RINA 5/2 | T47D cells | DTRPA |
| RINA 9/22 | T47D cells | DTRPA |
| SM3 | deglycos. mucin | PDTRP |
| F36/22 | MCF7 cells | RPAP |

Competition studies demonstrate a heterogeneity of the glycosylation pattern of the tandem repeat region of the breast mucin (Figure 1). When MoAb Mc5 was labeled with $^{125}$I, cold unlabeled Mc5 competed for binding to the native breast mucin, while cold BrE3 did not (Figure 1). In contrast, on a synthetic peptide of the tandem repeat, competition was seen between Mc5 and BrE3 (Figure 1). Analogous results are obtained when BrE3 is labeled and competed with BrE3 and Mc5 on the native mucin and synthetic peptide (results not shown). These results demonstrate a heterogeneity in the glycosylation pattern of the tandem repeat resulting in distinct epitopes for Mc5 and BrE3, some epitopes being more glycosylated and binding Mc5, while other regions are less glycosylated and bind BrE3.

Since both Mc5 and BrE3 bind strongly to breast carcinomas, they both were considered candidates for use in MoAb therapy. One advantage of the tandem repeat domain as a target for MoAb therapy is its polyepitopic nature. Because of the cell heterogeneity of expression of such epitopes on breast carcinoma cells, we have emphasized the use of radioimmunotherapy, since every cell need not bind the MoAb for achieving cytotoxicity for the localized tumor (Ceriani et al., 1988). Since Mc5 was shown to be highly effective in preclinical studies using human breast carcinomas transplanted in immunodefficient mice (Ceriani et al., 1990), it was prepared for the first human clinical imaging trials. Twelve breast cancer patients were injected with [131]I-labeled Mc5; however, with only one patient was there any significant imaging of the metastatic disease. In an effort to explain this lack of imaging, serum levels of the Mc5 epitope on circulating antigen were determined, and it was found that all patients had high levels of the Mc5 epitope in their serum. In contrast, in the same serum samples from these patients, the level of the BrE3 epitope was 5-10 fold lower (Table 2). Subsequently, clinical imaging trials were initiated with BrE3, but this time labeled with [111]In via a MXDTPA chelate (Kramer et al., 1993). In this case very successful imaging was obtained, where 86% of all known lesions were localized (Kramer et al., 1993). The most straight forward interpretation of these results is that the cell-associated mucin is less glycosylated than that which is released into circulation. Thus, BrE3, which identifies a less glycosylated mucin is better for therapy, while Mc5, which identifies the more glycosylated mucin that is released into circulation, is better as a diagnostic reagent for construction of serum assays (Ceriani et al., 1992).

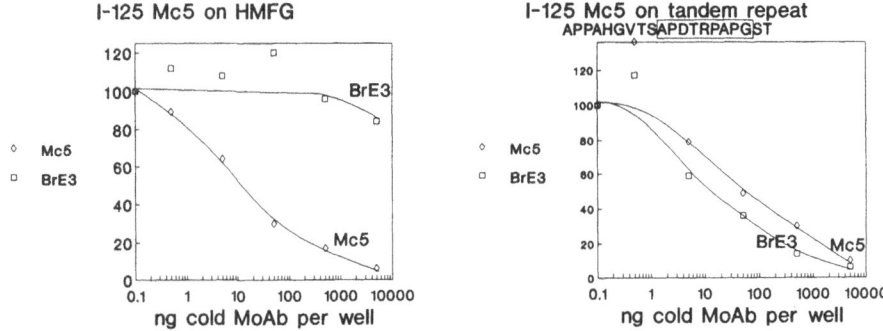

**Figure 1.** Competition between monoclonal antibodies Mc5 and BrE3 for binding to the fully glycosylated breast mucin in the human milk fat globule (HMFG) membrane and to a synthetic peptide of the 20 amino acid tandem repeat. MoAb Mc5 was labelled with [125]I and added to microtiter plates containing the respective antigens bound to the solid phase in the presence of different concentration of unlabeled Mc5 or BrE3 and incubated overnight. The plates were then washed and then the bound radioactivity determined.

Another difference between Mc5 and BrE3 epitopes is that the latter appears to be on a molecular form of the breast mucin that in internalized, while that of Mc5 is not. This is suggested by results from studies of toxin-conjugate MoAbs (Derbyshire et al., 1992). They compared the cytotoxicity of Ricin A chain-conjugated Mc5 and BrE3 on lung carcinoma cells and found that the BrE3 conjugate was highly toxic, while that of Mc5 was not. No toxicity was seen on a lymphoblastoid cell line. This is further evidence that there are different molecular forms of the breast mucin (possibly different mRNA splice variants of glycosylated forms), some that are internalized and some that are not. This ability of BrE3 to be internalized may also contribute to its ability to localize breast tumors in patients compared to Mc5 by increasing the retention time of the radiolabelled antibody chelate in the tumor.

**Table 2.** Comparison of levels of Mc5 and BrE3 epitopes in serum of breast cancer patients.

| Patient Sample | Epitope content ($\mu$g/ml) | |
| --- | --- | --- |
| | Mc5 | BrE3 |
| 001 | 260.0 | 20.6 |
| 002 | 86.7 | 0.54 |
| 003 | 6.9 | 0.12 |
| 004 | 3.2 | 0.36 |
| 005 | 117.0 | 10.8 |
| 006 | 15.2 | 0.24 |
| 007 | 5.6 | 1.2 |
| 008 | 319.5 | 59.5 |
| 009 | 9.6 | 4.7 |
| 010 | 1.92 | 0.42 |
| 011 | 82.9 | 10.2 |
| 012 | 15.3 | 4.8 |

## THE BA46 GLYCOPROTEIN IN BREAST CANCER THERAPY AND DIAGNOSIS

A novel antigen that we have identified in the human milk fat globule membrane and in breast epithelial cells is a 46 kDa glycoprotein that is recognized by four MoAbs: Mc3, Mc8, Mc15, and Mc16 (Peterson et al., 1990). We have isolated and sequenced a partial cDNA clone and found that it falls into a family of molecules with homology to the C1C2 domain of human coagulation factors V and VIII (43% and 38% respectively) (Larocca et al., 1991). Other proteins that have homology with the C1C2 domain of factors V and VIII include a neuronal recognition molecule (A5 antigen) of Xenopus (Takagi et al., 1991), discoidin I of *Dictyostelium discoideum* (Poole et al., 1981), a receptor tyrosine kinase with an extracellular discoidin I-like domain (Johnson et al., 1993), a 63/55 kDa glycoprotein of the mouse milk fat globule (Stubbs et al., 1990), and components 15/16 and GP55 of bovine and guinea-pig milk fat globule, respectively (Mather et al., 1993). The greatest homology is seen with the mouse milk fat globule antigen (63%), which was found to have an EGF-like sequence on the N-terminal end of the protein (Stubbs et al., 1990). The C1C2 domain of coagulation factors V and VIII appears to be involved in phospholipid binding, a necessary interaction involved in coagulation (Ortel et al., 1992). However, the function of the C-type domains in the other proteins is not known, though it may provide a novel means for association with cell membranes (Larocca et al., 1991).

MoAbs against BA46 were found to be useful in both breast cancer diagnosis and therapy in preclinical studies, but as with MoAbs against the breast mucin, they differed in their effectiveness. Both Mc3 and Mc8 recognized the antigen in circulation of breast cancer patients (Ceriani et al., 1982); however, Mc8 was more effective in recognizing immune complexes in such patients, where an increase in level correlated with tumor load (Salinas et al., 1987). With regard to breast cancer therapy, Mc3 was found to be highly effective in localizing breast tumors in immunodeficient mice, where as much as 72% dose per gram was found in the transplanted tumors. Also, in experimental radioimmunotherapy studies using $^{131}$I labelled MoAbs, Mc3 was much more effective than Mc8 (Figure 2). Furthermore, $^{90}$Y-labeled Mc3 was superior to the $^{131}$I conjugate, since 6/7 of the animals were cured of their transplanted tumors when injected with $^{90}$Y-Mc3, while none of the 6 animals treated with $^{131}$I-Mc3 were cured, though there was a significant reduction in tumor growth (Figure 2).

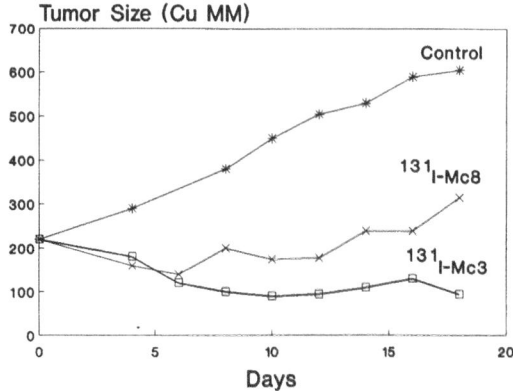

**Figure 2.** Comparison of radioimmunotherapy of human breast carcinomas transplanted in immunodeficient mice between two MoAbs, Mc3 and Mc8 against the BA46 glycoprotein. Groups of 6 mice carrying established tumors were each injected with 1500 microcuries of the $^{131}$I-labeled antibody and tumor volume (mm$^3$) measured. Control mice were uninjected.

Epitope mapping of the 53 amino acid sequence in the C2-like region of the derived amino acid sequence of BA46 cDNA (Larocca et al., 1991) identified the epitopes of Mc8 and Mc16 as DPRTG and SSKIF, respectively. Neither Mc3 nor Mc15 mapped in this region, thus they must bind to other portions of the molecule or to oligosaccharide structures of this glycoprotein. The BA46 antigen has 4 potential N-linked glycosylation sites and numerous O-linked glycosylation sites. Further epitope mapping of the entire BA46 cDNA is now underway to determine the epitope of the latter MoAbs.

These results demonstrate, that with two different breast epithelial antigens, the breast mucin and BA46 antigen, different epitopes on the same molecule can have considerable differences in their effectiveness as targets for radioimmunotherapy and also for development of serum assays for breast cancer diagnosis. In the case of the breast mucin, these differences are probably due to alterations in glycosylation that occur in breast carcinoma cells, but also can be due to the polymorphic nature of the mucin and its different mRNA splice variants. In the case of the BA46 glycoprotein, these difference could be also due to differential glycosylation; however, it can also be due to binding of the MoAbs to different functional domains of the molecule. Once the epitopic structures are determined that provide the best target for MoAb-guided therapy or detection of antigen in circulation, such structures can be made by either recombinant techniques or synthetically for production of new generation MoAbs.

# ACKNOWLEDGEMENTS

This work was supported in part by NIH grants CA39936, CA39932, and CA42767.

# REFERENCES

Burchell, J.M., Taylor-Papadimitriou, J., Boshell, M., Gendler, S.J., and Duhig, T., 1989, A short sequence, within the amino acid tandem repeat of a cancer-associated mucin, contains immunodominant epitopes, *Int. J. Cancer* 44:691.

Ceriani, R.L., Thompson, K., Peterson, J.A., and Abraham, S., 1977, Surface differentiation antigens of human mammary epithelial cells carried on the human milk fat globule, *Proc. Natl. Acad. Sci. USA* 74:582.

Ceriani, R.L., Sasaki, M., Sussman, H., Wara, W.M., and Blank, E.W., 1982, Circulating human mammary epithelial antigens in breast cancer, *Proc. Natl. Acad. Sci. USA* 79:5420.

Ceriani, R.L., Peterson, J.A., Lee, J.Y., Moncada, R., and Blank, E.W., 1983, Characterization of cell surface antigens of human mammary epithelial cells with monoclonal antibodies prepared against human milk fat globule, *Somatic. Cell Genet.* 9:415.

Ceriani, R.L., Peterson, J.A., and Blank, E.W., 1984, Variability in surface antigen expression of human breast epithelial cells cultured from normal breast, normal breast peripheral to breast carcinomas, and breast carcinomas, *Cancer Res.* 44:3033.

Ceriani, R.L. and Blank, E.W., 1988, Experimental therapy of human breast tumors with 131I-labeled monoclonal antibodies prepared against the human milk fat globule, *Cancer Res.* 48:4664.

Ceriani, R.L., Blank, E.W., Peterson, J.A., Battifora, H., and Singh, H., 1990, Immunotherapeutic preclinical evaluation of anti-human milk fat globule MoAbs Mc5 and BrE-1, *Antibody Immunoconj. Radiopharm.* 3:181.

Ceriani, R.L., Larocca, D., Peterson, J.A., Enloe, S., Amiya, R., and Blank, E.W., 1992, A novel serum assay for breast epithelial antigen using a fusion protein, *Anal. Biochem.* 201:178.

Derbyshire, E.J. and Wawrzynczak, E.J., 1992, An anti-mucin immunotoxin BrE-3-ricin A-chain is potently and selectively toxic to human small-cell lung cancer, *Int. J Cancer* 52:624.

Duwe, A.K. and Ceriani, R.L., 1989, Human milk fat globule membrane derived mucin is a disulfide-linked heteromer, *Biochem. Biophys. Res Commun.* 165:1305.

Gendler, S.J., Lancaster, C.A., Taylor-Papadimitriou, J., Duhig, T., Peat, N., Burchell, J.M., Pemberton, L., Lalani, E.N., and Wilson, D., 1990, Molecular cloning and expression of human tumor-associated polymorphic epithelial mucin, *J. Biol. Chem.* 265:15286.

Hareuveni, M., Wreschner, D.H., Kieny, M.P., Dott, K., Gautier, C., Tomasetto, C., Keydar, I., Chambon, P., and Lathe, R., 1991, Vaccinia recombinants expressing secreted and transmembrane forms of breast cancer-associated epithelial tumour antigen (ETA), *Vaccine* 9:618.

Hilkens, J. and Buijs, F., 1988, Biosynthesis of MAM-6, an epithelial sialomucin. Evidence for involvement of a rare proteolytic cleavage step in the endoplasmic reticulum, *J Biol Chem* 263:4215.

Johnson, J.D., Edman, J.C., and Rutter, W.J., 1993, A receptor Tyrosine kinase found in breast carcinoma cells has an extracellular discoidin I-like domain, *Proc. Natl. Acad. Sci. USA* 90:5677.

Kramer, E.L., DeNardo, S.J., Liebes, L., Kroger, L.A., Noz, M.E.G., Mizrachi, H., Salako, Q.A., Furmanski, P., Glenn, S.D., DeNardo, G.L., and Ceriani, R.L., 1993, Radioimmunolocalization of metastatic breast carcinoma using Indium-111-methyl benzyl DTPA BrE-3 monoclonal antibody: Phase 1 study, *J. Nucl. Med.* 34:1067.

Lan, M.S., Batra, S.K., Qi, W.N., Metzgar, R.S., and Hollingsworth, M.A., 1990, Cloning and sequencing of a human pancreatic tumor mucin cDNA, *J. Biol. Chem.* 265:15294.

Larocca, D., Peterson, J.A., Bistrain, A., Urrea, R., Kuniyoshi, J., and Ceriani, R.L., 1991, A 46 KDa human milk fat globule glycoprotein that is highly expressed in carcinoma cells has homology with human clotting factors V and VIII, *Cancer Res.* 51:4994.

Larocca, D., Peterson, J.A., and Ceriani, R.L., 1992, High level expression in E. coli of an alternate reading frame of pS2 mRNA that encodes a mimotope of human breast epithelial mucin tandem repeat, *Hybridoma* 11:191.

Ligtenberg, M.J.L., Vos, H.L., Gennissen, A.M.C., and Hilkens, J., 1990, Episialin, a carcinoma-associated mucin, is generated by a polymorphic gene encoding splice variants with alternative amino termini, *J. Biol. Chem.* 265:5573.

Mather, I.H., Banghart, L.R., and Lane, W.S., 1993, The major fat-globule membrane proteins, bovine components 15/16 and guinea-pig GP 55, are homologous to MGF-E8, a murine glycoprotein containing epidermal growth factor-like and factor V/VIII-like sequences, *Biochem. Mol. Biol Int.* 29:545.

Nicolini, A., Colombini, C., Luciani, L., Carpi, A., and Giuliani, L., 1991, Evaluation of serum CA15-3 determination with CEA and TPA in the post-operative follow-up of breast cancer patients, *Br. J. Cancer* 64:154.

Ortel, T., Devore-Carter, D., Quinn-Allen, M., and Kane, W.H., 1992, Deletion analysis of recombinant human factor V. Evidence for a phosphotidylserine binding site in the second C-type domain, *J Biol. Chem.* 267:4189.

Peat, N., Gendler, S.J., Lalani, N., Duhig, T., and Taylor-Papadimitriou, J., 1992, Tissue-specific expression of a human polymorphic epithelial mucin (MUC1) in transgenic mice, *Cancer Res.* 52:1954.

Peterson, J.A., Zava, D.T., Duwe, A.K., Blank, E.W., Battifora, H., and Ceriani, R.L., 1990, Biochemical and histological characterization of antigens preferentially expressed on the surface and cytoplasm of breast carcinoma cells identified by monoclonal antibodies against the human milk fat globule, *Hybridoma* 9:221.

Peterson, J.A., Larocca, D., Walkup, G., Amiya, R., and Ceriani, R.L., 1991, Molecular analysis of epitope heterogeneity of the breast mucin. *in:* "Breast Epithelial Antigens: Molecular Biology to Clinical Applications," R.L. Ceriani, ed., Plenum Publications, New York, p. 55.

Poole, S., Firtel, R.A., and Lamar, E., 1981, Sequence and expression of the discoidin I gene family in dictyostelium discoideum, *J. Mol. Biol.* 153:273.

Salinas, F.A., Wee, K.H., and Ceriani, R.L., 1987, Significance of breast carcinoma-associated antigens as a monitor of tumor burden: characterization by monoclonal antibodies, *Cancer Res.* 47:907.

Stubbs, J.D., Lekutis, C., Singer, K.L., Bui, A., Yuzuki, D., Srinivasan, U., and Parry, G., 1990, cDNA cloning of a mouse mammary epithelial cell surface protein reveals the existence of epidermal growth factor-like domains linked to factor VIII-like sequences, *Proc. Natl. Acad. Sci. USA* 87:8417.

Takagi, S., Hirata, T., Agata, K., Mochii, M., Eguchi, G., and Fujisawa, H., 1991, The A5 antigen, a candidate for the neuronal recognition molecule, has homologies to complement components and coagulation factors, *Neuron* 7:295.

Wreschner, D.H., Hareuveni, M., Tsarfaty, I., Smorodinsky, N., Horev, J., Zaretsky, J., Kotkes, P., Weiss, M., Lathe, R., Dion, A., and Keydar, I., 1990, Human epithelial tumor antigen cDNA sequences, *Eur. J. Biochem.* 189:463.

8

# PEPTIDE EPITOPES IN BREAST CANCER MUCINS

Pei-Xiang Xing, Vasso Apostolopoulos, Joe Trapani,
Julie Prenzoska, and Ian F.C. McKenzie

The Austin Research Institute
The Austin Hospital
Heidelberg VIC 3084
Australia

## INTRODUCTION

Major advances have occured in the structural analysis of mucins found in breast cancer following the isolation of cDNAs and the gene for MUC1 - which is the predominant mucin expressed in breast cancer[1-4]. In addition, other genes coding for mucins have been identified which are expressed in a variety of tissues, and are also found in breast tissue and to a lesser extent in breast cancer (particularly MUC2 and MUC3)[5,6]. It was of interest that these genes were isolated using polyclonal antibodies and bacterial expression libraries, indicating that the active antibodies were detecting a non-glycosylated linear peptide, and this prediction was proven by the finding that many existing anti-MUC1 monoclonal antibodies react with synthetic peptides. The focus of this review will be to determine whether: a) monoclonal antibodies made against tumors react with peptides and what epitopes are detected (particularly for MUC1); b) if anti-peptide antibodies can be made which react with cancers (MUC1, 2, 3); c) second generation antibodies can be made to fusion proteins (MUC1); d) and what epitopes are detected with all of these antibodies; e) finally, what are the implications of these new advances in the diagnosis and treatment of breast cancer.

## MATERIALS AND METHODS

Monoclonal antibodies were produced by standard procedure[7]; peptides were synthesized using either the solid phase ABI synthesiser[8], or using the pepscan method whereby 6 peptides are synthesized on polyethylene pins[9]. Using the solid phase method, the peptides can be made in large amounts, cleaved and used in various serological assays.

*Antigen and Antibody Molecular Engineering in Breast Cancer Diagnosis*
*and Treatment*, Edited by R.L. Ceriani, Plenum Press, New York, 1994

For the pepscan method, the peptides remain attached to the pin for an ELISA test (recently cleavage of these peptides has also been described). The testing of antibodies on peptides used an ELISA test with the peptides either bound to a microplate (solid phase) conjugated to bovine serum albumin using either solid phase or in solution as inhibition tests or using the peptides synthesised on the pins[9,10]. As has been noted in the past, slightly different results occur with each of these 4 methods[11]. Longer peptides were also made as fusion proteins wherein 5 VNTR repeats of MUC1 were made using the pGEX system[12]. Immunoperoxidase staining has been described elsewhere[5].

## RESULTS AND DISCUSSION

### Anti-Mucin1 Antibodies Can React With Synthetic Peptides

Our Laboratory participated in the First International Workshop on Mucins, wherein antibodies including (BC1, BC2, BC3, HMPV, 4B6, CC2, CC3 and 3E1.2) were tested for their reaction on synthetic peptides. These antibodies had been made either against breast cancer or HMFG. Of the 8, 5 (BC1, BC2, BC3, HMPV and 4B6) were found to react with the synthetic peptides - thus approximately, half the antibodies made to breast cancer mucin, and which react with HMFG, react with a linear peptide (Table 1). When epitope mapping studies were performed on these antibodies, either in our laboratory or elsewhere, it was demonstrated that the highly immunogeneic APDTRP epitope was detected by virtually all the Mabs (Table 1). By conventional hydrophilicity analysis this epitope was predicted to be the most immunogenic, and indeed has been proven so by the reactions of antibodies produced by many different immunizing regimes. It was of interest that we found no antibodies reacting with N-terminal or C-terminal peptides of MUC1. While the observations essentially proved that small linear peptides are immunogenic, the analysis of the existing anti-tumor antibodies - some of which are currently being used in serum tests, for imaging and for therapy, is some of the most sophisticated analysis of epitopes in cancer research. However, if this has any implications for improved diagnosis or therapy remains to be seen!

### Synthetic Peptides To Produce Second Generation Antibodies To MUC1

Two different types of experiments were performed, using synthetic peptides and a fusion protein[7,12]. A synthetic peptide C-p13-32 (CPAHGVTSAPDTRPAPGSTAP) was made. It will be noted that the APDTR sequence is in the centre of this peptide - a site we have found to be most immunogenic. The cysteine at the N-terminal end was used as a potential site for conjugation to a carrier, but also served as a site for the spontaneous formation of dimers[11]. Four antibodies (BCP7,8,9,10) were made and are described in detail elsewhere[7], the major features will be summarized here: a) only BCP-8 reacted with formalin fixed tissue - BCP7,9&10 reacted only with fresh tissue (a finding in keeping with the peptide nature of the epitopes which tend to be destroyed by formalin); b) in

**Table 1.** Epitopes recognised by mAbs tested by overlapping peptides.

| | IMMUNOGEN | P A H G V T S A P D T R P A P G S T A P |
|---|---|---|
| BCP7 | C-P13-32 | V T S A |
| BCP8 | C-P13-32 | D T R |
| BCP9 | C-P13-32 | G S T A P |
| BCP10 | C-P13-32 | R P A P |
| BC1 | HMFG | A P D T R |
| BC2 | HMFG | A P D T R |
| BC3 | HMFG | A P D T R |
| HMPV | HMFG AND p1-24 | A P D T R |
| 4B6 | HMFG | (P) D T R |
| OM1 | Ovarian Cancer Cells | D T R P (A) |
| SM3 | Stripped HMFG | P D T R P |
| HMFG1 | HMFG | P D T R (P A) |
| HMFG2 | HMFG | D T R |
| NCRC11 | | R P A P |
| ONC-M15 | | T R P A |
| EMA | | T R P A P |
| F36/22 | | R P A P |
| VA1 | Fusion protein | A P G |
| VA2 | Fusion protein | D T R P A |

**Table 2.** Reactivity of anti-peptide and fusion protein antibodies on breast tissue

| Antibodies | Imunogens | Breast cancer | Normal Breast | Epitopes detected |
|---|---|---|---|---|
| *MUC1* | | | | |
| BCP7 | C-p13-32[1] | ++++ | ++ | VTSA |
| BCP8 | C-p13-32 | ++++ | ++ | DTR |
| BCP9 | C-p13-32 | ++ | - | GSTAP |
| BCP10 | C-p13-32 | ++ | - | RPAP |
| VA1 | Fusion protein[2] | ++++ | ++ | APG |
| VA2 | Fusion protein | ++++ | - | DTRPA |
| *MUC2* | | | | |
| CCP31 | MI-29[3] | - | + | STTT |
| CCP37 | MI-29 | - | + | PTT |
| CCP38 | MI-29 | - | + | TGTQTP |
| *MUC3* | | | | |
| M3.1 | SIB-35[4] | ++ | + | SITTTE |
| M3.2 | SIB-35 | ++ | + | NOT KNOWN |
| M3.3 | SIB-35 | - | - | PSFTSS |

[1]MUC1 VNTR peptide:cPAHGVTSAPDTRPAPGSTAP.
[2]Containiing 5 VNTR repeats of MUC1.
[3]MUC2 VNTR peptide: KYPTTTPISTTTMVTPTPTPTGTQTPTTT.
[4]MUC3 VNTR peptide: CHSTPSFTSSITTTETTSHSTPSFTSSITTTETTS.

general, the antibodies resemble those made against breast cancer or native mucin in their tissue reactivity - particularly BCP8 (Table 2);  c) some of the antibodies gave a much stronger reaction on breast cancer tissue than on normal breast, and indeed, BCP9 and 10 were non-reactive on normal breast tissue. Whether this is a manifestation of low antibody affinity, or reflects the real distribution of the epitope, has yet to be established, but the finding is important, as these reagents differentiate between cancer and normal tissue better than most other anti-mucin antibodies. In this light, they resemble the reactions of the SM-3 antibody made to deglycosylated HMFG[13]; d) a variety of epitopes were detected including the APDTR with BCP8, and others summarized in Table 1. The significance of antibodies detecting different epitopes is not clear, for if one immunizes with a peptide, a whole range of epitopes can be detected.

In addition to these studies, we asked whether the threonine in the native APDTR was glycosylated. by examining synthetic peptides and determing whether threonine could be substituted with any of the other 19 amino acids, and still give reactivity with the anti-peptide antibody BCP8. Essentially, only one other substitution, Q for T, could be made; all other substitutions destroyed the activity and therefore it was clear that for BCP8, threonine (T) was a crucial amino acid in the epitope. By contrast, using an antibody made against native mucin and which also reacts with the APDTR peptide, virtually any amino acid could be used in place of T. Thus, for an anti-native mucin antibody, T was not a crucial part of the epitope - perhaps because it is glycosylated[11]. However, this evidence is indirect and it requires definitive studies on the direct glycosylation of threonine to prove this - studies that are in progress in other laboratories.

# A Fusion Protein To Produce Second Generation Antibodies To MUC1

Other laboratories have used the "MAP" technique where branches occur and a repeating peptide can be produced[14]. However, a limited number of repeats occur, and for this reason we produced a 5 repeat fusion protein using the pGEX system and immunised with this[12]. Two antibodies were produced, VA1 and VA2[12], their characteristics are summarised in Table 2. VA2 appeared to be specific for breast cancer and gave no reaction on normal tissues, whereas VA1 reacted strongly with breast cancer and gave a weaker reaction on normal breast. These antibodies react with different epitopes (Table 2) and could prove useful, particularly for imaging or therapeutic purposes.

# Second Generation Antibodies To MUC2

The cDNA encoding the variable number of tandem repeats (VNTR) from MUC2 was recently isolated[15], and using the translated sequence from this, a peptide was synthesised (Table 2) and ultimately monoclonal antibodies made (Table 2). The Northern analysis in the original report indicated predominant expression in gastrointestinal tract (the cDNA clone was isolated from a λgt11 library from the intestine), but some reaction with lung and breast RNA was described; our monoclonal antibodies confirm these reactions[16]. In gastrointestinal tract we noted some differential expression of MUC2 between cancer and normal tissue, but not as much as the 10-fold increase in MUC1 expression in breast cancer[17]. MUC2 was also found in normal breast tissue, but, there was no staining of breast cancer tissue. The epitopes of these antibodies were mapped using the pepscan method (Table 2). It is of interest to note that in contrast to MUC1 where the most highly immunogeneic epitopes were also the most hydrophilic, with MUC2, there was essentially no hydrophilic region[18]. Thus, MUC2 is found in breast tissue and the expression appears to be <u>decreased</u> in normal and malignant breast tissues.

# Second Generation Antibodies To MUC3

MUC3 is a distinct gene found on a different chromosome to MUC1 and 2, but having the same basic structure of VNTRs[19]. Similar studies were performed with MUC3 as described above for MUC2 ie. monoclonal antibodies made, the tissue distribution performed, and the epitopes mapped (Table 2). Again the predominant reaction was with gastrointestinal tract. There were weak reactions in breast tissue, with both malignant and normal breast tissues staining similarly.

Thus, normal breast tissue expresses MUC 1,2,3 as does malignant breast cancer, but, the increase in amount and distribution of the mucins in breast cancer is confined to MUC1.

## Immunotherapeutic Studies With Synthetic Peptides, Fusion Proteins, And HMFG

As the MUC1 peptides and fusion protein were highly immunogenic - as far as antibodies were concerned, it was concluded that the immunising material contained epitopes required to simulate T helper cells (for antibody production) and also led to antigen presentation by B cells for antibody production. Whether this immunogenicity could be translated into protection from tumor transplants was not clear, although other studies indicated protection of rats by immunising with MUC1+ tumors[20]. To examine the immunogenicity of peptides, fusion protein and HMFG we used 3T3 tumor cells of BALB/c origin expressing MUC1 after transfection (obtained from Dr. D. Wreschner). The 3T3 cells grew in BALB/c mice and were not rejected, whereas the MUC1 cells grew and were subsequently rejected by all mice; these mice resisted a challenge with MUC1+ 3T3 cells. In mice immunized with either synthetic peptides, fusion proteins or HMFG - good antibody production was noted. The immunized mice were challenged with the MUC1+ 3T3 cells; after the first few days it appeared that in the immunized mice, the tumour grew more slowly than in those immunized with the control peptide - however, there was little difference noted and the tumors were ultimately rejected at the same rate. It was of interest that the mice immunised with the control peptide, and which had rejected the tumour, did not produce antibodies against MUC1; nor did the mice immunised with peptide and other immunogens have an increase in titer after rejecting the tumor. We presume that tumor graft rejection is due to cell mediated mechanisms and that the tumour itself induces good cellular immunity - as the tumor is rejected, and a second challenge is resisted, whereas those immunised with the peptide, fusion protein or HMFG produce good humoral immunity and not cellular immunity. Methods therefore need to be designed to alter the immunizing agents or protocol so that the humoral immunity produced is converted into cellular immunity prior to use as an immunotherapeutic agent.

## CONCLUSIONS

Monoclonal antibodies can readily be produced to MUC1 peptides, and these react with breast cancer - either by immunising with synthetic peptides, fusion proteins, HMFG or breast cancer itself. For all of these immunisations, APDTR is the immunodominant epitope, but other epitopes can react with different antibodies - particularly when immunising with non-glycosylated peptides or fusion proteins. Several new antibodies are described - which, on tissue sections, appear to be specific for breast cancer. Antibodies were also produced to MUC2 and MUC3 peptides; and although MUC2 & 3 are predominantly expressed in the gastrointestinal tract, the antibodies also reacted with breast tissue (MUC2 & 3) and with breast cancer (MUC3). However, in contrast to MUC1, which is greatly over expressed in breast cancer, MUC2 & 3 have no increase in expression in cancer and are therefore of limited usefulness for the diagnosis of breast cancer. Synthetic peptides and fusion proteins could, theoretically, provide the basis of an immunising program for vaccination in breast cancer - particularly as females with breast cancer can mount an immune response to MUC1 (see elsewhere in this volume). On this basis, an immunising program was established in mice using MUC1$^+$ transfected 3T3 cells. Immunisation with peptides, fusion protein and HMFG gave rise to significant humoral immunity - but little protection from a tumor challenge, the peptides will have to be extensively modified for use as a vaccine.

## REFERENCES

1.  S. J. Genlder, J. M. Burchell, T. Duhig, D. Lamport, R. White, M. Parker , and J. Taylor-Papadimitriou, Cloning of partial cDNA coding differentiation and tumour-associated mucin glycoproteins expressed by human mammary epithelium, *Proc. Natl. Acad. Sci.* USA, 84:6060-6064 (1987).

2.  J. Siddiqui, M. Abe, D. Hayes, E. Shani, E. Yunis, and D. Kufe, Isolation and sequencing of a cDNA coding for the human DF3 breast carcinoma associated antigen, *Proc. Natl. Acad. Sci. USA*, 85:2320-2323 (1988).

3.  D. H. Wreschner, M. Hareuveni, I. Tsarfaty, N. Smorodinsky, J. Horev, J. Zaretsky, P. Kotkes, M. Weiss, R. Lathe, A. Dion, and I. Keydar, Human epithelial tumor antigen cDNA sequences - differential splicing may generate multiple protein forms, *Eur. J. Biochem.* 189:463-474 (1990).

4.  M. J. L. Lightenberg, H. L. Vos, A. C. M. Gennissen, and J. Hilkens, Episialin, a carcinoma-associated mucin, is generated by a polymorphic gene encoding splice variants with alternative amino-termini, *J. Biol. Chem.* 265:5573-5578 (1990).

5.  P.X. Xing, J. Prenzoska, G.T. Layton, P. Devine, and I.F.C. McKenzie, Second-generation monoclonal antibodies to intestinal MUC2 peptides reactive with colon cancer, *J. Natl. Cancer Inst.* 84: 699-703 (1992).

6.  V. Apostolopoulos, P.-X. Xing, and I.F.C. McKenzie, Second genration MUC3 peptide monoclonal antibodies reactive with colon cancer, *Gastroenterology.* (1992), (Submitted).

7.  P.X. Xing, J. Prenzoska, K. Quelch, and I.F.C. McKenzie, Second generation anti-MUC1 peptide monoclonal antibodies, *Cancer Res.* 52:2310-2317 (1991).

8.  R. S. Hodges, and R. B. Merrifield, Monitoring of solid phase peptide synthesis by an automated spectrophomeric picrate method, *Anal. Biochem.* 65:241-252 (1975).

9.  H. M. Geyson, S. J. Rodda, T. J. Mason, G. Tribbick, and P. G. Schoofs, Strategies for epitope analysis using peptide synthesis, *J. Immunol. Meth.* 102:259-274 (1987).

10. P. X. Xing, J. Prenzoska, and I.F.C. McKenzie, Epitope mapping of anti-breast and anti-ovarian mucin monoclonal antibodies, *Molecular Immunol.* 29: 641-650 (1991).

11. P. X. Xing, K. Reynolds, G. Pietersz, and I.F.C. McKenzie, Effect of variations in peptide sequence on anti-human milk fat globule membrane antibody reactions, *Immunology.* 72:304-311 (1991).

12. V. Apostolopoulos, P. X. Xing, J.A. Trapani, and I.F.C. McKenzie, Production of anti-breast cancer monoclonal antibodies using a glutathione-S-transferanse-MUC1 bacterial fusion protein, *Br.J Cancer.* 67: 713-729 (1993).

13. J. Burcell, S. Gendler, J. Taylor-Papadimitriou, A. Girling, A. Lewis, R. Millis and D. Lamport, Development and characterization of breast cancer reactive monoclonal antibodies directed to the core protein of the human milk mucin, *Cancer Res.* 47:5476-7482 (1987).

14. D. N. Posnett, H. McGrath, and J. P. Tam, A novel method for producing anti-peptide antibodies: Production of site-specific antibodies to the T cell antigen receptor ß- chain, *J. Biol. Chem.* 263:1719-1725 (1988).

15. J. R. Gum, J. C. Byrd, J. W. Hicks, N. W. Toribara, D. T. A. Lamport, and Y. S. Kim, Molecular cloning of human intestinal mucin cDNAs: Sequence analysis and evidence for genetic polymorphism, *J. Biol. Chem.* 264:6480-6487 (1989).

16. B. H. Jany, M. W. Gallup, P.-S. Yan, J. R. Gum, Y. S. Kim, Human brounchus and intestine express the same mucinm gene, *J. Clin. Invest.* 87 : 77-82 (1991).

17. J. Hilkens, M. J. L. Ligtenberg, H. Vos, and S. Litvinov, Cell membrane-associated mucins and their adhesion-modulating property. *TIBS.* 17:359-363 (1992).

18. T. P. Hopp, and K.R. Woods, A computer program for predicting protein antigenic determinants, *Mol. Immunol.* 20:483-493 (1983).

19. J. R. Gum, J. W. Hicks, D. M. Swallow, R. L., Lagace, J. E. Byrd, D. T. A. Lamport, B. Siddick, and Y. S. Kim, Molecular cloning of cDNAs derived from a novel human intestinal mucin gene, *Biochem. Biophy. Res. Comm.* 171:407-415 (1990).

20. M. Hareuveni, C. Gautier, M.-P.Kieny, D. Wreschner, P. Chambon, and R. Lathe, Vaccination against tumor cells expressing breast cancer epithelial tumor antigen, *Proc. Natl. Acad. Sci. USA.* 87:9948-9502 (1990).

# DOES A NOVEL FORM OF THE BREAST CANCER MARKER PROTEIN, MUC1, ACT AS A RECEPTOR MOLECULE THAT MODULATES SIGNAL TRANSDUCTION?

Daniel H. Wreschner, Sheila Zrihan-Licht, Amos Baruch, Dalit Sagiv, Mor-li Hartman, Nechama Smorodinsky and Iafa Keydar

Dept. of Cell Research and Immunology
Tel Aviv University, Ramat Aviv, Israel, 69978

## ABSTRACT

Molecular analysis of a protein highly expressed in human breast cancer, indicates the presence of a polymorphic tandem repeat domain that encodes a conserved 20 amino acid repeat motif rich in serine and threonine residues that in the mature protein, designated MUC1, are linked via O-glycosidic linkages to sugar residues. Recent studies performed in our laboratory have led to the molecular characterization of a novel MUC1 repeat array minus mRNA, generated by an alternative splicing event that deletes the central tandem repeat array and its flanking sequences. The conceptually derived amino acid sequence of the novel MUC1 protein shows that it is identical with the previously reported transmembrane MUC1 amino acid sequence except for the deletion of the central 20 amino acid tandem repeat array and sequences immediately flanking the repeat array. This indicates that the novel MUC1 protein, which is devoid of the "hallmark" feature of mucins, the tandem repeat array, may be functionally different to the much larger, heavily glycosylated polymorphic repeat array containing MUC1 proteins, that affect cell-cell interactions. Based on an analysis of its peptide sequence, we propose the hypothesis that the novel MUC1 protein may act as a receptor molecule that modulates signal transduction. Preliminary experimental data supports this hypothesis. It appears, therefore, that the MUC1 gene is multifunctional with regard to its protein products- the repeat array containing MUC1 proteins may alter cellular adhesion processes whereas the novel MUC1 protein could be acting as a receptor-like molecule participating in signal transmission.

## INTRODUCTION

A number of different monoclonal antibodies generated in various laboratories detect a protein that is highly abundant in human breast cancer tissue [1-9]. Molecular analyses [10-15] indicate that this protein, designated MUC1, is heavily glycosylated and although a constituent of normal secretory epithelium, its expression in breast cancer

*Antigen and Antibody Molecular Engineering in Breast Cancer Diagnosis and Treatment*, Edited by R.L. Ceriani, Plenum Press, New York, 1994

17

tissue is different both qualitatively and quantitatively (note should be taken that the MUC1 gene products have previously been referred to as PEM, EMA, episialin, MAM6,H23Ag, etc.). One of the MUC1 protein forms contains a transmembrane domain that anchors the protein in the cell membrane and bisects it into a large heavily glycosylated extracellular domain that contains a polymorphic tandem 20 amino acid repeat array and a smaller 69 amino acid cytoplasmic domain. The MUC1 protein can also be detected in the sera of breast cancer patients indicating the existence of a secreted MUC1 form [10].

A major feature of the MUC1 molecule is the central tandem repeat array that codes for a polymorphic 20 amino acid repeat motif that is rich in serine, threonine and proline residues [10-15]. This repeat array is heavily glycosylated via O-linked glycosylation on the serine and threonine residues, and the carbohydrate structures present may vary considerably between MUC1 protein synthesized in normal mammary tissue as compared to breast cancer tissue MUC1. The MUC1 protein is also rich in proline residues and this, in addition to the extensive glycosylation, may confer a rigid, extended structure to the cell surface located MUC1. These considerations indicate that one of the transmembrane forms of MUC1 may be involved in cell-cell interactions [16,17].

The transmembrane form of MUC1 is composed of *extracellular, transmembrane,* and *cytoplasmic* domains, and is highly reminiscent of a receptor protein, that may bind an as yet unidentified ligand and transduce signals into the cell from the external environment. The fact that the MUC1 cytoplasmic domain comprises a comparatively long 69 amino acid tail, that shows a very high degree of similarity with the mouse MUC1 homologue [18], supports this hypothesis.

Could it be that one form of MUC1 is involved in cell-cell interaction [16,17] whereas another novel MUC1 form acts as a membrane located receptor molecule?

Here we report the existence of a novel MUC1 protein that is devoid of the "hallmark" feature of mucins- the tandem repeat array. Evidence is presented suggesting that whereas the polymorphic repeat array containing MUC1 proteins may be involved in cell-cell adhesion/repulsion processes [16,17], the novel MUC1 protein may be acting as a receptor-like molecule participating in signal transmission.

## RESULTS AND DISCUSSION

### Novel MUC1 Splice Variants Minus The Tandem Repeat Array

We have recently reevaluated the expression of the MUC1 gene by probing Northern blots with the 60 bp repeat cDNA derived from the tandem repeat array, as well as with unique MUC1 nucleotide sequences located both 5' and 3' to the tandem repeat array. These studies not only confirmed the expression of polymorphic mRNAs, as observed following probing with the repeat 60bp sequence, but also showed that tumor tissues having high levels of MUC1 polymorphic mRNA expression, demonstrate an additional invariantly sized mRNA species of 1.2kb length, that specifically hybridizes to the MUC1 unique sequence probes, yet does not hybridize with a repeat array probe. The nucleotide sequence of this novel MUC1 mRNA demonstrated the deletion of the central tandem repeat array and its flanking sequences that had occurred by a differential splicing event. This alternative splice utilizes splice donor and acceptor sequences that are located upstream and downstream to the tandem repeat array, respectively. The amino acid sequence conceptually derived from the nucleotide sequences of the novel MUC1 mRNA shows that the sequences downstream of the alternative splice acceptor site are translated in the same reading frame as in the repeat array containing MUC1 mRNA. Distal to the splice site, all other splicing events present in the novel MUC1 molecule are identical with those reported for the transmembrane MUC1 repeat array positive sequence. It appears therefore, that by differential splicing, the MUC1 gene can generate an invariantly sized novel MUC1 mRNA and thereby protein, devoid of both the repeat array and its immediate flanking sequences, in addition to the MUC1 polymorphic, repeat array containing mRNAs (see Fig.1 for scheme of the polymorphic MUC1 protein and the novel MUC1 protein devoid of the tandem repeat array).

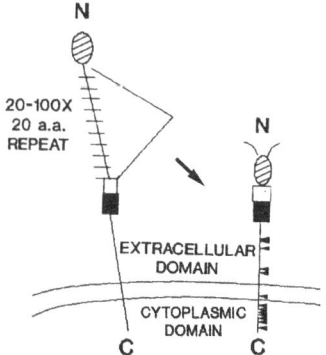

**Figure 1** *Scheme of the polymorphic repeat array containing MUC1 protein, the novel MUC1 protein and biased localization of tyrosine residues*

The polymorphic repeat array containing MUC1 protein is depicted on the left whereas the novel MUC1 protein lacking the tandem repeat array is shown on the right. The novel MUC1 protein is obviously derived from the novel repeat array minus mRNA - the part of the polymorphic MUC1 protein that is lacking in the novel MUC1 protein is bracketed by the two diagonal lines encompassing the repeat array. The biased localization of tyrosine residues (arrow heads) is shown in the novel MUC1 protein- they are identically distributed in the polymorphic repeat array containing MUC1 protein.

## Interspecies Conservation of Regions Retained in the Novel MUC1 Protein

The finding reported here of a novel MUC1 protein that is devoid of the "hallmark" feature of mucins- the tandem repeat array- introduces an additional level of complexity in MUC1 function. Interestingly, a comparison of the human MUC1/H23 amino acid sequence with the mouse MUC1/H23 homologue shows that whereas a tandem repeat structure rich in serine and threonine residues is also observed in the mouse protein, there is very little conservation of actual amino acid sequence in this region, indicating perhaps that the primary function of mucin tandemly repeated domains is to provide the "infrastructure" for extensive O-linked glycosylation, that may subsequently play a role in reduced cell adhesion.

Inspection of MUC1/H23 sequences in other species may provide further insights into functionally important regions of MUC1/H23 gene products. For example, the mouse MUC1/H23 homologue shows, in contrast to the lack of similarity within the tandem repeating sequence, a very high degree of amino acid sequence conservation with human MUC1/H23, in the cytoplasmic and transmembrane domains as well as in the 120 amino acids N-terminal to the transmembrane domain. This degree of amino acid sequence similarity is, in the cytoplasmic and transmembrane domains, almost 90%, indicating that these regions, as well as the 120 amino acids N-terminally adjacent to the transmembrane domain, may be functionally very important. In this regard, it seems very relevant that the amino acid sequences retained by the novel invariant repeat array minus MUC1 proteins are mostly those that are identical with the mouse MUC1 homolog- the cytoplasmic and transmembrane domains as well as the 120 amino acids adjacent N-terminally to the transmembrane domain.

## Biased Localization of Tyrosine Residues in the MUC1 Protein

Analysis of the amino acid distribution within the MUC1 sequence reveals the startling finding that all MUC1 tyrosine residues are located solely within the 69 amino acid cytoplasmic domain, the transmembrane domain and the 91 amino acids adjacent N-terminally to the transmembrane domain, which contain 7, 1 and 5 tyrosine residues, respectively (Fig. 1). Significantly all these tyrosine residues are retained within the novel MUC1 protein. No other tyrosine residues appear throughout the complete MUC1 molecule. As phosphorylation of tyrosine residues is an essential feature of the signal transmission pathway of several ligand/membrane receptor systems the biased localization, rather than random distribution, of tyrosine residues within the MUC1 protein may indicate that one or more MUC1 forms are participating in signal transduction.

## The MUC1 Cytoplasmic Domain Contains a Consensus Tyrosine Phosphorylation Site

An interesting system that may have relevance to the function of the transmembrane **MUC1** protein, is the CSF/CSF1-R (colony stimulating factor/colony stimulating factor receptor) interaction [19,20]. CSF binding to its receptor is known to induce, in addition to activation of the catalytic kinase domain, autophosphorylation of tyrosine residues in the kinase insert region of the cytoplasmic domain of the CSF receptor. Phosphorylation of specific tyrosine residues within this kinase insert region, is obligatory for the high affinity interaction of the CSF1-R with SH2 (sarc homologous region 2) sequences present in downstream second messengers in the signal transmission cascade, such as PI 3' kinase ( phosphatidyl inositol 3' kinase), phospholipase C gamma 1 and GAP (GTPase activating protein, [21,22]). It is interesting to note that the tyrosine phosphorylation sites within the CSF1-R kinase insert ( *DTYVEM*, *GGYMDH*, *VDYVPM*, *NEYMDM* and *EEYMPM*,, the phosphorylation site underlined is essential for interaction with the PI 3' kinase) are similar to the site *DTYHPM* located within the cytoplasmic domain of transmembrane **MUC1**. Furthermore, following ligand binding the PDGF-R (platelet derived growth factor receptor) undergoes autophosphorylation on a tyrosine (Tyr-751) residue present within the kinase insert domain that is obligatory for its specific interaction with downstream proteins such as PI 3' kinase [23]. This site, *IDYVPM*, is also remarkably similar (see below, A) to the above described MUC1 site.

A)

    PDGF-R    IDYVPM      Autophosphorylation site (Tyr 751)

    CSF1-R     DTYVEM      Autophosphorylation site

    MUC1        **DTYHPM**


As the **MUC1** cytoplasmic domain is 69 aa long, it probably does not have intrinsic kinase activity- yet it may undergo phosphorylation by interaction with a transphosphorylating kinase(s).

Our working hypothesis is that the cytoplasmic domain of the MUC1 protein may undergo transphosphorylation on tyrosine residues by other activated tyrosine kinases, and act as a "decoy" tyrosine kinase insert attracting to itself second messenger proteins that participate in the signal transduction pathway and thereby modulate signal transduction (Fig.2).


## Transphosphorylation May Modulate Signal Transduction- Homology Between the MUC1 Protein and the Acetylcholine Receptor

A computer search for other proteins that share the postulated MUC1 *DTYHPMS* transphosphorylation sequence, revealed that the sequence *TYHPMS* is contained within a subunit of the acetylcholine receptor. Interestingly this peptide sequence is located at the same position as the postulated MUC1 transphosphorylation sequence- adjacent to the transmembrane domain and just within the cytoplasmic domain (see Fig. 3). The activity

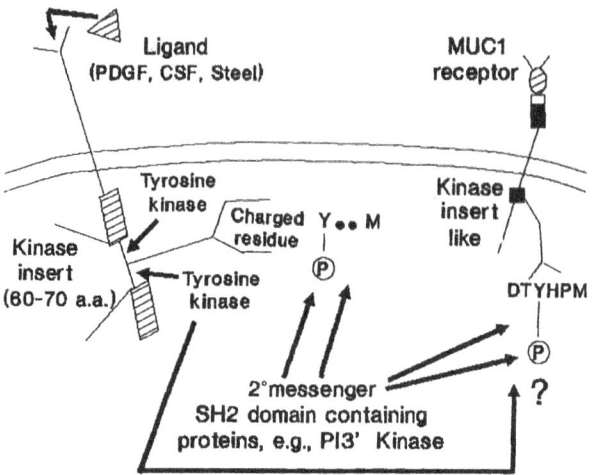

**Figure 2** *Scheme depicting modulation of signal transduction by the putative MUC1 receptor-* The signal transduction pathway for the PDGF, CSF-1 and Steel ligands and their respective receptors (PDGF-R, CSF-1-R and c-kit) is depicted on the left. Ligand binding induces autophosphorylation on cytoplasmic tyrosine residues of the receptor that include sites within the kinase insert domain. The tyrosine residue (Y-P) that when phosphorylated attracts to it the SH2 domain containing protein PI3' kinase is located within a site that invariably contains a charged residue one or two amino acids upstream and two amino acids downstream, a methionine residue (charged residueY-P..M). By analogy, the putative MUC1 receptor (to the right of the figure) consists of a kinase insert like cytoplasmic domain that contains a consensus tyrosine phosphorylation site (**DTYHPM**) that may undergo transphorylation and thereby attract to it second messenger proteins involved in signal transduction.

of the acetylcholine receptor is known to be modulated by transphosphorylation on tyrosine residues and although the actual tyrosine phosphorylation site has not as yet been defined, it is likely to occur on this *TYHPMS* sequence- by analogy, the MUC1 *TYHPMS* sequence may also undergo transphosphorylation and thereby modulate signal transduction (Fig. 3).

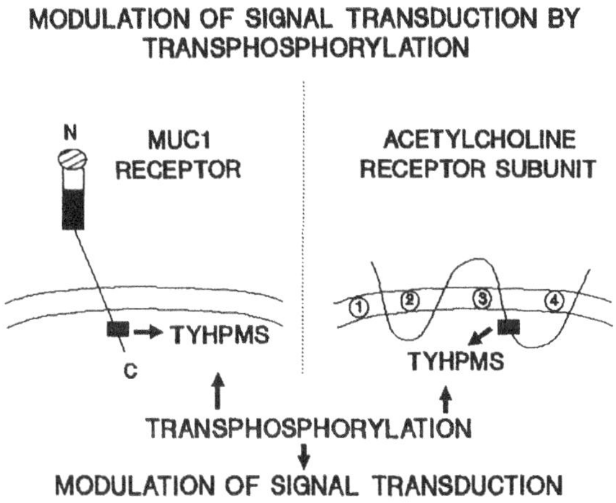

MODULATION OF SIGNAL TRANSDUCTION BY
TRANSPHOSPHORYLATION

**Figure 3** *Modulation of signal transduction by transphosphorylation of tyrosine residues in the cytoplasmic domain of the acetylcholine receptor- analogy with MUC1-* The novel MUC1 protein is depicted to the left of the figure and the acetylcholine receptor to the right. The acetylcholine receptor consists of 4 transmembrane domains thereby forming two cytoplasmic domains. The sequence **TYHPMS** is juxtaposed to the transmembrane domain just within the cytoplasmic domain, in both the novel MUC1 protein and the acetylcholine receptor. The acetylcholine receptor is known to undergo transphosphorylation that subsequently modulates its activity- by analogy the MUC1 receptor may also undergo transphosphorylation.

**MUC1 Expression Modulates Protein Tyrosine Phosphorylation**

To analyse experimentally whether the MUC1 protein participates in signal transduction via modulation of protein tyrosine phosphorylation, the total tyrosine phosphorylation patterns of cytoplasmic proteins prepared from either control neomycin (antibiotic resistance marker) transfected rat fibroblasts or the same cells transfected with an expression vector harboring the MUC1 cDNA, were compared. Western blotting of proteins derived from these 2 cell lines followed by reaction with anti-phosphotyrosine antibodies demonstrated that MUC1 expression both up and down regulates the tyrosine phosphorylation levels of specific proteins (Fig. 3 A, open and closed arrows, respectively). To assess the generality of this phenomenon the effect of MUC1 expression on protein tyrosine phosphorylation was assessed in mouse mammary cell MUC1 transfectants- MUC1 expression markedly influenced the protein tyrosine phosphorylation patterns both by up and down regulation (Fig. 3 B, open and closed arrows, respectively). These results demonstrate that MUC1 expression may modulate signal transduction processes.

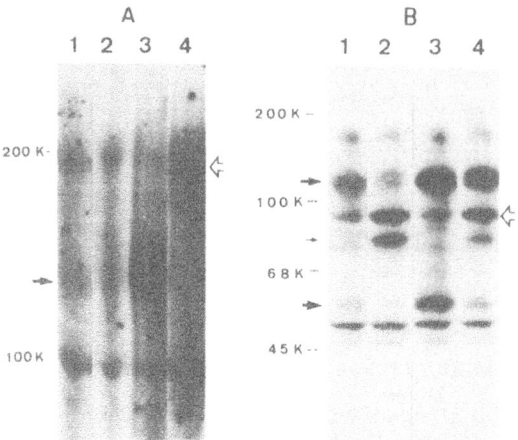

**Figure 4** *Changes in protein tyrosine phosphorylation patterns concomitant with MUC1 expression*- Ras transformed rat fibroblasts (A) and MM5 mouse mammary epithelial cells (B) were transfected either with the neomycin resistance gene alone (lanes 1 & 3) or with MUC1 cDNA (lanes 2 & 4) and stable transfectants selected. Cell lysates prepared after 2 or 3 days of cell growth in culture (lanes 1,2 and 3,4 respectively) were analyzed by SDS-PAGE, Western blotted and probed with antiphosphotyrosine antibodies. Both up and down regulation of protein tyrosine phosphorylation (open and closed arrows respectively) was observed in the MUC1 transfectants.

**Conclusions and Perspectives**

We and others have previously demonstrated that expression of the polymorphic repeat array containing MUC1 proteins in cell transfectants markedly alters cell morphology and cellular aggregation processes, that is likely mediated by expression of the highly glycosylated, negatively charged tandem repeat array [16,17]. As presented here, we have recently found that a novel 1.2kb MUC1 mRNA species is expressed that lacks the tandem repeat array and its immediate flanking sequences, and therefore codes for a smaller non-polymorphic transmembrane protein- the novel MUC1 protein. The following features suggested that the novel MUC1 protein likely plays a role distinct to that of the polymorphic repeat array positive MUC1 protein, and, specifically, that it may act as a receptor like molecule participating in signal transduction- **a)** it contains a relatively long 69 aa cytoplasmic tail that has extensive homolgy between the human and mouse **MUC1** proteins, **b)** it demonstrates biased localization of tyrosine residues in the **MUC1** sequence, **c)** it has similarity between tyrosine phosphorylation sites in receptor tyrosine kinase insert regions and tyrosine containing sequences in the **MUC1** cytoplasmic domain and **d)** there is marked similarity between a putative transphosphorylation site in the acetylcholine receptor that modulates its signal transducing properties and a sequence in the cytoplasmic domain of the novel MUC1 protein. The hypothesis that one of the MUC1 protein forms may be modulating signal transduction is supported experimentally by the demonstration of changes in protein tyrosine phosphorylation patterns concomitant with MUC1 expression, thereby strongly implicating MUC1 participation in signal transduction. It appears, therefore, that the MUC1 gene is multifunctional with regard to its protein products- the polymorphic repeat array containing MUC1 proteins may alter cellular adhesion processes via expression of the highly glycosylated, negatively charged tandem repeat array, whereas the novel MUC1 proteins lacking the tandem repeat array may be acting as receptor-like molecules participating in signal transmission. The relationship between these seemingly diverse MUC1 functions is presently being investigated.

**Acknowledgements:** This work was supported in part by the Israel Cancer Association, the Israel Cancer Research Fund and the Naftali Foundation (D.H.W.), Simko Chair for Breast Cancer Research, Frederico Fund for Tel Aviv University, Barbara Friedman Fund and The Washington Friends of T.A.U. (I.K.).

# REFERENCES

1. Ceriani, R.L., Peterson, J.A. and Blank, E.W. (1984). Cancer Res. 44, 3033-3039.
2. Keydar, I., Chou, C.S., Hareuveni, M., Tsarfaty, I., Sahar, E., Seltzer, G., Chaitchik, S. and Hizi, A. (1989) Proc. Natl. Acad. Sci. USA, 86, 1362-1367.
3. Abe, M. and Kufe, D. J. Cell Physiol. (1986) 126, 126-136.
4. Bramwell, M.E., Bhavanandan, V.P., Wiseman, G. and Harris, H. (1983) Br. J. Cancer 48, 177-183.
5. Burchell, J., Gendler, S., Taylor-Papadimitriou, J., Girling, A., Lewis, A., Millis, R. and Lamport, D. (1987) Cancer Res. 47, 5476-5482.
6. Hilkens, J., Buijs, F., Hilgers, J., Hageman, P., Calafat, J., Sonnenberg, A. and van dar Valk, M. (1984) Cancer 34, 197-204.
7. Johnson, V.G., Schlom, J., Paterson, A.J., Bennett, J., Magnani, J.L. and Colcher, D. (1986) Cancer Res. 46, 850-857.

8. Lan, M.S., Finn, O.J., Fernsten, P.D. and Metzgar, R.S. (1985) Cancer Res. 45, 305-310.

9. Tjandra, J.J. and McKenzie, I.F.C. (1988) Br. J.Surg. 75, 1067-1075.

10. Wreschner, D.H., Tsarfaty, I., Hareuveni, M., Zaretsky, J., Smorodinsky, N., Weiss, M., Horev, J., Kotkes, P., Zrihan, S., Jeltsch, J-M., Green, S., Lathe, R., and Keydar, I. (1989) In: Breast Cancer: Progress in biology , clinical management and prevention, pp 41-59, Eds. Rich, M.A., Hager, J.C. and Keydar, I., Boston: Kluwer Academic Publishers.

11. Wreschner, D.H., Hareuveni, M., Tsarfaty, I, Smorodinsky, N., Horev, J., Zaretsky, J., Kotkes, P., Weiss, M., Lathe, R., Dion, A.S., and Keydar, I. (1990). Eur. J. Biochem. 189: 463-473.

12. Abe, M., Siddiqui, J. and Kufe, D. (1989) Biochem. Biophys. Res. Commun. 165, 644-649.

13. Gendler, S.J., Lancaster, C.A., Taylor-Papadimitriou, J., Duhig, T., Peat, N., Burcheli, J., Pemberton, L., Lalani, E-N. and Wilson, D. (1990) J. Biol. Chem. 265, 15286-15293.

14. Ligtenberg, M.J.L., Vos, H.L., Genissen, A.M.C. and Hilkens, J. (1990) J. Biol. Chem. 265, 15573-15578.

15. Lan, M.S., Batra, S.K., Qi, W-N, Metzgar, R.S. and Hollingworth, M.A. (1990) J. Biol. Chem. 265, 15294-15299.

16. Ligtenberg, M.J.L., Buijs, F., Vos, H.L., and Hilkens, J. (1992) Cancer Res. 52, 2318-2324.

17. Hartman, M., Tsarfaty,I., Hareuveni, M., Keydar,I. and Wreschner, D.H. (1992). In: "Senology" L. Ioannidou-Mouzaka, N.J. Agnantis and I. Karydas (Eds.) Elsevier Science Publishers, pp 379-383.

18. Spicer, A.P., Parry, G., Patton, S. and Gendler, S.J. (1991) J.Biol. Chem. 266, 15099-15109.

19. Shurtleff, S.A., Downing, J.R., Rock, C.O., Hawkins, S.A., Roussel, M.F. and Sherr, C.J. (1990) EMBO J. 9, 4215-4221.

20. Reedijk, M. Liu, Y. and Pawson, T. (1990). Mol. Cell Biol. 10, 5601-5608.

21. Anderson, D., Koch, C.A., Grey, L., Ellis, C., Moran, M.F. and Pawson, T. (1990) Science 250, 979-982.

22. Moran, M., Koch, C.A., Anderson, D., Ellis,C., England, C., Martin, G.S. and Pawson, T. (1990) Proc. Natl. Acad. Sci. USA 87, 8622-8626.

23. Escobedo, J.A., Kaplan, D.R., Kavanaugh, W.M., Turck, C.W. and Williams, L.T. (1991) Mol. Cell. Biol. 11, 1125-1132.

# CANCER METASTASIS DETERMINED BY CARBOHYDRATE-MEDIATED CELL ADHESION

Tatsuro Irimura

Department of Chemical Toxicology and Immunochemistry
Faculty of Pharmaceutical Sciences, The University of Tokyo
Hongo, Bunkyo-ku, Tokyo 113, Japan

During the progression of cancer to advanced stages, highly malignant and metastatic tumor cells are thought to arise within primary tumors and become predominant. On the basis of this hypothesis, surgical specimens from patients at various clinical stages of colorectal carcinomas were compared for a variety of molecular phenotypes possibly related to metastasis. As a result, colorectal carcinomas with increased metastatic potential and with poor prognosis have been characterized by the increased expression of sialyl-Le$^X$ antigens. Human colon carcinoma cell lines were selected for their high or low expression of sialyl-Le$^X$ antigens on the cell surfaces. These cells differ in their metastatic behavior in nude mice. The high expresser cells strongly adhere to activated endothelial cells in vitro. Retrospective studies with immunohistochemical technique have revealed that these molecules could be used as a predictive marker for colorectal cancer metastasis.

## I. INTRODUCTION

Adenocarcinomas of the colon and rectum are the second most prevalent cause of cancer death in the United States. The incidence has recently been increasing in Japan corresponding to the changes in the eating habit. The presence or absence of metastasis is the most critical factor in determining a patient's prognosis in colorectal cancer, since primary tumors can be successfully treated by surgery[1]. Colorectal carcinoma is staged according to the presence or absence of metastasis[2-3] and the patient survival rate after surgery differs among different stages. The biology of human colorectal carcinoma metastasis seems to be unique. Our work[4] and work by Wolmark et al.[5], indicate that the size of the colorectal carcinoma and, therefore, tumor burden has no relationship to a tumor's metastatic potential. Thus, biochemical differences unrelated to the tumor growth at the primary sites may account for differences in metastatic behavior. We assumed that metastatic colorectal carcinoma cells, which may be predominant in primary and metastatic tumors of advanced stages, express different phenotypes from non-metastatic carcinoma cells predominant in tumors of early stages. During the

*Antigen and Antibody Molecular Engineering in Breast Cancer Diagnosis and Treatment*, Edited by R.L. Ceriani, Plenum Press, New York, 1994

27

progression of colorectal carcinoma, such alterations should occur in subpopulations of tumor cells. The changes are probably not directly related to the genetic changes occurring at the time of colorectal tumorigenesis (Fig. 1, Fig. 2).

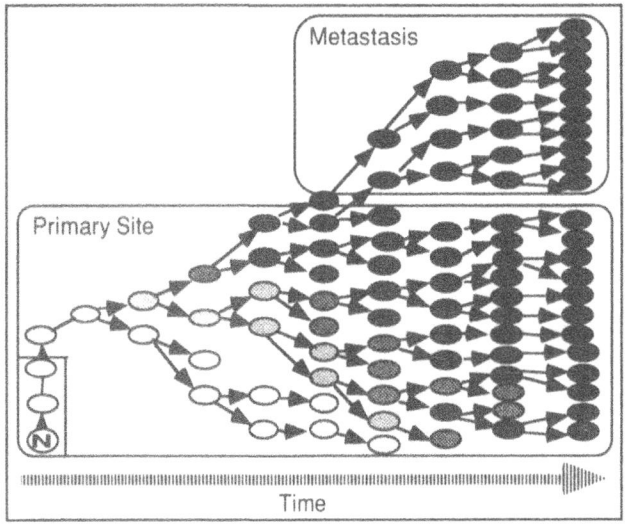

**Figure 1.** A hypothetical drawing of the generation of metastatic tumor cells within a primary tumor during the cancer progression.

On the basis of this assumption, we compared biochemical properties associated with colorectal primary carcinomas at various stages and metastases obtained at surgery. If there is a molecule associated with metastatic colorectal carcinoma cells, such a molecule should be useful as a prognostic indicator for colorectal carcinoma recurrence and metastasis, independent of clinical staging. Because approximately 50% of the stage B2 patients may develop recurrence, which often present as liver metastasis, it will be critical to define the group of patients at higher risk of recurrence and metastasis within B2 patients to improve post-operative management of the primary colorectal cancer.

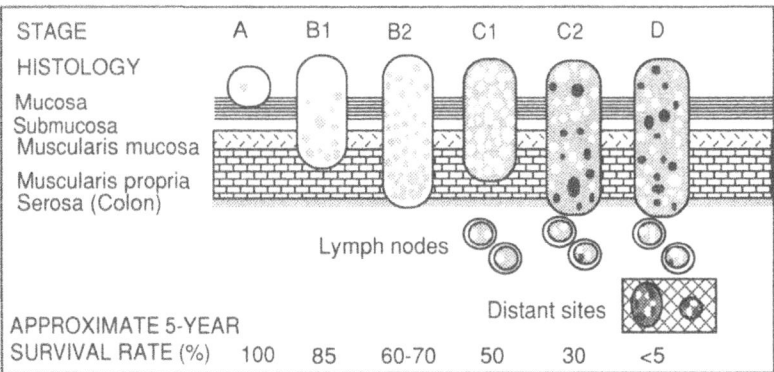

**Figure 2.** Morphological staging of colorectal carcinoma. The staging is based on the presence or absence of metastasis and on the depth of tumor invasion. The metastatic tumor cells are shown by dark spots.

## II. CORRELATION BETWEEN sLe[X] EXPRESSION AND CLINICAL STAGES

We have focused our work on cell surface and extracellular molecules produced by colorectal carcinoma cells because the metastatic behavior of carcinoma cells depends on their interaction with surrounding cells and tissues. We have developed a comprehensive data base of patient records and of pathological observations of the tumors. The clinical relevance of the biochemical data has been assessed using this data base. We have compared the differential expression of molecules between primary tumors and metastases and among primary tumors classified at different clinical stages. The expression of four different high-$M_r$ glycoproteins, probably mucins, decreased or increased during tumor progression and metastasis[7-13]. While the expression of these molecules changed in a relatively consistent manner, changes in secreted collagenolytic enzymes did not show differences[14]. All these glycoproteins distinguished by their carbohydrate chains had characteristics of having high $M_r$. One of the most remarkable phenotypes found in the advanced and metastatic tumors was an increase in the amount of mucins bearing sialyl-Lewis X antigens (sLe[X]).

**Table 1.** *Molecules in colorectal carcinoma surgical specimens differentially expressed between primary tumors at different stages or between primary tumors and metastases.*

| Phenotypes | Advanced vs early stage | Metastasis vs primary | Reference |
|---|---|---|---|
| MUC1 sialomucin | ↗ | ↗ | Irimura et al., 1988; Nakamori et al, 1992 |
| Sulfomucin | ↘ | ↘ | Yamori et al., 1987, 1989 |
| Sialyl-Lewis X antigen | ↗ | ↗ | Hoff et al., 1989, 1990; Matsushita et al, 1990 |
| UEA-1-reactive mucin | ↘ | → | Irimura et al., 1987 |

As shown in Table 1, we reported in 1987 that the expression of a high molecular weight mucin-like molecule with type-2 blood group H and/or Le[Y] antigens was decreased at the advanced stages in carcinomas of distal colon and rectum[7]. These findings led us to believe that specific changes in ABO blood group-related carbohydrate chains occur during the progression of colorectal carcinoma cells to the metastatic phenotype. We investigated other variants of blood group type-2 carbohydrate chains expressed by colorectal carcinoma tissues and cells. Monoclonal antibody (mAb) to glycolipid antigens with poly-(N-acetyllactosamine) backbones purified from colon adenocarcinoma were used in these studies. Some of these antigens are known to accumulate in the sera of carcinoma patients and are considered as serum markers for diagnosis[15-16]. However, the relationship of these molecules to the biological behavior of tumors was not previously known. We found increased expression of sLe[X] in primary colorectal carcinomas that had already developed metastases compared with primary tumors that had not metastasized[11-12].

Subsequent immunohistochemical studies made it clear that the increased expression of sLe[X] in metastatic tumors was due to the increased percentage of cells producing this antigen[13]. Examinations of serial sections indicated that areas within an individual tumor that were stained with one mAb specific for an Le[X]-related structures were not always reactive with another mAb, although these mAb identify closely related structures and these antigens are biosynthesized through closely related pathways. After examination of cytoplasmic, membrane-associated, and secreted antigens, the degree of mAb reactivity with carcinoma sections was classified by percentage of positive carcinoma cells. When primary tumors and metastases from the same patients were compared, an equivalent or higher proportion of carcinoma cells in the metastatic lesions was reactive with mAb FH6 than in the primary colon carcinomas, but such correlation was not seen with the other antigenic structures [13].

## III. SELECTION AND CHARACTERIZATION OF HUMAN COLON CARCINOMA sLe[X] VARIANT CELLS

The biological role of sLe[X] antigens expressed by colon carcinoma cells has been investigated using variant cell lines selected by cell sorting[17-18]. KM12-HX and KM12-LX, high and low expresser variant cells, were assessed for their metastatic potential in nude mice after intrasplenic injection[19]. All mice injected with KM12-HX or KM12-LX cells developed splenic tumors. The size of splenic tumors did not differ between those animals injected with KM12-HX and KM12-LX cells. The incidence of liver metastases in mice injected with KM12-HX cells was significantly greater than that in mice injected with KM12-LX cells. Also, KM12-HX cells produced more metastatic nodules than KM12-LX cells did.

The results of northern blotting analysis indicated that KM12-HX cells contained higher levels of polyA+ mRNA for $\alpha(1, 3/1, 4)$fucosyltransferase than KM12-LX cells, strongly suggesting that the levels of this glycosyltransferase played key roles in the differential sLe[X] levels between KM12-HX and KM12-LX cells (Fig. 3).

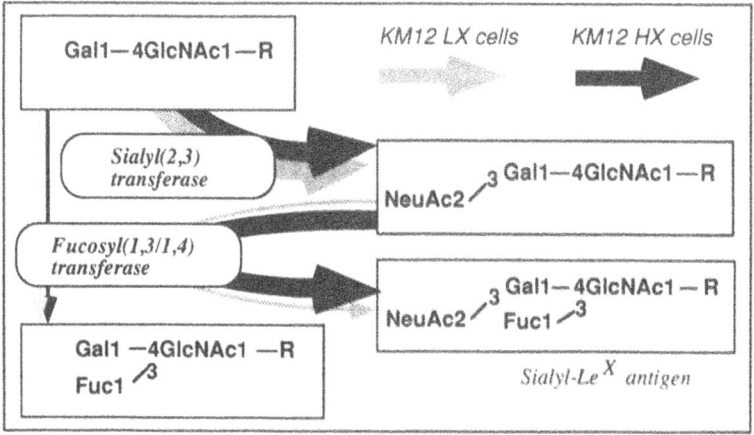

**Figure 3.** Putative differences in the biosynthetic pathways of sLe[X] antigens between KM12-HX cells and KM12-LX cells.

Furthermore, difference in the polyA+ mRNA for so-called metastasis-related genes such as urokinase, type IV collagenase, nm23, laminin-binding protein, and ribosomal phosphoprotein P2 was not observed between these cell lines, strongly suggesting that the difference in their metastatic potential was due to the cell surface carbohydrate antigens[19]. On KM12-HX cells, sLe$^X$ antigenic carbohydrate chains were attached to mucins as well as glycoproteins with various molecular weights[18].

## IV. BIOLOGICAL BEHAVIOR OF sLe$^X$ VARIANT CELLS IN VITRO

An obvious next question was whether the different metastatic behavior of these cells was mediated by cell surface carbohydrates. It is well-known that the adherence of specific tumor cells to capillary endothelial cells of the target organs may contribute to distant metastasis. The significance of several adhesion molecules, such as laminin receptors, carcinoembryonic antigens and a molecule homologous to N-CAM, in colon carcinoma pathogenesis was described[20-24]. None of these adhesion molecules described in these reports have been rigorously assessed for either their contribution to the adhesion of colon carcinoma cells to endothelial cells or their correlation with metastatic potentials in vivo. Recent studies on the role of neutrophil cell surface carbohydrates have clearly shown that the cell surface sLe$^X$ acts as a ligand to endothelial cell surface lectin-like adhesion molecules, such as E-selectin[25-27]. We have tested such a possibility and demonstrated that KM12-HX cells adhered more strongly than KM12-LX cells to human umbilical vein endothelial cells treated with tumor necrosis factor-$\alpha$ (Fig. 4). Thus, sLe$^X$ antigens seemed to function as an ectopic adhesion ligand that promotes metastatic tumor cell implantation.

It was reported that antibodies against E-selectin blocked the adhesion of human and mouse melanoma cells and human colon carcinoma cells to activated endothelial cells[28]. Direct interaction of various carcinoma cells and E-selectin or P-selectin was also demonstrated[29-30]. The adhesion of KM12-HX cells was partially inhibited by antibodies specific for E-selectin.

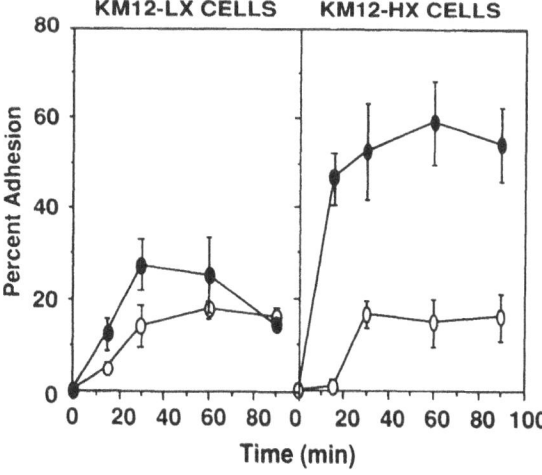

*Figure 4.* Adhesion of human colon carcinoma cells to HUVEC. HUVEC was untreated or treated with 20 ng/ml of human TNF-$\alpha$ for 3 h prior to adhesion assays. TNF-$\alpha$ was not added during the adhesion assays. Mean ± S.D. from triplicate experiments is shown. (—●—):TNF-$\alpha$-treated HUVEC; ( —O—): untreated HUVEC.

Information is not available regarding the specificity of mouse selectins, although KM12-HX cells were more metastatic to the liver than KM12-LX cells in nude mice that is presumably mediated by mouse endothelial cell-human tumor cell interactions. Our preliminary results indicated that KM12-HX cells and KM12-LX cells differentially adhered to mouse hepatic sinusoidal endothelial cells. Furthermore, the adhesion of KM12-HX cells to mouse hepatic sinusoidal endothelial cells was dependent on the cell surface sLe$^X$ structure. KM12-HX cells were also more adhesive to activated human platelets than KM12-LX cells. Such a mechanism may assist these cells to colonize in distant organs. Tumor cell-endothelial cell interactions and tumor cell-platelet interactions may lead to the extensive damage of vascular walls induced by neutrophils and other inflammatory cells.

## V. THE sLe$^X$ EXPRESSION AND PROGNOSIS OF COLON CARCINOMA PATIENTS

We histochemically scored mAb FH6-reactivity within primary carcinoma according to the percentage of positively stained cells. An advantage of immunohistochemical methods was that we could use archived specimens suitable for retrospective survival studies. In this experiment the degree of mAb reactivity with carcinoma sections was classified by percentage positive carcinoma cells after examining cytoplasmic, membrane-associated, or secreted antigens. Colon carcinoma tissues were classified into 4 categories according to the score based on the percentage of positive carcinoma cells. As shown in Fig. 5, death due to early recurrence and metastasis was seen with colorectal carcinoma patients with a high degree of mAb FH6 reactivity. Therefore, this antibody seems to be useful for identifying the group of patients with high and low risk of recurrence and metastasis. More than 80% of those who had recurrent diseases had distant metastases.

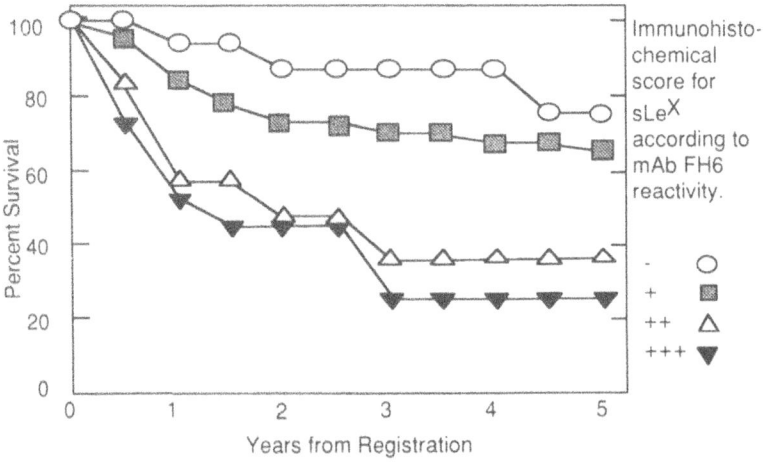

**Figure 5.** *Five-year survival of a total of 92 colon carcinoma patients divided into four groups based on the percentage of tumor cells expressing sLe$^X$ antigens within primary tumor specimens. The patient survival was recorded every two month.*

## VI.  CONCLUSIONS

A carbohydrate antigen, sLe$^X$, is one of the metastatic phenotypes of human colorectal cancer.  It apparently acts as ligands for carbohydrate-specific adhesion molecules expressed on endothelial cells and platelets.  The levels of sLe$^X$ in primary colorectal carcinoma may be useful as a prognostic indicator for post surgical recurrence and metastasis.

## REFERENCES

1.  Sugarbaker PH, Gunderson L, Wittes RE (1985) Colorectal cancer.  DeVita VT,Jr., Hellman S, Rosenberg SA (eds),  Cancer: Principles and Practice of Oncology, 2nd ed, pp 795-884.  J. B. Lippincott, Philadelphia.

2.  Astler VA, Coller FA (1954) The prognostic significance of direct extension of the colon and rectum. Ann Surg 139: 846-852.

3.  Dukes CE (1932) The classification of cancer of the rectum.  J Pathol Bacteriol 35: 323-332.

4.  Miller W, Ota DM, Giacco G, Guinee V, Irimura T, Nicolson GL, Cleary KR (1985) Absence of relationship of size of primary colon carcinoma with metastasis and survival. Clin Exp Metastasis 3: 189-196.

5.  Wolmark N, Cruz I, Redmond CK, Fisher B, Fisher ER, contributing NSABP investigators (1983) Tumor size and regional lymph node metastasis in colorectal cancer: Primary analysis from the NSABP clinical trials.  Cancer 51: 1315-1322.

6.  Fearon ER, Vogelstein B (1990) A genetic model for colorectal tumorigenesis. Cell 61: 759-767.

7.  Irimura T, Ota DM, Cleary KR (1987) *Ulex europeus* agglutinin-I reactive high-molecular-weight glycoproteins of adenocarcinoma of distal colon and rectum and their possible relationship with metastatic potential. Cancer Res 47: 881-889.

8.  Yamori T, Kimura H, Stewart K, Ota DM, Cleary KR, Irimura T (1987) Differential production of high molecular weight sulfated glycoproteins in normal colonic mucosa, primary colon carcinoma and metastases.  Cancer Res 47: 2741-2747.

9.  Irimura T, Carlson DA, Yamori T, Price J, Giavazzi R, Ota DM, Cleary KR (1988) Differential expression of a sialoglycoprotein with an approximate molecular weight of 900,000 on metastatic human colon carcinoma cells growing in culture and tumor tissues. Cancer Res 48: 2353-2360.

10.  Yamori T, Ota DM, Cleary KR, Hoff S, Hager LG, Irimura T (1989) Monoclonal antibody against human colonic sulfomucin: Immunochemical detection of its binding sites in colonic mucosa, colorectal primary carcinoma, and metastasis. Cancer Res 49: 887-894.

11.  Hoff S, Matsushita Y, Ota DM, Cleary KR, Yamori T, Hakomori S, Irimura T (1989) Increased expression of sialyl-dimeric Le$^X$ antigen in advanced primary colorectal carcinomas and liver metastases.  Cancer Res 49: 6883-6888.

12.  Hoff SD, Irimura T, Matsushita Y, Ota DM, Cleary KR, Hakomori S (1990) Metastatic potential of colon carcinoma: Expression of ABO/Lewis-related antigens.  Arch Surg 125: 206-209.

13.  Matsushita Y, Cleary KR, Ota DM, Hoff SD, Irimura T (1990) Sialyl-dimeric Le$^X$ antigen expressed on mucin-like glycoproteins in colorectal cancer metastases. Lab Invest 63: 780-791.

14.  Irimura T, Yamori T, Bennett SC, Ota DM, Cleary KR (1987) The relationship of collagenolytic activity to stage of human colorectal carcinoma.  Int J Cancer 40: 24-31.

15.    Kannagi R, Fukushi Y, Tachikawa T, Noda A, Shin S, Shigeta K, Hiraiwa N, Fukuda Y, Inamoto T, Hakomori S (1986) Quantitative and qualitative characterization of human cancer-associated serum glycoprotein antigens expressing fucosyl or sialyl-fucosyl type 2 chain polylactosamine. Cancer Res 46: 2619-2626.

16.    Magnani JL, Nilsson B, Brockhaus M, Zopf D, Steplewski Z, Koprowski H, Ginsburg V (1981) A monoclonal antibody-defined antigen associated with gastrointestinal cancer is a ganglioside-containing sialylated lacto-N-fuco-pentaose II. J Biol Chem 257: 14365-14369.

17.    Matsushita Y, Hoff SD, Nudelman ED, Ohtaka M, Hakomori S, Ota DM,, Cleary KR, Irimura T. (1991) Metastatic behavior and cell surface properties of HT-29 human colon carcinoma variant cells selected for their differential expression of sialyl-dimeric Le$^X$ antigen. Clin Exp Metastasis 9: 283-299.

18.    Matsushita Y, Nakamori S, Seftor EA, Hendrix MJC, Irimura T. (1991) Human colon carcinoma cells with invasive capacity obtained by selection for sialyl-dimeric Le$^X$ antigen. Exp Cell Res 196: 20-25.

19.    Irimura T, Nakamori S, Shinha S, Matsushita Y, Smith C W, Hakomori S, Fidler IJ.   Tumor cell adhesion and metastasis mediated by sialyl Lewis-X carbohydrate antigen. submitted.

20.    Mafune K, Ravikumar TS, Wong JM, Yow H, Chen LB, Steel GD. (1990) Expression of a $M_r$ 32,000 laminin-binding protein messenger RNA in human colon carcinoma correlates with disease progression. Cancer Res, 50: 3888-3891.

21.    Cioce V, Castronovo V, Shmookler BM, Garbisa S, Grigioni WF, Liotta LA, Sobel ME. (1991) Increased expression of the laminin receptor in human colon cancer. J Natl Cancer Inst 83: 29-36.

22.    Nicolson GL. (1982) Cancer metastasis. Organ colonization and cell-surface properties of malignant cells. Biochem Biophys Acta 695: 113-176.

23.    Fearon ER, Cho KR, Nigro JM, Kern SE, Simons JW, Ruppert JM, Hamilton SR, Presinger AC, Thomas G, Kinzler KW, Vogelstein B. (1990) Identification of a chromosome 18q gene that is altered in colorectal cancers. Science 247: 49-56.

24.    Benchimol S, Fuks A, Jothy SM, Beauchemin N, Shirota K, Stanners CP. (1989) Carcinoembryonic antigen, a human tumor marker, functions as an intercellular adhesion molecule. Cell 57: 327-334.

25.    Lowe JB, Stoolman LM, Nair RP, Larsen RD, Berhend TL, Marks RM. (1990) ELAM-1-dependent cell adhesion to vascular endothelium determined by a transfected human fucosyltransferase cDNA. Cell 63: 475-484.

26.    Phillips ML, Nudelman, Gaeta FCA, Perez M, Singhal AK, Hakomori S, Paulson JC. (1990) ELAM-1 mediates cell adhesion by recognition of a carbohydrate ligand, sialyl-Le$^X$. Science 250: 1130-1132.

27.    Walz G, Aruffo A, Kolanus A, Bevilacqua D, Seed B. (1990) Recognition by ELAM-1 of the sialyl-Le$^X$ determinant on myeloid and tumor cells. Science 250: 1132-1135.

28.    Rice, GE., and Bevilacqua, MP. (1989) An inducible endothelial cell surface glycoprotein mediates melanoma adhesion. Science 246: 1303-1306.,

29.    Takada A, Ohmori K, Takahashi N, Tsuyuoka K, Yago K, Zenita K, Hasegawa A, Kannagi R. (1991) Adhesion of human cancer cells to vascular endothelium mediated by a carbohydrate antigen, sialyl Lewis A. Biochem. Biophys Res Commun 179: 713-719.

30.    Aruffo A, Dietsh MT, Wan H, Hellstrom E, Hellstrom I. (1992) Granule membrane protein 140 (GMP140) binds to carcinomas and carcinoma-derived cell lines. Proc Natl Acad Sci USA 89: 2292-2296.

# EXPERIMENTAL IMMUNOTHERAPY OF BREAST CANCER USING ALPHA INTERFERON CONJUGATED TO MONOCLONAL ANTIBODY Mc5

Luciano Ozzello,[1] Carolyn M. De Rosa ,[1] Edward W. Blank,[2]
Kari  Cantell,[3] Roberto L. Ceriani,[2]  and David V. Habif, Sr.[1]

[1]College of Physicians and Surgeons , Columbia University
New York, NY  10032
[2]Cancer Research Fund of Contra Costa, Walnut Creek, CA 94596
[3]National Public Health Institute, SF-00280 Helsinki, Finland

## INTRODUCTION

In recent years, rapidly advancing knowledge on biological response modifiers and the advent of monoclonal antibodies (MoAbs) have provided renewed incentives for immunotherapy of malignant neoplastic diseases.  Indeed, important progress has been made in the management of several solid tumors and leukemias through a variety of immunological manipulations,[1,2] while other tumors, including carcinomas of the breast, have thus far been regarded as poor candidates for immunotherapy.  Nevertheless, some encouraging local results have been obtained in breast cancer recurrences and metastases treated with intralesional (i.l.) injections of interferons (IFNs).[3-5]  A recent study has shown that natural interferon-$\alpha$ combined to natural interferon-$\gamma$ (nIFN-$\alpha$/nIFN-$\gamma$) delivered i.l. to recurrences and metastases of carcinomas of the breast can effectively eradicate the tumor cells apparently through direct antineoplastic effects and enhancement of cell-mediated immunological responses.[5]

At the present time, complete eradication of breast cancer cells in patients can be achieved when the IFNs are injected i.l., but not when they are delivered systemically.[4,5] Likewise, experiments *in vivo* using human breast cancer xenografts growing in nude mice have shown that complete and lasting regressions of the tumors can be obtained with i.l. injections of nIFN-$\alpha$/nIFN-$\gamma$,[6] whereas only partial regressions are observed when the IFNs are delivered systemically.[6,7]

*Antigen and Antibody Molecular Engineering in Breast Cancer Diagnosis
and Treatment,* Edited by R.L. Ceriani, Plenum Press, New York, 1994

35

It is thus apparent from clinical and experimental evidence that IFNs can eradicate breast cancer cells when their concentrations in the tumor tissue are elevated. Therefore, in order to enhance the efficacy of IFN-therapy, it is advisable to envision modalities to deliver the IFNs selectively to the neoplastic cells and to retain them within the tumor for as long as possible. This might be accomplished by delivering IFNs conjugated to MoAbs recognizing breast cancer-associated antigens. To test this hypothesis we have carried out experiments using an immunoconjugate composed of nIFN-α and Mc5, a MoAb raised against a breast epithelial mucin,[8] to treat human breast cancer xenografts growing in nude mice. Mc5, together with other MoAbs of the same group (Mc1, Mc3 and Mc8) have been shown to actively bind to human mammary carcinoma cells and to exert a growth inhibitory activity on human breast cancer xenografts,[9] an activity that was enhanced when [131]I was bound to the same MoAbs.[10]

Results to date indicate that the antitumor effects of immunoconjugate nIFN-α/Mc5 are greater than those of nIFN-α and of Mc5 used separately. Preliminary findings have been reported earlier.[11] In this essay we wish to present evidence supporting the conclusion that the enhanced antitumor action of nIFN-α/Mc5 is the result of a combination of interrelated mechanisms including targeting of the IFN by Mc5, impeded elimination of the IFN, and IFN-mediated up-regulation of antigenic expression by the carcinoma cells.

## IMMUNOCONJUGATE

Human nIFN-α was conjugated in a noncleavable manner to MoAb Mc5 in a 1:1 molecular ratio. The nIFN-α[12] was purified by immunoadsorption on sepharose containing mouse NK2 MoAb anti-human IFN-α[13] and had a specific activity of $2 \times 10^8$ IU/mg of protein. In the preparation of nIFN-α to be used in the conjugate, the albumin stabilizer was omitted to avoid interference in the conjugation. Mc5, an IgG$_1$ murine MoAb prepared against human milk fat globule proteins, recognizes a mucin molecule on the cell surface of normal and neoplastic human mammary epithelium.[8] nIFN-α was conjugated to Mc5 or to irrelevant mouse IgG$_1$ via the noncleavable homobifunctional imidoester dimethyladipimidate (DMA, Pierce, Rockford,IL).[14] The reaction was terminated by adding 1.0 M glycine in phosphate buffered saline (PBS). The final mixture was diluted in PBS containing 0.5% bovine serum albumin (BSA) and frozen at -80°C. The conjugation procedure did not affect the specific activity of the nIFN-α as tested by its antiviral activity.

## EXPERIMENTAL DESIGN

Xenografts of the human mammary carcinoma cell line MCF-7 were transplanted bilaterally in the s.c. tissue of the dorso-lateral regions of female nude mice as previously described.[15] For optimal growth of these estrogen-dependent tumors a pellet of 1.25 mg of 17β-estradiol was implanted s.c. in all animals prior to transplantation. Treatment was initiated when the tumors reached a size of 60-70 $mm^3$. The experimental substances were injected in 1 of the 2 tumors in 0.04 ml of PBS containing 0.5% BSA. Control animals were given injections of 0.04 ml PBS with 0.5% BSA. The injected tumors received 4 cycles of 5 daily injections separated by 2 days of rest. Injected and noninjected tumors were excised 24 hours after the 20th injection. When the tumors regressed completely, the tumor bed including skin and s.c. tissue was excised *en bloc*. Specimens were fixed in 10% buffered formalin and embedded in paraffin for histological examination. If enough tissue was available a portion of the tumor was also fixed in Bouin's solution and part was frozen at -80°C. Paraffin sections were stained with hematoxylin and eosin. Immunohistochemical staining with biotinylated MoAb Mc5 was done on paraffin sections using the avidin-biotin technique (Vectastain ABC Kit, Vector Laboratories, Burlingame, CA). Incubation with the primary antibody at concentrations ranging from 0.1 μg to 5 μg/ml was carried out overnight at 4°C.

The therapeutic response was assessed as described earlier[6] by monitoring the evolution of the tumor volumes at the beginning of each 5-day treatment cycle and at the time of sacrifice, and by calculating the growth increment (GInc) of each tumor. In addition, the percentage of inhibition of growth (%IG) was determined[16] to corroborate the GInc. Student's *t* test and Wilcoxon rank-sum test were used for statistical evaluation at a significance level of 0.05 and were found to yield equivalent results.


## GROWTH INHIBITORY EFFECTS

### Effects of nIFN-α/Mc5

Table 1 and Fig. 1 show the effects on the growth of MCF-7 xenografts of nIFN-α and Mc5 injected singly or conjugated. It can be seen that treatment with nIFN-α (2 x $10^5$ IU per injection), when compared to the PBS controls, resulted in a lower GInc and a 30.6% IG (p<0.001) in the injected tumors, whereas Mc5 (50 μg per injection) had no growth inhibitory effects. With the immunoconjugate (nIFN-α, 2 x $10^5$ IU/Mc5, 5 μg per injection) a much greater growth inhibition was observed (p<0.025). The tumors decreased progressively in size and at the end of therapy showed a striking decrease in the number of tumor cells and of their mitotic activity, together with interstitial fibrosis. None of these tumors, however, underwent complete regression. It is of interest to note that when nIFN-α and Mc5 were injected in combination, but not conjugated, the growth inhibition was significantly less than that achieved with the immunoconjugate (p<0.0025). The noninjected tumors of animals treated with the immunoconjugate showed significant growth inhibitions although of lesser magnitude than those of the corresponding injected tumors. This growth inhibition was over twice as much as that caused by nIFN-α (p<0.025).

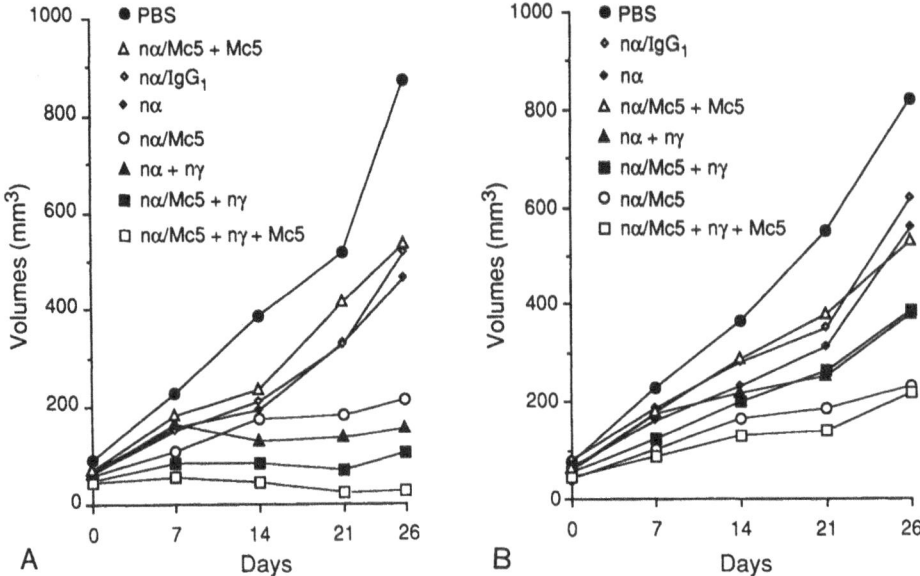

**Fig. 1.** Growth curves for selected control and experimental groups. A, injected tumors; B, noninjected tumors.

**Table 1.** Antitumor effects of immunoconjugate nIFN-α/Mc5 on MCF-7 xenografts (4 cycles of i.l. injections).[1]

|  |  | Injected Tumors | | Non-injected tumors | |
| --- | --- | --- | --- | --- | --- |
| Treatment | N | GInc | % IG | GInc | % IG |
| PBS | 5 | 3.8 ± 0.3 | - | 4.2 ± 0.7 | - |
| nIFN-α | 5 | 2.5 ± 0.3 | 30.6 ± 10.3 | 3.2 ± 0.2 | 21.3 ± 5.9 |
| Mc5 | 5 | 4.9 ± 0.6 | 0 | 4.2 ± 0.8 | 0 |
| nIFN-α /Mc5 | 6 | 1.4 ± 0.1 | 62.4 ± 3.8 | 2.2 ± 0.3 | 46.1 ± 8.5 |
| nIFN-α + Mc5 | 5 | 2.9 ± 0.2 | 23.3 ± 6.1 | 3.8 ± 0.3 | 7.3 ± 7.7 |
| nIFN-α /IgG₁ | 5 | 3.2 ± 0.7 | 15.7 ± 19.9 | 2.9 ± 0.2 | 27.9 ± 6.8 |

[1] Mean ± S.E.

To test whether the action of nIFN-α/Mc5 was simply due to the immunoglobulin component of the conjugate, nIFN-α was conjugated to an irrelevant murine IgG$_1$ (5 µg per injection) which resulted in a modest growth inhibition of the injected tumors. This inhibition was significantly less than that produced by nIFN-α/Mc5 (p<0.005), whereas the difference between the growth inhibitions caused by nIFN-α/IgG$_1$ and nIFN-α alone was small and not statistically significant (p>0.2). In the noninjected tumors, the growth was inhibited more by nIFN-α/Mc5 than by nIFN-α/IgG$_1$, but the difference was of marginal significance (p=0.055).

## Supplementation of nIFN-α/Mc5 with nIFN-γ

In view of the known synergism between type I (α, β) and type II (γ) IFNs it was interesting to determine whether and to what extent nIFN-γ could enhance the anti-tumor action of the immunoconjugate. The human nIFN-γ used in these experiments was prepared as described earlier[17] and was free of tumor necrosis factor or interleukins.[18] It had a specific activity of $2 \times 10^7$ IU/mg of protein and was used at the dose of $1 \times 10^5$ IU per injection. Table 2 and Fig. 1 illustrate that i.l. injections of nIFN-γ alone did not inhibit the growth of injected and noninjected xenografts. On the contrary, when nIFN-γ was injected in combination with nIFN-α/Mc5, the resulting anti-neoplastic effects on the injected tumors were significantly greater than those of nIFN-α/Mc5 alone (p<0.025). This appeared to be due to the marked synergistic action of the 2 IFNs since the differences in the effects of nIFN-α/Mc5 + nIFN-γ and nIFN-α + nIFN-γ were small and

**Table 2.** Effects of nIFN-γ on the antitumor action of nIFN-α/Mc5 on MCF-7 xenografts (4 cycles of i.l. injections).[1]

| Treatment | N | Injected Tumors | | Non-injected tumors | |
|---|---|---|---|---|---|
| | | GInc | % IG | GInc | % IG |
| PBS | 5 | 3.8 ± 0.3 | - | 4.2 ± 0.7 | - |
| nIFN-γ | 5 | 3.8 ± 0.4 | 0 | 4.4 ± 0.7 | 0 |
| nIFN-α /Mc5 | 6 | 1.4 ± 0.1 | 62.4 ± 3.8 | 2.2 ± 0.3 | 46.1 ± 8.5 |
| nIFN-α /Mc5 + nIFN-γ | 10 | 0.7 ± 0.2 | 80.0 ± 4.3 | 2.6 ± 0.3 | 34.6 ± 8.8 |
| nIFN-α + nIFN-γ | 5 | 0.8 ± 0.2 | 75.9 ± 5.2 | 2.3 ± 0.3 | 43.3 ± 9.3 |

[1]Mean ± S.E.

not statistically significant. No stimulatory action was observed in the noninjected tumors presumably because of the limited systemic effect of nIFN-γ.

### Supplementation of nIFN-α/Mc5 with Mc5

Since the amount of Mc5 in the immunoconjugate was very small (5 µg per injection) it was of interest to investigate the effects of higher doses of free Mc5 (50 µg/injection) administered in combination with the immunoconjugate or with each IFN (Table 3, Fig. 1). As indicated above, Mc5 alone had no growth inhibitory effects on the injected and noninjected tumors. In fact, the GInc of the tumors injected with Mc5 was greater than that of the control tumors injected with PBS, although the difference was not statistically significant (p>0.05). Likewise, supplementation with Mc5 did not cause any statistically significant enhancement of the antitumor activity of nIFN-α, nIFN-γ, nIFN-α + nIFN-γ and nIFN-α/Mc5. On the contrary, in mice treated with nIFN-α/Mc5 + nIFN-γ + Mc5 the growth inhibition was greater than with nIFN-α/Mc5 + nIFN-γ in both injected (p<0.01) and noninjected (p<0.05) tumors. Histologically, the estimated number of residual carcinoma cells at the end of therapy was smaller than in any other groups and complete eradication of neoplastic cells was seen in 1 of the 9 injected tumors.

Table 3. Antitumor effects of immunoconjugate nIFN-α/Mc5 supplemented with free Mc5 (4 cycles of i.l. injections)[1].

| Treatment | N | Injected Tumors | | Non-injected tumors | |
|---|---|---|---|---|---|
| | | GInc | % IG | GInc | % IG |
| PBS | 5 | 3.8 ± 0.3 | - | 4.2 ± 0.7 | - |
| Mc5 | 5 | 4.9 ± 0.6 | 0 | 4.2 ± 0.8 | 0 |
| nIFN-α /Mc5 + Mc5 | 9 | 2.9 ± 0.3 | 22.7 ± 9.3 | 3.1 ± 0.3 | 23.8 ± 8.3 |
| nIFN-α + nIFN-γ + Mc5 | 9 | 0.2 ± 0.1 | 94.0 ± 2.1 | 1.7 ± 0.3 | 56.9 ± 7.7 |
| nIFN-α /Mc5 | 6 | 1.4 ± 0.1 | 62.4 ± 3.8 | 2.2 ± 0.3 | 46.1 ± 8.5 |
| nIFN-α + Mc5 | 5 | 2.9 ± 0.2 | 23.3 ± 6.1 | 3.8 ± 0.3 | 7.3 ± 7.7 |
| nIFN-γ + Mc5 | 5 | 3.2 ± 0.5 | 17.5 ± 13.9 | 4.4 ± 0.6 | 0 |
| nIFN-α + nIFN-γ + Mc5 | 5 | 0.5 ± 0.1 | 87.0 ± 4.0 | 1.7 ± 0.3 | 57.7 ± 6.6 |

[1] Mean ± S.E.

The findings described above indicate that nIFN-α delivered as a noncleavable immunoconjugate with Mc5 causes marked growth inhibitory effects that are much greater than those produced by nIFN-α and Mc5 delivered singly or combined in a nonconjugated form. Furthermore, it is apparent that supplementation with nIFN-γ enhances the growth inhibiting activity of the immunoconjugate, most likely as a result of synergism between nIFN-α and nIFN-γ. The effects of the supplementation with Mc5 are unclear. In a previous study,[9,10] Mc5 delivered i.p. at the dose of 600 μg every other day for 6 weeks, was found to inhibit the growth of breast cancer xenografts MX-1 and MCF-7. In the present experiments, free Mc5 was used at a lower dose (50 μg) and did not exert any growth inhibitory action, nor did it have any appreciable enhancing effects on the activity of nIFN-α and of nIFN-α/Mc5. It is possible that when delivered together with nIFN-α/Mc5, the excess free Mc5 competed with the conjugated Mc5 impeding the action of the latter. However, the enhancement of growth inhibition which occured when free Mc5 was administered together with nIFN-α/Mc5 + nIFN-γ remains unexplained.

## BIODISTRIBUTION STUDIES

Radiolabeled nIFN-α was used to investigate the localization of the IFN alone or conjugated. Radiolabeling was done with $^{125}$I to a specific activity of 53.6 mCi/mg by the chloramine T method.[10] $^{125}$I-nIFN-α was then conjugated with Mc5 or IgG$_1$ using the same technique as for the unlabeled immunoconjugates. Nude mice bearing bilateral MCF-7 xenografts were divided into 3 groups of 6 mice each. They received 1 unilateral i.l. injection of 20 μCi of $^{125}$I-nIFN-α/Mc5, $^{125}$I-nIFN-α/IgG$_1$ or $^{125}$I-nIFN-α unconjugated. Three mice from each group were sacrificed 4 and 24 hours after injection. Samples of injected and noninjected MCF-7 tumors, s.c. peritumoral tissue, blood, skin, liver and kidney were counted in a Multi-Prias gamma counter (Packard, Downers Grove, IL). The uptake was expressed as % injected dose (% ID) per gram of tissue. Statistical significance was checked with Student's $t$ test (0.05 significance level).

At 4 hours after injection (Table 4) a much larger % ID of $^{125}$I-nIFN-α/Mc5 was present in the injected tumors and in the surrounding s.c. tissue than in any other location. The amount of $^{125}$I-nIFN-α was greater when the IFN was conjugated to Mc5 than when it was injected as a single agent, although the difference was not statistically significant. A greater difference was observed between the % ID of $^{125}$I-nIFN-α/Mc5 and $^{125}$I-nIFN-α in the peritumoral tissue on the injected side (p<0.025) suggesting that the former was released from the injected tumors at a slower rate. Furthermore, the % ID of $^{125}$I-nIFN-α/ Mc5 was significantly greater than that of $^{125}$I-nIFN-α in the peripheral blood and in all other tissues including the noninjected tumors (p<0.025). These observations suggest that conjugation of the IFN to Mc5 enhances its uptake in the tissues and delays its release. These effects are not due primarily to the immunoglobulin part of the immunoconjugate since the % ID for $^{125}$I-nIFN-$\alpha$/Mc5 was much greater than that of $^{125}$I-nIFN-$\alpha$/IgG$_1$. At 24 hours after injection (Table 5) small measurable amounts of IFN were still present in all samples, more so in the injected tumors, but the differences between conjugated and free IFN were not statistically significant.

**Table 4.** Biodistribution of $^{125}$I-labeled nIFN$\alpha$ injected i.l. alone or conjugated to Mc5 or IgG$_1$ (% ID per gram of tissue at 4 hours).[1]

| Tissues | $^{125}$I-nIFN$\alpha$/Mc5 | $^{125}$I-nIFN$\alpha$ | $^{125}$I-nIFN$\alpha$/IgG$_1$ |
|---|---|---|---|
| Injected tumors | 16.85 ± 9.09 | 11.73 ± 5.19 | 4.89 ± 0.82 |
| Noninjected tumors | 2.65 ± 0.12 | 0.79 ± 0.58 | 1.07 ± 0.08 |
| Peritumoral (inj. side) | 11.75 ± 2.52 | 3.41 ± 1.06 | 5.40 ± 3.36 |
| Peritumoral (noninj. side) | 1.68 ± 0.09 | 0.28 ± 0.02 | 0.48 ± 0.05 |
| Blood | 2.16 ± 0.39 | 0.77 ± 0.07 | 1.20 ± 0.17 |
| Skin | 4.04 ± 0.70 | 0.82 ± 0.10 | 0.94 ± 0.17 |
| Liver | 1.03 ± 0.19 | 0.29 ± 0.08 | 0.56 ± 0.06 |
| Kidney | 6.45 ± 0.66 | 1.89 ± 0.21 | 2.54 ± 0.72 |

[1] Mean ± S.E.

**Table 5.** Biodistribution of $^{125}$I-labeled nIFN$\alpha$ injected i.l. alone or conjugated to Mc5 or IgG$_1$ (% ID per gram of tissue at 24 hours).[1]

| Tissues | $^{125}$I-nIFN$\alpha$/Mc5 | $^{125}$I-nIFN$\alpha$ | $^{125}$I-nIFN$\alpha$/IgG$_1$ |
|---|---|---|---|
| Injected tumors | 2.58 ± 0.85 | 3.01 ± 0.90 | 0.72 ± 0.26 |
| Noninjected tumors | 0.27 ± 0.03 | 0.18 ± 0.01 | 0.02 ± 0.01 |
| Peritumoral (inj. side) | 1.11 ± 0.49 | 2.47 ± 1.65 | 0.34 ± 0.17 |
| Peritumoral (noninj. side) | 0.20 ± 0.08 | 0.10 ± 0.01 | 0.03 ± 0.02 |
| Blood | 0.31 ± 0.08 | 0.22 ± 0.03 | 0.03 ± 0.01 |
| Skin | 0.29 ± 0.05 | 0.49 ± 0.18 | 0.07 ± 0.02 |
| Liver | 0.19 ± 0.04 | 0.14 ± 0.01 | 0.02 ± 0.01 |
| Kidney | 1.47 ± 0.16 | 0.63 ± 0.11 | 0.38 ± 0.16 |

[1] Mean ± S.E.

## IMMUNOLOGICAL EFFECTS

In the experimental model used in these studies a human tumor growing in a
murine host was treated with human IFNs. Under these circumstances, because of the
species specificity of nIFNs, the effects of the IFNs on the immunologically competent
cells of the host cannot be evaluated. Nevertheless, it is possible to evaluate the
modulatory effects of the IFNs on the antigenic expression of the carcinoma cells. This
was done immunohistochemically using biotinylated Mc5. Immunostaining of sections
from the MCF-7 xenografts with Mc5 at a concentration of 5 µg/ml showed

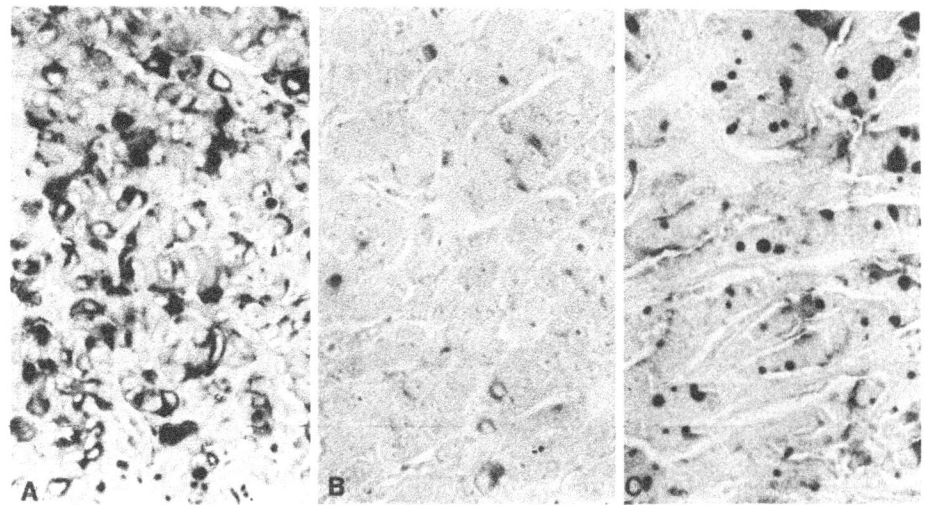

**Fig. 2.** A. Immunostaining of a PBS-injected MCF-7 tumor with Mc5 at a concentration
of 5 µg/ml. B. Same PBS-injected tumor stained with Mc5 at an end-point concentration of
0.1 µg/ml. C. MCF-7 tumor injected with nIFN-α/Mc5 stained with Mc5 (0.1 µg/ml).

immunoreactivity in most tumor cells. Reactivity was mainly localized on the cell
membranes and to a lesser extent in the cytoplasm, either in a diffuse manner or in
intracytoplasmic lumens (Fig 2A). Using Mc5 at an end-point dilution (0.1 µg/ml), only
a weak immunoreactivity was still present in rare cells of the control tumors (Fig 2B),
whereas a moderate to marked immunostaining was shown by the IFN-treated tumors
(Fig 2C). However, no appreciably greater reactivity could be detected in tumors treated
with the immunoconjugate as compared to those exposed to unconjugated preparations.
It is therefore apparent that nIFN-α up-regulated the expression of an antigen recognized
by Mc5 in the carcinoma cells.

## CONCLUSIONS

In these experiments we have shown that nIFN-α can destroy mammary carcinoma cells more effectively when it is conjugated to a MoAb than when it is used non-conjugated. Multiple mechanisms are likely to contribute to the enhanced antitumor activity of the immunoconjugate.

The biodistribution findings support both targeting of nIFN-α by Mc5 and its impeded elimination. Both of these effects are most likely the consequence of the binding of Mc5 to a specific antigen. On the one hand, Mc5 could not produce any antitumor effect of its own because of the very small dose contributed by the immuno-conjugate. On the other hand, these effects could not be ascribed merely to the immunoglobulin component of the conjugate through its large molecular weight (Mc5 150,000 and nIFN-α 20,000) since in all tissues examined, including kidneys, the amount of [125]I-nIFN-α/Mc5 was significantly larger than that of [125]I-nIFN-α/IgG$_1$.

The up-regulation of antigenic expression by the carcinoma cells caused by nIFN-α is not surprising as it is in keeping with previous observations by others[19,20] and by us.[5] It is tempting to speculate that targeting of the IFNs to the tumor and the antigenic up-regulation in the carcinoma cells acted in an interrelated fashion potentiating each other's effects. It is also possible that targeting of the IFN enhanced the antigenic up-regulation which in turn led to greater binding of nIFN-α/Mc5 and further direct action of nIFN-α on the carcinoma cells, both effects being favored by the delayed elimination of the IFN.

At the present time, the systemic effects of nIFN-α/Mc5, as judged by the response of noninjected tumors, are less than the local effects. It should be kept in mind, however, that in our experimental model, the IFN was presumably utilized in part by the injected tumors before being released into the surrounding tissues, thereby lessening the amount available systemically. Nevertheless, it is encouraging to observe that the immuno-conjugate did act at the systemic level, which justifies pursuing this line of investigation in order to optimize the composition and effectiveness of immunoconjugates in selectively delivering high concentrations of IFNs to carcinoma cells.

## ACKNOWLEDGEMENTS

Partial support was received from the Winfield Baird Foundation, William J. and Mary F. Cooper Research Fund, Jerome E. Goldman Cancer Research Fund, Margaret Milliken Hatch Foundation, Milstein Medical Research Foundation, Ambrose Monell Foundation, Mrs. Mary K. Monell, Mr. and Mrs. Anthony K. Moulton, Mr. and Mrs. George Shapiro, Theodore and Renee Weiler Foundation, the Weissman Charitable and Educational Fund and NIH/NCI Grant PO1-CA 42767 to R.L. Ceriani. We are grateful to H.-L. Kauppinen at the Finnish Red Cross Blood Transfusion Service for the purification of the interferon by immunoadsorption and to R. Gaslonde for his assistance in the statistical analyses.

# REFERENCES

1.  D. Goldstein, and J. Laszlo, Interferon therapy in cancer: from imaginon to interferon, *Cancer Res.* 46:4315 (1986).

2.  S.A. Rosenberg, The immunotherapy and gene therapy of cancer, *J. Clin. Oncol.* 10:180 (1992).

3.  G.P. Murphy, Current report on the interferon program at Rosewell Park Memorial Institute, *J. Surg. Oncol.* 17:99 (1981).

4.  R. Rosso, M.T. Nobile, M.R. Sertoli, A. Giannitelli, P.L. Santi, R. Volpe, and G. Nicolo, Antitumoral activity of human fibroblast interferon administered intranodularly, *Oncology* 42:86 (1985).

5.  L. Ozzello, D.V. Habif, C.M. De Rosa, and K. Cantell. Cellular events accompanying regression of skin recurrences of breast carcinomas treated with intralesional injections of natural interferons $\alpha$ and $\gamma$, *Cancer Res.* 52:4571 (1992).

6.  L. Ozzello, D.V. Habif, C.M. De Rosa, and K. Cantell, Treatment of human breast cancer xenografts using natural interferons-$\alpha$ and -$\gamma$ injected singly or in combination, *J. Interferon Res.* 8:679 (1988).

7.  F.R. Balkwill, E.M. Moodie, V. Freedman, and K.H. Fantes, Human interferon inhibits the growth of established human breast tumors in the nude mouse, *Int. J. Cancer* 30:231 (1982).

8.  R.L. Ceriani, J.A. Peterson, J.Y. Lee, R. Moncada, and E.W. Blank, Characterization of cell surface antigens of human mammary epithelial cells with monoclonal antibodies prepared against human milk fat globule, *Somat. Cell Genet.* 9:415 (1983).

9.  R.L. Ceriani, E.W. Blank, and J.A. Peterson, Experimental immunotherapy of human breast carcinomas implanted in nude mice with a mixture of monoclonal antibodies against human milk fat globule components, *Cancer Res.* 47:532 (1987).

10. R.L. Ceriani, and E. W. Blank, Experimental therapy of human breast tumors with [131]I-labeled monoclonal antibodies prepared against the human milk fat globule, *Cancer Res.* 48:4664 (1988).

11. L. Ozzello, C.M. De Rosa, E.W. Blank, K. Cantell, D.V. Habif, and R.L. Ceriani, Potentiation of anti-tumor efficacy resulting from the combined administration of interferon $\alpha$ and of an anti-breast epithelial monoclonal anibody in the treatment of breast cancer xenografts, *in:* "Breast Cancer Immunodiagnosis and Immunotherapy," R.L. Ceriani, ed., Plenum Press, New York (1989).

12. K. Cantell, S. Hirvonen, H-L. Kauppinen, and G. Myllyla, Production of interferon in human leukocytes from normal donors with the use of Sendai virus. *Methods Enzymol.* 78:29 (1981).

13. H-L. Kauppinen, S. Hirvonen, and K. Cantell, Effect of purification procedures on the composition of human leukocyte interferon preparations, *Methods Enzymol.* 119:27 (1986).

14. J.L. Dickerson, J.J. Cornuc, and D.C. Rees, Complex formation between flavodoxin and cytochrome C, *J. Biol. Chem.* 260:5175 (1985).

15. L. Ozzello, and M. Sordat, Behavior of tumors produced by transplantation of human mammary cell lines in athymic nude mice, *Eur. J. Cancer* 16:553 (1980).

16. K. Inoue, S. Fujimoto, and M. Ogawa, Antitumor efficacy of seventeen anticancer drugs in human breast cancer xenograft (MX-1) transplanted in nude mice, *Cancer Chemother. Pharmacol.* 10:182 (1983).

17. K. Cantell, S. Hirvonen, and H-L. Kauppinen, Production and partial purification of human immune interferon. *Methods Enzymol.* 119:54 (1986).

18. H-L. Kauppinen, B. Bang, J. Eronen, R. Majuri, G. Myllyla, H. Tolo, S. Hirvonen, and K. Cantell, Preparation of natural human gamma interferon for clinical use. *in:* "The Biology of the Interferon System", W.E. Stewart and H. Schellekens eds., Elsevier, Amsterdam (1986).

19. R. Tran, P. Horan Hand, J.W. Greiner, S. Pestka, and J. Schlom, Enhancement of surface antigen expression on human breast carcinoma cells by recombinant human interferons, *J. Interferon Res.* 8:75 (1988).

20. J.A. Leon, R. Mesa-Tejada, C.M. Gutieriez, A. Estabrook, J.W. Greiner, J. Schlom, and P.B. Fisher, Increased surface expression and shedding of tumor associated antigens by human breast carcinoma cells treated with recombinant human interferons or phorbol ester tumor promotors, *Anticancer Res.* 9:1639 (1989).

# CIRCULATING AND TISSUE MARKERS IN THE LONGITUDINAL MANAGEMENT OF BREAST CANCER PATIENTS

Morton K. Schwartz

Department of Clinical Chemistry
Memorial Sloan Kettering Cancer Center
New York, NY 10021

## INTRODUCTION

In the United States in 1992 there will be 180,000 cases of breast cancer and more than 45,000 deaths from that disease. It has been suggested that more than 90% of the deaths could be avoided if there was early detection and treatment[1]. Breast self-examination, clinical examination and mammography are the current screening procedures for breast cancer. There are no tumor markers or other laboratory tests that are useful in this regard. The mortality rate from breast cancer in women who avail themselves of screening programs is 50% lower at 5 years than women who have not been screened[2].

There are two very important questions in the management of breast cancer patients where tumor marker assays may play an important role. The first use is as a prognostic marker to be used following primary surgery to answer the question of recurrence particularly in the group of women with small cancers who do not exhibit positive lymph nodes but who will experience a recurrence in a short time. The second use of the markers is in monitoring patients and to use the values to evaluate response to therapy and to predict impending recurrence before there are clinical signs.

## SERUM MARKERS
## CEA

CEA levels have been shown to be elevated in about 50% of patients with breast cancer. However, the elevations are related to tumor burden and elevations are not observed in patients with early disease. In a review of the literature, elevations were seen in 9% of 194 patients with Stage I disease, 23% of 237 patients with Stage 2 disease, 45% of patients with Stage 3 disease and 58% of 2171 patients with Stage 4 breast cancer. Patients with bone or liver metastases had elevation more frequently than women with soft tissue metastases. There are conflicting reports concerning the role of CEA in monitoring patients with recurrent breast cancer. In a literature review of 10 reports in which serum CEA and recurrence were studied there were a total of

*Antigen and Antibody Molecular Engineering in Breast Cancer Diagnosis and Treatment*, Edited by R.L. Ceriani, Plenum Press, New York, 1994

47

1626 patients of whom 312 (19%) had recurrence. Of these 107 (34%) had an elevated or rising CEA level one to 31 months preceding documented clinical recurrence. In 120 other patients there was elevated CEA with no clinical evidence of recurrence. Thus in the 227 patients with an elevated CEA there was a false positive rate of 53%.[3] The confusion in use of CEA in monitoring may be related to the clearance kinetics during therapy. In a study of CEA in patients receiving therapy four distinct patterns were observed. Two patterns represented the expected picture, an immediate and linear fall during response or a continued linear rise reflecting failure of therapy. However, two other patterns were also recorded. In some responding patients there was an acute surge followed by a decline and in some patients who failed therapy there was a rapid decline followed by a progressive increase in CEA levels. The kinetic patterns are mathematically different and the authors suggest that knowledge of the paradoxical pattern will permit more effective use of CEA in monitoring.[4] It has been suggested that CEA monitoring during chemotheapy becomes useful if a baseline CEA value is obtained during the first 3 courses of chemotherapy (3 months) and that evaluation is begun after the reference value is obtained.[5] Despite reservations, Mughal and his associates have been very positive in the use of CEA in monitoring patients receiving therapy. In their study of 84 patients with metastatic breast cancer who had pretreatment elevated CEA values, the CEA decreased in 94% of the patients who responded to therapy (66/70). There was a duration of response of 22 months in those in whom the CEA returned to normal levels and nine months in those women in whom the CEA decreased but never returned to normal. Increases in CEA correlated with disease progression in 87% of the patients and rises in CEA proceeded evidence of progression in 77%.[6]

MUCIN MARKERS

During the past few years there have been a large number of mucin-type antigens proposed as breast cancer markers. Monoclonal antibodies have been prepared to many of these and diagnostic kits have been made available on an "investigational use only" basis for CA 15-3, CA 549, CA M26, CA M29, MSA, BCM and BR 27.29. The question has been raised whether any of these alone or in combination with each other and/or CEA can be useful in the management of the patient with breast cancer.

CA 15-3 is the earliest of these markers and the most widely studied. This high molecular weight protein reacts with two monoclonal antibodies 115D8 (anti milk fat globule membrane) and DF3 (anti membrane-enriched extract of a breast cancer cell line). In the initial report of CA 15-3, elevations were observed in 6/31 (14%) patients with non-metastatic disease.[7] In these same patients none exhibited elevations of CEA. Neither CA 15-3 or CEA was useful in identifying women with non-metastatic breast cancer. CA 15-3 was elevated in 99/158 (63%) of patients with either local or distant metastases and in 43/58 (76%) of the women with extensive metastases. When the total group was considered CEA was elevated in a slightly smaller percentage of women. In the women with metastases to bone CA 15-3 was elevated in 24/51 (71%) of the women compared to CEA elevations in only 15/34 (44%). CA 15-3 was extremely useful in monitoring patients. In 19/21 (91%) of women with recurrence there was at least a 25% increase in CA 15-3 and in 7/9 (78%) who had regression of the cancer there was at least a 50% decrease in the circulating CA 15-3.

There have been many other studies of CA 15-3 and CEA.[8-10]  The consensus of opinion is that neither marker is useful for the detection of early breast cancer, but they may be extremely useful in monitoring therapeutic response since antigen levels correlate closely with disease status.  In most patients CA 15-3 is the most demonstrative marker, but this is not always the case and it is necessary to measure both markers if monitoring is to be useful.

In another study, CA 15-3 was elevated in 18/35 (51%) of patients with a single metastatic site compared to 112/138 (81%) of women with multiple metastatic sites.  Again, the highest percentage of elevations was seen in women with bone metastases (31/44 (77%).  In patients with a single metastatic site, elevations of CA 15-3 were not significantly higher than elevations of CEA.  There was a significant correlation between the extent of disease and CA 15-3 levels.  An important observation in this and many other studies is that CA 15-3 is elevated in 30% to 50% of patients with ovarian cancer.

In a prospective study of 671 breast cancer patients who did not have metastases at the time of entry into the study, metastases occurred in 205 women within 8 to 314 months (median 51 months).  At the time of recurrence neither CEA nor CA 15-3 was elevated in 46 (22%) patients;  CA 15-3 alone in 56 (27%); CEA alone in 10 (5%); and both markers were elevated in 93 (45%).  In 466 patients who did not have metastases over an observation period of from 8 to 216 months (median observation 42 months), none had levels of CA 15-3 > 50 U/mL, and 63 had levels > 25 U/mL.  Seventy-seven of the 205 patients wtih recurrence were treated with tamoxifen citrate.  In 29 there was regression of disease associated with a decrease in the marker level.  In 48 of the patients there was progressive disease and continued rise in CA 15-3.

In our studies of women at high risk for recurrence after primary therapy or undergoing treatment of metastastic disease we observed at the time of recurrence elevated CA 15-3 in 23/33 (70%) of patients compared to elevations of CEA 19/33 (58%).[11]  We followed 39 patients sequentially and arbitrarity defined a significant change as a 25% rise or fall from baseline.  CEA and CA 15-3 seemed to provide comparable data in patients who responded to therapy with decreased levels of CEA in 6/9 (67%) of patients and CA 15-3 in 5/6 women (56%).  CEA remained unchanged in 2 responding patients and increased in 1 while CA 15-3 remained unchanged in 4 patients.  In 8 individuals with stable disease, 7 (88%) had unchanged CEA and 6 (75%) had no change in CA 15-3.  However, in patients with progressive disease CA 15-3 was clearly superior in monitoring the clinical course.  CA 15-3 increased in 21/22 (95%) patients and in the other patient the CA 15-3 rose but not 25% from the baseline.  CEA increased in only 14/22 (64%) of the women, decreased in 7 and remained unchanged in the other.  We feel that CA 15-3 has a substantial advantage over CEA in monitoring disease progression.  It must be stated that in an occcassional case monitoring with CEA may be superior to CA 15-3 in predicting therapeutic failure and clinical progression of disease and therefore both markers are recommended in the management of breast cancer patients.

Another high-molecular weight mucin proposed as a circulating breast cancer marker is CA 549 which reacts with two specific monoclonals; BC4E549 derived from a breast cancer cell line and BC4N154 from a milk fat globule.[12-16]  With an appropriate normal/abnormal cutoff point, abnormal CA 549 was found in 19/25 (76%) patients with advanced breast cancer. Elevations were not recorded in 100 normal persons nor in 22 women with benign breast disease. In another study, elevations were found in 40/80 (50%) patients with advanced breast cancer, 1/30 (3%) patients with early breast cancer, and 3/79 (4%) patients with benign breast disease. Elevations were observed in 11/88 (13%)patients with other forms of cancer. The proposed advantage of CA 549 is its high degree of specificity (about 98%) despite a sensitivity of only 50% in advanced breast cancer.

In our studies we have not observed elevations in any of 30 women with Stage I-III breast cancer, 2/4 women with Stage IV cancer but in 40/56 (71%) of women with recurrent metastatic disease.[17] In this same population CA 15-3 was elevated 3/32 (9%) women with Stage I-III disease, each of the four women with Stage IV cancer and 44/56 (79%) women with metastatic disease. CEA was abnormal in 7/32 (22%) patients with Stage I-III breast cancer; 3/4 with Stage I cancer and in 38/56 (68%) of women with recurrent disease. CA 549 was elevated in 3/52 (6%) women with benign disease compared to 7/52 (13%) who had elevations in CA 15-3 and 7/52 (13%) who expressed CEA elevations. When combined CEA and CA 15-3 had a sensitivity of 88% and a specificity of 77% compared to a sensitivity of 86% and was 83% when CA 549 was combined with CEA.

CA M26 and CA M29 are also mucin type markers.[18] Neither marker is elevated in most patients with early stage cancer, but CA M26 was abnormal in 47/80 (59%) women with metastatic disease and CA M29 in 57/80 (71%). In these same women CA 15-3 was elevated in 63 (79%) and CEA in 54 (68%).[19] These markers were less sensitive then either CEA or CA 15-3 in identifying breast cancer, but they have a superior specificity. CA M29 was elevated in 86% of women with advanced breast cancer and modestly elevated in 9% of women with benign disease. As a pair, these antigens may be useful in monitoring patients receiving chemotherapy.

CA M26 and CA M29 have been compared to BCM-EIA.[20] BCM-EIA is a mucin identified by two monoclonal antibodies; M85 which reacts with i/l oligosaccharide antigen sequences expressed on O-glycoside linkages and F26/22 which reacts with a glycoprotein called ductal carcinoma antigen. None of the markers were elevated in normal women or those with benign breast disease when the mean + 2SD was used as the cutoff. In women with primary breast cancer, CA M26 was elevated in 4/22 (18%), CA M29 in 2/15 (13%) and BCM in 3/22 (14%). In patients with recurrent disease CA M26 was abnormal in 4/31 (13%) patients, CA M29 in 8/31 (26%) and in BCM 13/31 (42%). The sites of recurrence were not described. In longitudinal studies, elevations in BCM greater than 25% above the base line value were observed in 27/32 (84%) of the patients 0-99 days before recurrence compared to 17/32 (53%) for CA M26 and 14/32 (44%) for CA M29. BCM and/or CA M26 elevations were observed as many as 299 days prior to clinical recurrence. The authors conclude that individually or together the 3 markers are unable to identify primary or recurrent breast cancer patients. In longitudinal measurements BCM and CA M29 can be helpful in providing a significant lead time before clinical evidence of recurrence.

Another breast related mucin, MSA has been studied by several workers. In one study an abnormal/normal cutoff point was used in which 20% of normal women had abnormal values, as did 13% of pregnant women. With this inappropriately low cutoff, elevations were found in 9/12 (75%) patients with Stage I breast cancer, 8/9 (89%) patients with Stage II disease, and 53/57 (93%) patients with Stage IV cancer. MSA showed increasing values in 7/8 patients who had progressive disease and decreasing values in 6/6 patients who had regressing disease. MSA was stated to be a superior marker to CEA. Elevations were seen in 2/12 (17%) patients with benign breast tumors, 35/62 (57%) of individuals with liver disease, 30% of those with gastrointestinal disorders, and 43% of women with pancreatic disease. In addition, 70% of women with ovarian cancer, 60% of individuals with colon cancer, 70% of persons with lung cancer and 59% of persons with kidney cancer had elevations.

CA 27.29 is a mucin type breast antigen similar to CA 15-3.[23] The antigen reacts with an antibody, B 27.29, with similar epitope binding as DF3, the antibody used in the CA 15-3 assay. In a comparative study with CA 15-3 of 100 women with Stage I-IV breast cancer a regression equation, $y = 12.8824 + 0.9343X (y = CA 15-3)$ $r = 0.95$ was obtained. There was a 95.2% concordance in 146 samples. Neither CA 27.29 or CA 15-3 was elevated in early stage breast cancer, but CA 27.29 was elevated in 83% of patients with metastatic disease compared to only 69% who demonstrated CA 15-3 elevations.[23]

Although it is not a mucin, preliminary evidence has been presented that TPS (Tissue proliferative antigen) is a useful adjunct to the mucin markers. Van Dalen has compared TPS with CEA and CA 15-3.[24] In patients with Stage I-III breast cancer CEA was elevated in 12/129 (9%) patients; CA 15-3 in 17/129 (13%) and TPS in 24/129 (19%). In 10 Stage IV cancer patients TPS was elevated in 8, CEA in 4 and CA 15-3 in 7. TPS appeared to useful in monitoring. Additional studies are needed to establish the role of TPS.

## PROGNOSTIC MARKERS

There has been a concerted effort to elucidate prognostic indicators which can assist in identifying patients who will have a recurrence. Tumor size, the number of positive nodes, age, menopausal status, histology as well as grade, lymphocyte infiltration, lymphatic or blood vessel invasion and DNA ploidy have all been useful.[25] The most extensive laboratory evaluation of tissue prognostic factors has been related to estrogen receptor protein (ERP) and progesterone receptor protein (PRP). In a summary of a large number of patient studies, 25% of ERP positive patients recurred in 5 years compared to 34% of ERP negative patients. ERP but not PRP was a highly significant discriminant for recurrence in almost 2000 node-negative patients. However, most studies have concluded that in node negative patients despite a statistically significant relationship to recurrence, receptors are not a major indicator of prognosis and do not provide sufficient information to permit identification of poor prognosis patients who may be administered aggressive adjuvant therapy. There is considerable difference in opinion concerning the prognostic significance of other tissue markers. These markers include epidermal growth factor (EGF), C-erb B-2 oncogene, cathepsin D, S2 gene, plasminogen activators and other markers of proliferation and membrane breakdown. Long term studies are neecded to establish the true role of these indicators and what if any is their clinical application.

## REFERENCES

1. M.K. Schwartz. The role of the laboratory in the prevention and detection of chronic disease, Clin Chem 38:1539 (1992).

2. S. Shapiro, W. Venet, L. Strax and R. Roesser, Selection, follow up and analysis in the Health Insurance Plan Study: A randomized trial with breast cancer screening, Natl Cancer Inst Monogr 67:65 (1985).

3. D. B. Beard and C. M. Haskell, Carcinoembryonic antigen in breast cancer; Clinical Review; Am J Med 80:241-245 (1986).

4. D.T. Kiang, L.J. Greenberg and B.J. Kennedy, Tumor marker kinetics in the monitoring of breast cancer, Cancer 65:193-199 (1989).

5. A. Quentmeir, P. Schlag, P. Hohenberger et al Assessment of serial carcinoembryonic antigen: Determinations to monitor the therapeutic progress and prognosis of metastatic liver disease treated by regional chemotherpy. J Surg Oncol 40:112-118 (1989).

6. A.W. Mughal, G.H. Hortobaygi, H.A. Fritsche et al, Serial plasma carcinobmbryonic antigen measurements during treatment of metastatic breast cancer. JAMA 249:1881-1885 (1983).

7. D.F. Hayes, V.R. Zurawski, D.W., Kufe, Comparison of circulating CA 15-3 and carcinoembryonic antigen levels in patients with breast cancer. 4:1542-1550 (1980).

8. C. Todini, D.F. Hayes, R. Gelman et al. Comparison of CA 15-3 and carcinoembryonic antigen in monitoring the clinical course of patients with metastatic breast cancer. Cancer Res. 48:4107-4112 (1988).

9. M.J. Kerin, O.J. McAnena, V.P. O'Malley et al. CA 15-3: Its relationship to clinical stage and progression to metastatic disease in breast cancer. Br J. Surg 76:838-839 (1981).

10. R. Colomer, A. Ruibal, L. Salvador. Circulating tumor marker levels in advanced breast carcinoma correlated with the extent of metastatic disease 64:1675-1681 (1989).

11. A.M. Dnistrian, M.K. Schwartz, E.J. Greenberg et al. CA 15-3 and carcinoembryonic antigen in the clinical evaluation of breast cancer, Clin Chim Acta 200:81-94 (1991).

12. K.R. Bray, J.E. Koda, P.K. Gaur. Serum levels and biochemical characteristics of cancer-associated antigen CA 549 a circulating breast cancer marker. Cancer Res 47:5853-60 (1987).

13. R.A. Beveridge, D.W. Chan, D. Bruzek et al. A new biomarker in monitoring breast cancer: CA 549. J Clin Oncol 6:1815-21 (1988).

14. L.M. Demers, H.A. Harvey, J.D. Glenn et al. CA 549 a new marker for patients with advanced breast cancer. J Clin Lab Anal 2:168-73 (1988).

15. D.W. Chan, R.A. Beveridge, D.J. Bruzek et al. Monitoring breast cancer with CA 549. Clin Chem 34:2000-4 (1988).

16. M.S. Shurbaji, R.A. Beveridge, D.W. Chan et al. CA 549: Immunohistochemistry and serum levels in breast carcinoma and other neoplasma. Anal Clin Lab Sci 19:408-14 (1989).

17. A.M. Dnistrian, M.K. Schwartz, E.J. Greenberg et al. CA 549 as a marker in breast cancer. Int J. Biol Markers 6:139-145 (1991).

18. P.S. Lingley, J.P. Brown, J.L. Magnani et al. Monoclonal antibodies reactive with mucin glycoproteins found in sera from breast carcinoma patients. Cancer Res 48:2138-2148 (1988).

19. A.M. Dnistrian, M.K. Schwartz, E.J. Greenberg et al. Evaluation of CA M26, CA M29, CA 15-3 and CEA as circulating tumor markers in breast cancer patients. Tumor Biol 12:82-90 (1991).

20. D. Ricketts, L. Hadcocks, M. Fitzek et al. Serum markers for primary and recurrent breast cancer: BCM-EIA, CA M27 and CA M29. Tumor Biol 13:189-248 (1992).

21. S.A. Stacker, N.P.N. Sacks, J. Golder et al. Evaluation of MSA as a serum marker in breast cancer: A comparison with CEA. Br. J Cancer 57:298-303 (1988)

22. J.J. Tjandra, I.S. Russell, J.P. Collins et al. Application of mammary serum antigen assay in the management of breast cancer: A preliminary report. Br. J Surg 75:811-817 (1988).

23. M.A. Reddish, N. Helbricht, A.F. Almeida et al. Epitope mapping of Mab B27.29 within the peptide core of the malignant breast carcinoma associated mucin antigen codes for the human MUC 1 Genl J. Tumor Marker Oncol 7:1-10 (1992).

24. A. Van Dahlen. TPS in breast cancer-A comparative study with carcinoembryonic antigen and CA 15-3. Tumor Biol 13:10-17 (1992).

25. C.K. Osborne. Prognostic factors in breast cancer, PPO Updates 4:1-11, (1990).

26. E.W. Hubbard. Breast tumor markers. Diagnostics and Clinical Testing 28:14-17 (1990).

# ENGINEERING OF ANTIBODIES FOR BREAST CANCER THERAPY: CONSTRUCTION OF CHIMERIC AND HUMANIZED VERSIONS OF THE MURINE MONOCLONAL ANTIBODY BrE-3

Joseph R. Couto[1], Edward W. Blank[1], Jerry A. Peterson[1], Radwan Kiwan[1], Eduardo A. Padlan[2], and Roberto L. Ceriani[1]

[1]Cancer Research Fund of Contra Costa
2055 North Broadway, Walnut Creek, California 94596
[2]Laboratory of Molecular Biology, National Institute of Diabetes and Digestive and Kidney Diseases, National Institutes of Health, Bethesda, Maryland 20892

The use of murine monoclonal antibodies as targeting agents for the treatment of malignancies is ironically precluded by the patient's own antimouse antibody (HAMA) response[1-3]. Human monoclonal antibodies should be tolerated, but unfortunately, they have not been forthcoming because of various technical difficulties. A number of recent advances, however, should circumvent these difficulties. Promising antibodies expressed by unstable human hybridomas or produced in low amounts, can now be salvaged by cloning their variable region-encoding cDNAs and splicing them into vectors encoding human constant regions. These are then transfected into stable murine myeloma cell lines. Another possibility for the production of useful human monoclonal antibodies is by panning phage display libraries[4], a process that requires no immunization. A new generation of human monoclonal antibodies should not, however, displace good murine antibodies that have resulted from years of arduous labor and minutious characterization since these murine antibodies may have uniquely useful binding properties, and since they can be humanized.

BrE-3 is one of our most promising murine monoclonal antibodies. It is an IgG1,k immunoglobulin that binds to the tandem repeat of the polypeptide core of human breast mucin[5-6]. It has been extensively characterized and its radioconjugates have been tested both in animal models and in human clinical trials (see reference 7, and papers by Kramer et al. and by DeNardo et al. in this publication). BrE-3 was the first of a series of murine monoclonal antibodies that we decided to humanize. Its sucessful humanization is briefly summarized here.

To humanize BrE-3, we first cloned the cDNAs encoding its variable regions. Due to sequence conservation it is possible to clone antibody variable regions by PCR [8-10], which is much faster than the traditional cloning methods. Thus, we

*Antigen and Antibody Molecular Engineering in Breast Cancer Diagnosis and Treatment*, Edited by R.L. Ceriani, Plenum Press, New York, 1994

55

extracted polyadenylated RNA from the BrE-3 hybridoma, reverse-transcribed it and amplified the resulting cDNA by PCR, using commercially available primers specific for leader peptide and constant region-encoding sequences. We sequenced several independent clones. The sequences encode bona fide VKII and $V_H$IIIC variable regions, as defined by Kabat et al.[11]. Notably, CDR H3 contains only 4 amino acids. These results have been published[12].

The next step towards humanization was the construction of a chimeric antibody (ChBrE3) by fusing the murine variable regions with human constant regions. While this step was not absolutely necessary, it both established the authenticity of the isolated cDNAs and provided a fallback option had efforts to humanize the antibody failed. To construct a chimeric version of BrE-3 we inserted the cDNAs into vectors pAG4622 and pAH4604, which encode human kappa and gamma 1 constant regions respectively. These vectors were developed[13] and kindly provided by S.L. Morrison (Dept. of Microbiology and Molecular Genetics, UCLA, Los Angeles, CA). The vector constructs were transfected into SP2/0-Ag14 mouse myeloma cells and the secreted chimeric antibody was purified and characterized. The authenticity of chimeric BrE-3 is unquestionable given that its affinity constant for the human breast mucin is indistinguishable from that of BrE-3, and that it competes with BrE-3 binding to its antigen in an identical fashion as BrE-3[12].

Several algorithms for the humanization of murine antibodies can be applied depending on individual objectives and preferences. We had two priorities for the humanization of the variable regions of ChBrE3. The first priority was to preserve the antibody's original binding affinity. The second was to diminish immunogenicity as much as possible. To satisfy our first priority we preserved the original murine CDRs as well as all framework (FR) amino acids that might affect the conformation and orientation of the CDRs. These FR residues, which we call important, include those that either interact with the CDRs or with the opposite chain, those that are buried, and finally, those that are either adjacent to the CDRs or close to the N-termini, since they often form a surface that is contiguous with the antigen binding surface. The positions of these important residues, in several antibodies whose structures have been determined to a high degree of resolution, are often invariant. Thus, we applied this spatial consensus to determine which amino-acids of BrE-3 could be important. These important murine amino acids were left intact while the others were changed to the identities found in the target human sequence.

To satisfy our second priority we chose, as target human sequences, the consensus sequences of human KII and HIII subclasses[11] respectively, rather than the sequences of a particular human antibody. We found that the numbers of important amino acids to be retained and of those to be mutated were small because of the similarity between human and mouse variable regions. We found, moreover, that many of the retained amino acids, while different from the human consensus sequences, in fact exist in a great proportion of specific human sequences.

There were only, respectively, 14 and 17 differences between the $V_L$ and the $V_H$ frameworks of BrE-3 and the KII and HIII human consensus frameworks. Of these, we changed (humanized) 8 positions in the $V_L$ and 8 positions the $V_H$ murine frameworks, thus, leaving behind 6 $V_L$ and 9 $V_H$ murine residues. The amino acid changes were implemented with several successive rounds of mutagenesis and the mutagenized cDNAs were inserted into the same expression vectors used to construct chimeric antibody genes[12-13].

The Kabat database[11] lists 11 VkII and nearly 80 $V_H$III complete sequences. If we disregard the CDRs and compare the $V_L$ and $V_H$ frameworks of HuBrE3 with the consensus sequences of the human VK and $V_H$ frameworks we find 93% and 90%

sequence identities respectively. This means that approximately 1/3 of all known VKII and $V_H$III human frameworks are less similar to their own consensus sequences than are the frameworks of HuBrE. For example, a few human HIII frameworks show more than 20 differences from their consensus, compared to 9 differences in HuBrE3 $V_H$. Furthermore, all of the 9 $V_H$ murine amino acids retained in HuBrE3 exist in the same positions in a number of human antibodies ranging from one to 31. Thus, strictly from a sequence similarity perspective, HuBrE3 is closer to an ideal human antibody than many human antibodies themselves are. The sequences of the humanized variable regions of HuBrE3v2 are shown in Fig. 1.

HuBrE3v2 $V_L$

```
ATG AAG TTG CCT GTT AGG CTG TTG GTG CTG TTG TTC TGG ATT CCT GCT TCC ATC AGT GAT GTT GTG ATG ACC CAA TCT CCA CTC TCC CTG
 m   k   l   p   v   r   l   l   v   l   L   F   W   I   P   A   S   I   S  Dl   V   V   M   T   Q   S   P   L   S   L

CCT GTC ACT CCT GGA GAG CCA GCT TCC ATC TCT TGC AGA TCT AGT CAG AAC CTT GTA CAC AAC AAT GGA AAC ACC TAT TTA TAT TGG TTC
 P   V   T   P   G   E   P   A   S   I   S   C   R   S   S   Q   N   L   V   H   N   N   G   N   T   Y   L   Y   W   F

CTG CAG AAG CCA GGC CAG TCT CCA AAG CTC CTG ATT TAT AGG GCT TCC ATC CGA TTT TCT GGG GTC CCA GAC AGG TTC AGT GGC AGT GGA
 L   Q   K   P   G   Q   S   P   K   L   L   I   Y   R   A   S   I   R   F   S   G   V   P   D   R   F   S   G   S   G

TCA GGG ACA GAT TTC ACA CTC AAG ATC AGC AGA GTG GAG GCT GAG GAT GTG GGA GTT TAT TTC TGC TTT CAA GGT ACA CAT GTT CCG TGG
 S   G   T   D   F   T   L   K   I   S   R   V   E   A   E   D   V   G   V   Y   F   C   F   Q   G   T   H   V   P   W

ACG TTC GGT GGA GGC ACC AAG CTG GAA ATC AAA C

 T   F   G   G   G   T   K   L   E   I   K
```

HuBrE3v2 $V_H$

```
ATG TAC TTG GGA CTG AAC TAT GTC TTC ATA GTT TTT CTC TTA AAA GGT GTC CAG AGT GAA GTG CAG CTT GTG GAG TCT GGA GGA GGC TTG
 m   y   l   g   l   n   y   v   f   I   V   F   L   L   K   G   V   Q   S   El  V   Q   L   V   E   S   G   G   G   L

GTG CAA CCT GGA GGA TCC ATG AGA CTC TCT TGT GCT GCT TCT GGA TTC ACT TTT AGT GAT GCC TGG ATG GAC TGG GTC CGC CAG TCT CCA
 V   Q   P   G   G   S   M   R   L   S   C   A   A   S   G   F   T   F   S   D   A   W   M   D   W   V   R   Q   S   P

GGG AAG GGC CTT GAG TGG GTT GCT GAA ATT AGA AAC AAA GCC AAT AAT CAT GCA ACA TAT TAT GAT GAG TCT GTG AAA GGG AGG TTC ACC
 G   K   G   L   E   W   V   A   E   I   R   N   K   A   N   N   H   A   T   Y   Y   D   E   S   V   K   G   R   F   T

ATC TCA AGA GAT GAT TCC AAA AGT ACT GTG TAC CTG CAA ATG AAT AGC TTA AGA GCT GAA GAC ACT GCC CTT TAT TAC TGT ACT GGG GAG
 I   S   R   D   D   S   K   S   T   V   Y   L   Q   M   N   S   L   R   A   E   D   T   A   L   Y   Y   C   T   G   E

TTT GCT AAC TGG GGC CAG GGG ACT CTG GTC ACT GTC TCT TCT G
 F   A   N   W   G   Q   G   T   L   V   T   V   S   S
```

FIGURE 1. $V_L$ and $V_H$: Nucleotide and Derived Protein Sequences of HuBrE3v2. The CDR amino acid residues are underlined and were assigned in accordance with reference 11. The leader peptide residues that are shown in lower case are not necessarily correct since they correspond to PCR primers. The mature chains begin at D1 and E1, respectively. Underlined nucleotides indicate mutagenized (humanized codons).

Overall, we constructed three progressivelly more human-like versions of BrE-3. First, we constructed a chimeric antibody (ChBrE3) that has unchanged murine Vk and $V_H$ regions fused to human Ck and C-gamma-1 regions respectively. Second, we constructed the humanized version HuBrE3v1, which is like ChBrE3 but possessing 8 "human" amino-acids in the Vk framework. Third, we constructed HuBrE3v2, which is like HuBrE3v1 but with 8 "human" aminoacids in the $V_H$ framework. All three versions have been expressed in SP2/0-Ag14 mouse myeloma cells, purified and characterized. All versions stain human breast tumors in histological paraffin-embedded sections as deeply and specifically as the original murine BrE-3 monoclonal antibody (not shown).

Figure 2 shows the results of binding competition experiments. The cold antibody to be tested competed with radioiodinated murine BrE-3, for binding to antigen attached to a microtiter plate. Cold ChBrE3 and cold murine BrE-3 compete equally well. Both humanized versions, however, compete better than murine BrE-3 for antigen. While we do not understand the reasons for this increase in binding competition we can rule out the possibility that an N-linked glycosylation site was removed by the humanization procedure since no such sites were found in the amino acid sequence of either variable region. On the other hand, differences in O-linked glycosylation of the chimeric and humanized forms could be possible since some of the amino acid changes involved serines and threonines.

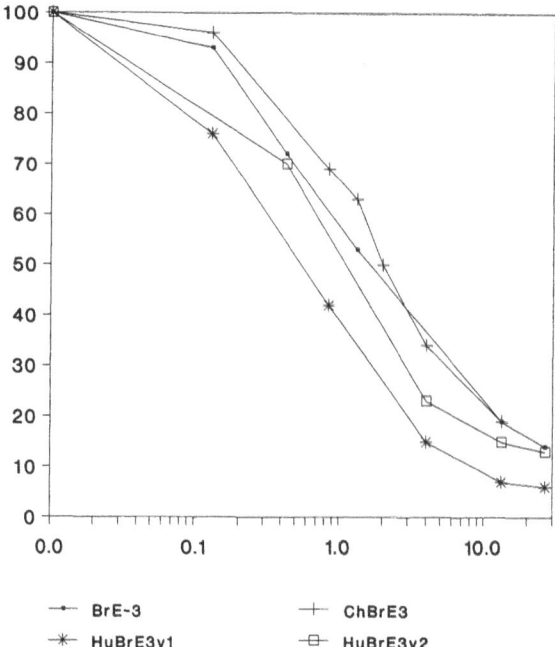

- BrE-3
- + ChBrE3
- * HuBrE3v1
- HuBrE3v2

FIGURE 2. Inhibition of Binding of Radiolabeled BrE-3 by Competing Unlabeled BrE-3, ChBrE3, HuBrE3v1 and HuBrEv2 Antibodies. Y axis (linear): % counts of bound radiolabeled murine BrE-3 antibody. X axis (log) nanomolar (nM) concentration of competing unlabeled antibody estimated either by radioimmunodetection, by a Lowry assay or by both. Microtiter plates were prepared using successive layers of methylated BSA, glutaraldehyde, anti-$\beta$-galactosidase and the fusion protein 11-2 (a hybrid of $\beta$-galactosidase and a fragment of human breast mucin containing the tandem repeat[14,15]. To each well we added [125]I-BrE-3 and competed with the tested antibody.

In conclusion, we have been successful in the construction of one chimeric and two humanized versions of the important murine monoclonal antibody BrE-3, without diminishing the ability of the variable regions to bind to the human breast mucin. The resulting engineered versions are very similar to human antibodies and should, therefore, elicit fewer or no HAMA responses in human patients.

## REFERENCES

1. Schroff, R.W., Foon, K.A., Beatty, S.M., Oldham, R.K., and Morgan, A.C. Jr., Human anti-murine immunoglobulins responses in patients receiving monoclonal therapy. Cancer Res.,45:879-885 (1985).
2. Shawler, D.L., Bartholomew, R.M., Smith, L.M., and Dillman, R.O. Human immune response to multiple injections of murine monoclonal IgG. J. Immunol., 135:1530-1535 (1985).

3. Courtenay-Luck, N.S., Epenetos, A.A., Moore, R., Larche, M., Pectasides, D., Dhokia, B. and Ritter, M.A. Development of primary and secondary immune responses to mouse monoclonal antibodies used in the diagnosis and therapy of malignant neoplasms. Cancer Res., 46:6489-6493 (1986).

4. Marks JD; Hoogenboom HR; Griffiths AD; Winter G., Molecular evolution of proteins on filamentous phage. Mimicking the strategy of the immune system. J. Biol Chem. 267:16007-16010 (1992).

5. Peterson, J.A., Zava D.T., Duwe, A.K., Blank, E.W., Battifora, H., and Ceriani R.L. Biochemical and histological characterization of antigens preferentially expressed on the surface and cytoplasm of breast carcinoma cells identified by monoclonal antibodies against the human milk fat globule. Hybridoma, 9:221-235 (1990).

6. Peterson, J.A., Larocca D., Walkup G., Amiya R., and Ceriani R.L. Molecular analysis of epitope heterogeneity of the breast mucin. In: Breast epithelial antigens: Molecular biology to clinical applications. Ceriani R.L. (ed). Plenum Publications, New York (1991).

7. Blank, E.W., Pant, K.D., Chan, C.M., Peterson, J.A., and Ceriani, R.L. A novel anti-breast epithelial mucin MAb (BrE-3). Characterization and experimental biodistribution and immunotherapy. Cancer J., 5:38-44 (1992).

8. Orlandi, R., Gussow, D.H., Jones, P.T., and Winter, G. Cloning immunoglobulin variable domains for expression by the polymerase chain reaction. Proc. Natl. Acad. Sci. USA, 86:3833-3837 (1989).

9. Coloma, M.J., Larrick, J.W., Ayala, M., and Gavilondo-Cowley, J.V. Primer design for the cloning of immunoglobulin heavy-chain leader-variable regions from mouse hybridoma cells using the PCR. BioTechniques, 11:152-156 (1991).

10. Gavilondo-Cowley, J.V., , M., Vazquez, J., Ayala, M., Macias, A., Fry, K.E., and Larrick, J.W. Specific amplification of rearranged immunoglobulin variable region genes from mouse hybridoma cells. Hybridoma, 9:407-417 (1990).

11. Kabat, E.A., Wu, T.T., Perry, H.M., Gottesman, K.S., and Foeller, C. Sequences of proteins of immunological interest. U.S. Dept. Health and Human Services, NIH publication No. 91-3242, 5th Edition (1991).

12. Couto, J.R., Blank, E.W., Peterson, J.A., and Ceriani, R.L., Cloning of cDNAs encoding the variable domains of antibody BrE-3 and construction of a chimeric antibody. Hybridoma, 12(1):15-23 (1993).

13. Coloma, M.J., Hastings, A., Wims, L.A., and Morrison, S.L. Novel vectors for the expression of antibody molecules using variable regions generated by PCR. J. Immunol. Methods, 152:89-104 (1992).

14. Ceriani, R.L., Larocca, D., Peterson, J.A., Enloe, S., Amiya, R., and Blank, E.W. A novel serum assay for the breast epithelial antigen using a fusion protein. Anal Biochem., 201:178-184 (1992).

15. Larocca, D., Peterson, J.A., Walkup, G., and Ceriani, R.L., High level expression in E. coli of an alternate reading frame of pS2 mRNA that encodes a mimitope of human breast epithelial mucin tandem repeat. Hybridoma, 11:191-201 (1992).

# HUMANIZATION OF AN ANTI-MUCIN ANTIBODY FOR BREAST AND OVARIAN CANCER THERAPY

T. S. Baker, C. C. Bose[1], H. M. Caskey-Finney, D. J. King,
A. D. G. Lawson, A. Lyons, A. Mountain, R. J. Owens[2], M. R. Rolfe,
M. Sehdev, G.T. Yarranton and J. R. Adair

Oncology Biology, [1]Oncology Chemistry,
[2]Inflammation Biology,
Celltech Research Division
Celltech Ltd.,216 Bath Rd., Slough, Berks.
U. K. SL1 4EN

## SUMMARY

Antibody-drug conjugates utilize the targetting potential of antibodies to improve the potential of cytostatic or cytocidal drugs. One such murine monoclonal antibody, CTM01 (mCTM01), which recognizes an epitope on breast epithelial mucin, has potential for the treatment of breast and ovarian cancers. We examine in this paper the comparative properties of mCTM01 against a number of other anti-mucin antibodies. We then describe the humanization and high level re-expression of humanized CTM01 (hCTM01), a process designed to avoid the immune response to administered murine antibodies in human patients and to produce sufficient material for clinical studies. We show that the humanized form has properties superior to mCTM01 in terms of binding affinity to antigen presented on tumour cells.

## INTRODUCTION

### Antibodies for treatment of breast and ovarian tumours

The use of antibodies as targetting agents relies on the presence on the tumour of tumour associated antigens (TAAs). The utility of these TAAs is determined by several factors including the level of expression on the tumour cells, homogeneity of expression throughout the tumour, restriction of expression in non-tumour tissues, ability to be shed from the surface of the cells and ability to be internalized after binding by the antibody. For breast cancer a number of such markers have been described including the epidermal growth factor receptor (EGFR), the HER2 antigen (p185$^{HER2}$) and polymorphic epithelial mucin (PEM)

*Antigen and Antibody Molecular Engineering in Breast Cancer Diagnosis and Treatment*, Edited by R.L. Ceriani, Plenum Press, New York, 1994

61

(Thor et al., 1989). PEM is a cell surface glycoprotein, variously known as episialin, epithelial membrane antigen and MUC1 (reviewed in Hilkens et al., 1992, see also Ceriani, 1991 and references therein).

A number of antibodies have been described which recognize and bind to PEM including HMFG1, HMFG2, (Taylor-Papadimitriou et al., 1981), C595 (Price et al., 1990c), SM3 (Burchell et al., 1987). Another antibody, CTM01, initially known as 7F11C7 (Aboud-Pirak, et al., 1988), was raised against the membrane fraction of human milk fat globule (HMFG) and believed to recognize an epitope within PEM. The antibody has an affinity, $K_D$ of $1.4 \times 10^{-8}$ M for antigen presented on MCF-7 cells, a human metastatic breast carcinoma cell line. mCTM01 specifically immunoprecipitates two molecules of approx. Mr 350 kDa and 400 kDa from labelled MCF-7 cells. The antigen appears to be a non-mannose containing glycoprotein with O-linked oligosaccharides of sialic acid in the epitope. On binding of the antibody to the antigen on MCF-7 cells, mCTM01 is internalized and transported to the lysosomes for breakdown. mCTM01 reacts homogeneously with all tumour cells present in breast primary carcinomas as well as with derived metastases.

Rodent Mabs of themselves have in general proven very ineffective in cancer therapy, (reviewed in Catane and Longo, 1988). Alternative effectors (e.g. enzymes, toxins, drugs, radionuclides) can be used which can be attached to the antibody by genetic means or by chemical coupling. In the last few years several types of cytotoxic drugs have been identified which have greatly superior potency than the commonly used chemotherapeutic agents and which may prove to be more suitable for MAb-targetted cancer therapy. These include the enedienes (reviewed by Nicolaou et al., 1992). Suitable linkages and procedures for MAb conjugation have been developed for one of the most promising of these new agents, the enediene calicheamicin (Lee et al., 1987a and b) which cleaves DNA after binding in the minor groove (Drak et al., 1991), and mCTM01-calicheamicin conjugates have been shown to be very efficient *in vitro* in killing breast cancer cells and *in vivo* in inducing tumour regression of tumour xenografts in nude mice (Hinman, 1990).

A major disadvantage of the use of rodent MAbs, however, is the development by the patient of an immune response to the administered antibody, the HAMA (human anti-murine antibody) response. Chimeric (mouse variable region-human constant region) (Morrison et al., 1984) antibodies have been developed to reduce this problem and several have been tested in the clinic (reviewed in Adair, 1992). In most cases a response to the murine variable region still emerges (Table 1) and therefore fully humanized forms of rodent MAbs with therapeutic potential have been constructed (reviewed in Adair, 1992).

In this paper we compare mCTM01 with a panel of established anti-PEM antibodies. We describe the humanization of mCTM01 as a means of reducing the probable HAMA response to the murine MAb in vivo, and we show that the humanized form of the antibody is superior to the murine antibody in its recognition and binding to tumour derived PEM.

## MATERIALS AND METHODS

### Reagents

Breast tumour material was obtained from Dr. M. Dowsett, Department of Academic Biochemistry, Royal Marsden Hospital. U. K. Ovarian tumour material was obtained from Dr. S. Mather, ICRF, London, U. K. and from Dr. J. Crocker, Department of Histopathology, East Birmingham Hospital.

Antigen preparations were made from human milk and human urine, obtained from healthy volunteers, was used to prepare antigen according to the method of Price et al., (1987). Briefly, antigen was purified by affinity chromatography following initial treatment as follows: the urine was filtered (0.45μm) and a skim milk fraction of human milk was

**Table 1.** HAMA Response to chimeric antibodies - Current clinical situation

| ANTIBODY | INVESTIGATOR | SOURCE | ISOTYPE | RESPONSE | FREQUENCY | REFERENCE |
|---|---|---|---|---|---|---|
| c17-1A | LoBuglio (Alabama) | Centocor | IgG1 | 1/25 | 4% | LoBuglio et al., 1989; 1991; Trang et al., 1990; Meredith et al, 1991; 1992a |
| cB72.3 | Begent (Charing Cross) | Celltech | IgG4 | 7/14 | 50% | Baker et al, 1991; Begent et al., 1990; R. H. J.Begent pers. comm. |
| cB72.3 | LoBuglio | Celltech | IgG4 | 16/24 | 67% | Khazaeli et al., 1991; LoBuglio et al., 1991; Meredith et al., 1992a; 1992b: A. F. LoBuglio pers. comm. |
| cAnti-GD2 | LoBuglio | Abbott | IgG1 | 8/13 | 56% | Saleh et al., 1992 |
| cAnti-CD4 | Knox (Stanford) | Becton-Dickinson | IgG1 | 2/7 | 29% | Knox et al., 1991 |
| cL6 | Goodman (Seattle) | Bristol Myers | IgG1 | 4/17[§] | 24-50% | DeNardo et al., 1991a; 1991b; Goodman, 1991 |

[§] Some of these patientswere followed for only two-three weeks, response rate in those studied up to 11 weeks was approx. 50%.

isolated by an initial low speed centrifugation (30 min. at 1300g) followed by a high speed centrifugation (60 min. at 10000g) and filtration (0.45μm). Affinity columns were prepared by coupling mCTM01 to a cross-linked agarose support (Immunopure Antigen/Antibody Immobilisation Kit, Pierce Warriner Ltd. Cheshire, U. K.) according to the manufacturers instructions, at 5 mg antibody per 1 mL of gel. Skim milk fraction (25 column volumes) or urine (45 column volumes) were applied to the affinity columns followed by at least 50 column volumes of buffer (0.5% (v/v) Brij-35 in phosphate buffered saline (PBS)). Antigen was eluted in at least 8 column volumes of either 0.1M diethylamine or 0.1M glycine/hydrochloric acid pH2.8 and fractions adjusted immediately to pH7 with 1M sodium dihydrogen phosphate or 1M Tris-HCl pH9.5 respectively. Following extensive dialysis against deionized water pooled antigen containing fractions were lyophilized and the mass of recovered antigen estimated gravimetrically.

MCF-7 cells (Soule et al., 1973), grown in Dulbecco's Modified Eagles medium (DMEM) (Gibco Ltd) supplemented with 10% heat inactivated foetal calf serum (FCS), were used as a source of cell bound antigen for use in flow cytometry assays. Cells were grown attached to plastic in culture and were removed from the plastic support by trypsin/EDTA treatment prior to use in the assays.

Peptides were prepared by FMOC-solid phase peptide synthesis (Atherton et al., 1989).

Antibodies HMFG1 (IgG1/κ) and HMFG2 (IgG1/κ) (Taylor-Papadimitriou et al., 1981) were obtained from Unipath Ltd. Basingstoke, U.K. Antibody C595 (IgG3/κ) (Price et al., 1990c) was obtained from Dr. M. R. Price, CRC Laboratories, University of Nottingham U.K. Antibody SM3 (IgG1/κ) (Burchell et al., 1987) was obtained from Imperial Cancer Research Technology, London, U. K., courtesy of Dr. S. Mather. Antibody EMA (IgG2a/κ) was obtained from Dakopatts A/S Denmark. The hybridoma line expressing mCTM01 (IgG1/κ) was obtained from IRE-Celltarg SA, Brussels, Belgium (Aboud-Pirak et al., 1988).

Antibodies were biotinylated by reacting a 20 fold molar excess of biotin-ε amino caproic acid N-hydroxy succinimide ester (Calbiochem Inc.) with the antibody (1 to 10 mg/mL) at pH 7.5 for 30 min. Low molecular weight by-products were removed by PD10 column (Pharmacia Ltd.) chromatography.

Antibodies were fluorescein labelled by reacting 1 mL of a 1 mg/mL solution of antibody in 0.1M sodium bicarbonate pH8.5 with 30 μL of a freshly prepared 30 mg/mL solution of fluorescein isothiocyanate (FITC) (Sigma Chemical Co., Poole, U. K.) in dimethyl sulphoxide. Reaction was allowed to proceed for 3 h in the dark with gentle mixing. FITC-labelled antibody was purified from the reaction mixture by PD10 column chromatography run in 0.1M bicarbonate buffer and stored in the dark at $4^{\circ}C$.


## Assays

**Assembly assay.** An assembly enzyme linked immunosorbent assay (ELISA) assay for quantifying yields of intact IgG used microwell plates coated with a goat $F(abU)_2$ anti-human IgG Fc (Jackson Immunoresearch Inc.). Transfected culture supernatants were incubated for 1 h in the wells then washed extensively with tap water. Bound humanized antibody was revealed with a horse radish peroxidase (HRP)-conjugated murine anti-human Ig Kappa antibody (The Binding Site, Birmingham, U. K.) by incubation for 1 h followed by a further wash stage and colour development using a mixture of 0.005% (v/v) hydrogen peroxide and 0.01% (w/v) tetramethyl benzidine as the substrate (TMB reagent). Absorbance measurements were made at $A_{630nm}$ using a Biotech EL300 plate reader. Concentrations of humanized antibody in the samples were interpolated from a calibration curve generated from serial dilutions of purified chimeric B72.3(γ4) antibody (King et al., 1992).

**Direct binding ELISA.** A direct binding ELISA for determining the antigen binding activity of anti-PEM antibodies used affinity purified human urine or human milk antigen passively adsorbed onto microwell plates (200 μL per well) at approximately 0.4 μg/mL (milk antigen) or 0.6 μg/mL( urine antigen). Alternatively the microwell plates were coated with a 1 μM solution of a 29mer peptide (CTSAPDTRPAPGSTAPPAHGVTSAPDTRP). The microwells were then incubated for 1 h with serial dilutions of antibody after which the plates were washed extensively with tap water. Binding of hCTM01 was revealed and quantified as for the assembly assay except using the alternative conjugate: HRP-goat anti-murine IgG Fc antibody (Jackson Immunoresearch).

**Competition binding ELISA.** A competition ELISA, also employing affinity purified antigens as above, was used to compare the relative antigen binding potencies of various hCTM01 constructs and the above anti-PEM antibodies. Biotinylated mCTM01 at 2.5 μg/mL was competed against varying concentrations (0.01 to 100 μg/mL) of unlabelled mCTM01, hCTM01 or anti-PEM antibodies in the antigen coated microwells for 1h at 20°C. Unbound antibody was removed from the wells by four 400μL washes of 0.5% Tween-20 in PBS. The presence of antigen bound biotinylated mCTM01 was revealed by incubation (30 min at 20°C) with 1 μg/mL of a streptavidin-HRP conjugate (Celltech Ltd., Slough, U.K.) followed by washing as above, and colour development using the TMB reagent as for the assembly ELISA. Absorbance at 630nm was read at 30 min. and plotted against antibody concentration. The relative potency of a test antibody was calculated as the percentage dose of test antibody relative to the dose of unlabelled mCTM01 antibody, required to generate a 50% reduction of biotinylated mCTM01 binding to antigen.

**Two-site ELISA assays.** A two-site ELISA format was used to test the immunoreactivity of PEM from different tumour samples against different combinations of solid phase and biotinylated anti-PEM antibody pairs run in the same experiment. mCTM01 or various anti-PEM antibodies (SM3, C595, HMFG1) were coated onto microwells by passive adsorption at 2 μg/mL (200μL). Tumour samples were prepared as tissue homogenates, diluted to 5% (w/v) in PBS containing 20% Nonidet P40, and filtering (0.45 μm). These were further diluted 10 to 3162 fold in assay diluent, comprising 0.5% (w/v) bovine serum albumin, 0.1% (w/v) polyvinylpyrrolidine, 0.1% (w/v) thiomersol, 0.1% (v/v) mouse serum, 0.5% Tween-20 (v/v) in PBS. Titrations of diluted tumour extracts or affinity purified antigen (200 μL) were incubated in the coated microwells for 2 h at 20°C. Wells were washed as for the competition ELISA and were incubated with 200 μL of biotinylated antibody (2.5 μg/mL) for 2 h at 20°C. Following a further wash stage the presence of immuno-adsorbed biotinylated antibody was revealed as for the competition ELISA. For a given sample titration curves of absorbance versus the reciprocal of the sample dilution were plotted for the various combinations of solid-phase antibody-labelled antibody pairs. The relative position of the linear region of each titration curve on the reciprocal dilution axis was expressed as a percentage of that of the titration curve for the biotinylated mCTM01 antibody.

In order to measure the relative potency of different anti-PEM antibodies (unlabelled and in solution phase) to immuno-extracted PEM, from different tumour samples the two-site ELISA was also adapted to competition format. For each combination of solid phase anti-PEM antibody/ biotinylated CTM01, and for each tumour sample tested, a dilution was selected of between 316 and 3162 fold which would yield a sufficiently high signal (>0.5 absorbance units). Multiple wells coated with the chosen anti-PEM antibody were incubated with this single dilution of sample as for the two site ELISA up to and including the first wash stage. They were then incubated with 100 μL of unlabelled test antibody, including mCTM01, (0.031 to 10 μg/mL) and 100 μL of biotinylated mCTM01 (2.5 μg/mL). Bound biotinylated antibody was revealed as previously described. Relative potency for each test antibody was expressed as the dose of antibody giving 25% inhibition of signal as a percentage of the dose of unlabelled mCTM01 also giving 25% inhibition of signal.

**Flow cytometry assays.** A trypsinized cell suspension of MCF-7 cells in 12 mL of culture medium was centrifuged and resuspended three times (on ice) in equivalent volumes of cold FACS buffer (5% (v/v) FCS, 0.1% sodium azide in PBS). After the final wash the buffer volume was adjusted to give approximately $2 \times 10^5$ cells/mL. hCTM01 or anti-PEM antibody was diluted in the range 31 to 316200 ng/mL in FACS buffer containing a constant level of FITC-mCTM01 (20µg/mL). Aliquots (250µL) of dilutions were added to 250µL aliquots of suspended ice-cold MCF-7 cells. The cells and antibody were incubated for 2 h at $0^\circ$C or for 18 h at $4^\circ$C. The cells were pelleted by low speed centrifugation, washed in FACS buffer (14 mL) and re-centrifuged. Finally the cells were resuspended in 0.5 mL of FACS buffer and the fluorescence intensity measured in a fluorescence activated cell analyzer (FACScan, Becton Dickinson).

## Molecular biology procedures

**Cloning and sequencing of CTM01 variable regions.** DNA coding for the heavy chain variable domain ($V_H$), including the signal sequence for secretion, of mCTM01 was cloned using the Polymerase Chain Reaction (PCR) (Saiki et al., 1988). Polyadenylated RNA (poly A+ RNA) was isolated from the mCTM01 hybridoma cell line using the guanidinium isothiocyanate/lithium chloride method and double stranded cDNA was synthesised (Maniatis et al., 1982), and used as a template for PCR amplification of the $V_H$ gene (Jones and Bendig, 1991). The PCR amplified $V_H$ fragment was cloned in a pEE6 based (Stephens and Cockett, 1989) eukaryotic expression vector to give a chimeric mouse V region-human IgG4P constant region (Angal et al., 1992) gene which can be expressed by transcription from the human Cytomegalovirus major immediate early promoter/enhancer. The IgG4P constant region differs from the natural IgG4 sequence at a single amino acid position in the hinge region where serine 241 has been changed to a proline. This alteration allows complete disulphide bridge formation at the hinge during the assembly of IgG4 based antibody (Angal et al., 1992).

The light chain variable domain ($V_L$) of mCTM01 was obtained from a cDNA library constructed in the commercially available plasmid pSP64 (Amersham International Plc.), using cDNA from the mCTM01 hybridoma cell line. A fragment of the light chain cDNA, which encodes the signal sequence and $V_L$ was recovered by PCR amplification and fused to the human kappa constant region DNA sequences in a similar eukaryotic expression vector to that used for the heavy chain cloning.

The deduced amino acid sequence for the mature light and heavy chain variable region sequences matched that obtained from N terminal peptide sequencing of mCTM01.

The chimeric genes were expressed in CHO L761h cells (Cockett et al., 1991) in a transient expression experiment (Bebbington, 1991) to demonstrate that the resultant chimeric antibody competed for the same binding sites as the mCTM01 and hence confirmed that the cloned sequences coded for the same antibody (data not shown).

**Humanization of CTM01 variable region sequences.** The variable regions of the chimeric CTM01 genes were humanized by reconstructing the DNA sequences such that the antigen binding site from mCTM01 was substituted into the variable domains of a human recipient antibody, EU (Kabat et al., 1987), using methodology described in Adair et al., (1991).

Single strand DNA sequences of between 60 and 100 nucleotides were identified from the DNA sequences coding for the required variable region amino acid sequences such that they alternated on the sense and anti-sense strands and would overlap at their 5U and 3U extremities on annealing to form short double stranded sections. These oligonucleotides were produced by conventional chemical synthesis using a commercial machine (Applied Biosystems Inc. USA). These oligonucleotides were then assembled into V regions by a PCR based assembly procedure. (A similar methodology has been described by Lewis and Crowe, 1991, and Daugherty et al., 1991). A feature of the design is the inclusion of sites for appropriate restriction enzymes immediately before the start and at the end of the V regions (Hind3 and Apa1 for the heavy chain, and BstB1 and Spl1 for the light chain, respectively, see Figure 1). These sites enable the assembled regions to be cloned directly into separate expression vectors (M. R. R. and J. S. Emtage unpublished) which contain the human constant region genes, suitable transcriptional signals and selectable markers allowing immediate characterization by expression of humanized antibody genes.

The humanized genes, on separate expression vectors, were co-expressed in CHO L761h cells (Cockett et al., 1991) in transient expression experiments (Bebbington, 1991) to demonstrate that the humanized antibody bound to antigen with affinity similar to that of the mCTM01, as measured by competition binding with mCTM01 for PEM binding sites.

**Cell line development**. A single vector for long term, high level expression of hCTM01 in NS0 cells was assembled by transferring the promoter and heavy chain gene into the light chain vector to give pAL55 (Figure 1).

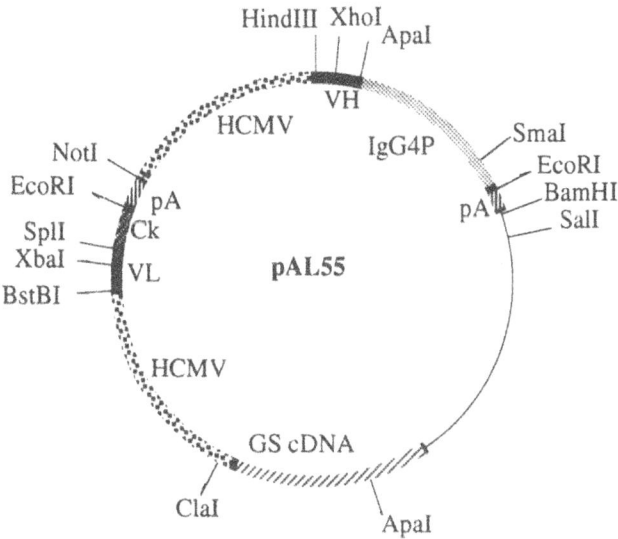

**Figure 1.** Diagram of expression plasmid pAL55.

The plasmid pAL55 has the following features: 1. the gene for the hCTM01 light chain; 2. the gene for the hCTM01 heavy chain; 3. two copies of the major immediate early promoter/enhancer region from the human Cytomegalovirus (hCMV-MIE). In the expression vector these promoters allow the transcription of the antibody genes; 4. Downstream of the constant region coding sequence of each antibody gene is a sequence, derived from the SV40 genome, which directs polyadenylation of mRNA; 5. a bacterial origin of replication and an ampicillin resistance marker; 6. a cDNA gene coding for the enzyme glutamine synthetase (GS cDNA) expressed from the SV40 early promoter. Glutamine synthetase is used as a means of vector selection when the expression vector is transfected into mammalian cells (Bebbington et al., 1992; reviewed in Bebbington, 1991). Downstream of the GS cDNA is a further SV40 polyadenylation sequence

From these lines several were taken for a round of subcloning. Cell line 18D8 was selected which yielded 700-1000 mg/L in serum free medium in shake flask experiments and 1L stirred fermentors, and 600-1000 mg/L post-purification in 30L-200L air-lift fermentors.

## RESULTS

### Specificity and epitope recognition of mCTM01

An initial series of experiments was designed to confirm that mCTM01 had immuno-reactivity to PEM. A panel of well characterized anti-PEM antibodies (HMFG1, HMFG2, SM3, C595 and EMA) showed specific binding in the direct binding ELISA (Figure 2) to solid phase antigen where the antigen had been extracted from human milk or human urine using a mCTM01 immunoadsorbent. In this assay system mCTM01, not surprisingly, showed high reactivity compared to members of the panel; with the following rank orders: mCTM01 (100%), HMFG1 (65%), HMFG2 (14%), C595 (7%), SM3 (0.1%) for milk derived antigen and mCTM01 (100%), HMFG2 (19%), HMFG1 (8%), C595 (1%), EMA (0.9%) SM3 (0.5%) for human urine derived antigen. The low binding of SM3 observed is consistent with the fact that it poorly binds PEM from non tumour sources (Burchell et al., 1987).

Peptides based on the the variable number of tandem repeat (VNTR) of the PEM core peptide (Briggs et al., 1991; Dion et al., 1991) were passively adsorbed onto plastic wells in the direct binding ELISA in order to determine whether mCTM01 was a member of the anti-PEM core peptide family. The 20mer peptide (PDTRPAPGSTAPPAHGVTSA) only gave a positive result with HMFG2 (data not shown), possibly due to restrictions imposed on a plastic adsorbed peptide (Dion et al., 1991). However when the longer peptide (CTSAPDTRPAPGSTAPPAHGVTSAPDTRP) was employed (Figure 3) antibodies bound with the following rank order of relative potency: C595 (316%), HMFG2 (277%), CTM01 (100%), SM3 (22%) and HMFG1 (19%), thus providing strong evidence that CTM01 had anti-PEM core peptide reactivity.

### Tumour specificity and relative affinity of mCTM01

In a series of experiments using tumour extracts and non-tumour antigen mCTM01 was compared to other anti-PEM antibodies: C595 (Price et al., 1990c; I. M. Symonds, personal communication), and HMFG1 (Burchell et al., 1987), reported to have good tumour binding and pan-specificity and SM3 (Girling et al., 1989; Van Dam et al., 1991)with somewhat reduced binding affinity but a high degree of tumour specificity.

Figure 4 shows the relative potencies of mCTM01, SM3 and C595 as determined by two site ELISA using either affinity purified antigen from human milk and urine or individual cytosols from two breast tumour homogenates. Each antibody was in turn used as the solid phase capture antibody to delineate any bias on affinity comparisons due to potential immuno-adsorption of discrete sub-populations of PEM. Since each biotinylated antibody was used as the revealing reagent, a total of 9 permutations for each antigen source were examined where relative potency was compared to mCTM01 as 100% for eachsolid phase. In all permutations the relative potency of C595 was less than 10%. Similarly, with one

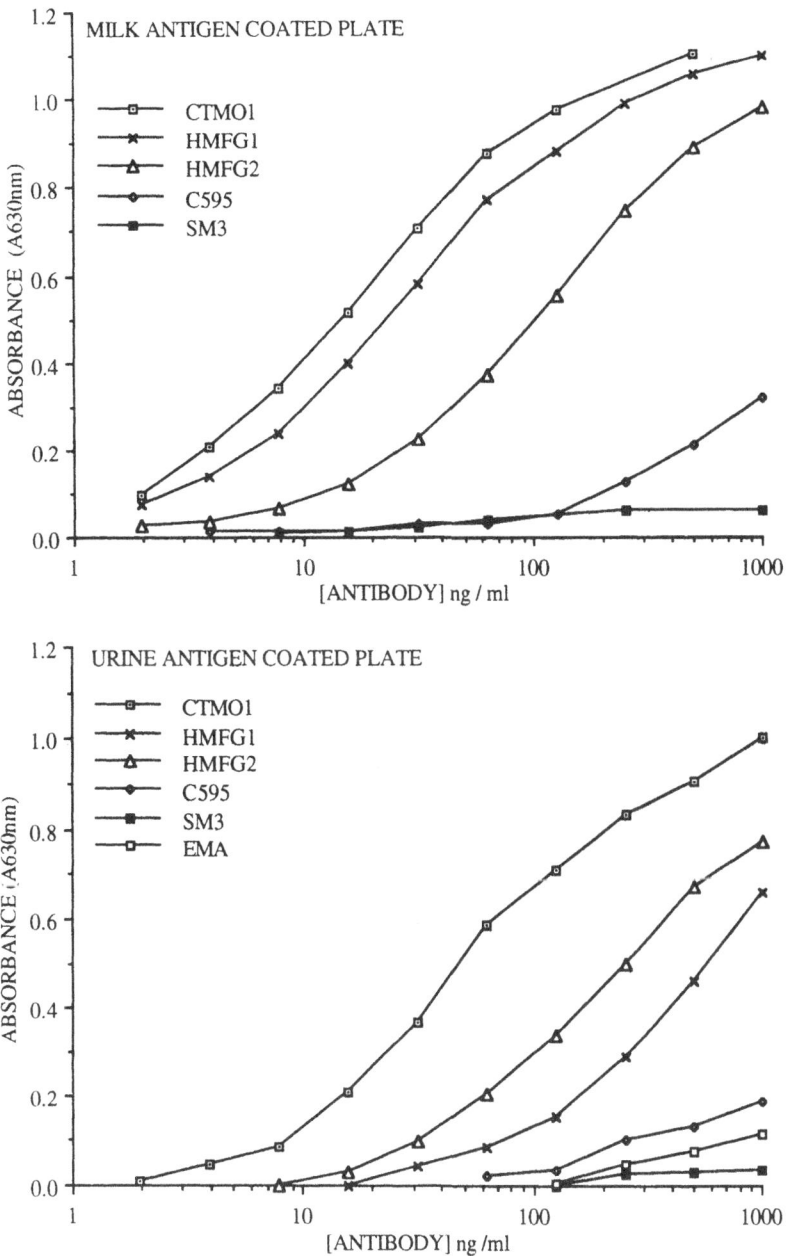

**FIGURE 2** Titration of anti-PEM antibodies showing binding to milk and urine antigen.

Titration curves for mCTM01 and a panel of anti-PEM MAbs, showing binding of each to affinity purified (via mCTM01 affinity column) human milk antigen (top panel) and human urine antigen (lower panel) as determined by direct binding ELISA.

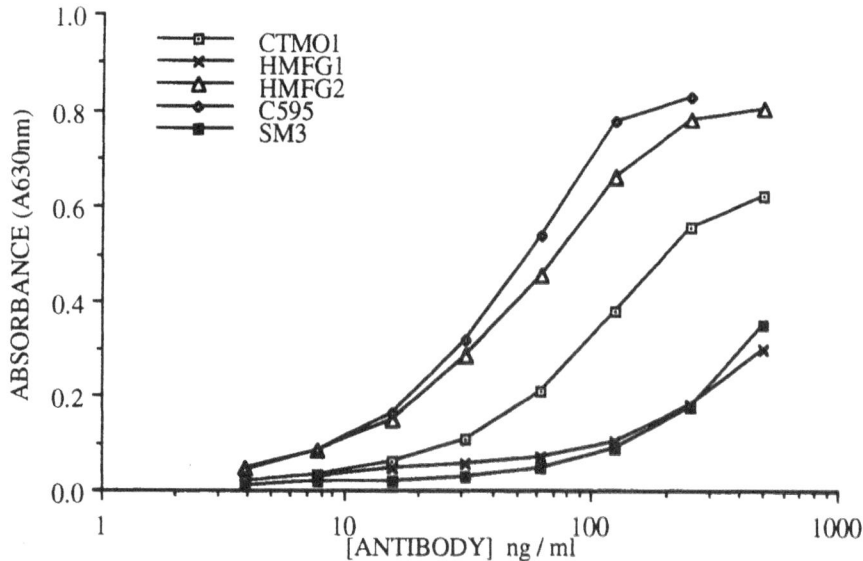

**FIGURE 3** Titration of anti-PEM antibodies showing binding to PEM core peptide analogues.
Titration curves for mCTM01 and a panel of anti-PEM MAbs, showing binding to a plastic adsorbed PEM core peptide analogue of sequence CTSAPDTRPAPGSTAPPAHGVTSAPDTRP (single amino acid code) as determined by direct binding ELISA.

exception, the relative potency of SM3 was 1% or less. These relative potencies broadly reflect the relative affinities of the three antibodies. Comparing normal to tumour sources of PEM, C595 exhibited similar relative potency values, whereas SM3 had approximately 10 fold greater relative potency values for the tumour PEM, suggesting that SM3 recognized a sub-population of PEM which may be tumour specific. The results show further evidence of PEM heterogeneity in that immuno-extraction of tumour PEM with either C595 or SM3 (compared to mCTM01) resulted in an increase of relative potency of 2.7 and 27 fold respectively when bound PEM was subsequently revealed with the respective homologous antibody. This data is consistent with the presence of discrete sub-populations of PEM within tumour PEM where immuno-adsorption with SM3 or C595 leads to enrichment of a particular sub-population of PEM. mCTM01 appears to be relatively pan-reactive and to have a higher affinity than the other two antibodies.

In a second series of studies the relative potency of mCTM01 was compared to HMFG1. Using the two-site ELISA format for the four combinations of solid phase and biotinylated reagents, on a total of six breast and one ovarian tumour samples, relative potencies were determined (Figure 5). Whichever antibody was used to immuno-capture sample antigen the relative potency with HMFG1 as the revealing antibody, with one exception (246%) was always lower (<3 to 33%) than with biotinylated CTM01 suggesting a higher affinity for the latter.

Immuno-adsorption of antigen by HMFG1 gave very low or undetectable binding in 8/14 cases compared to only 3/13 cases using CTM01 as solid phase antibody, suggesting that the latter has broader specificity than HMFG1. Interestingly the combination of HMFG1 as both solid phase and revealing antibody resulted in very low relative potency for tumour samples in contrast to milk and urine antigen at 154% and 20% relative potency respectively. Since heterologous combinations of HMFG1 and CTM01 show higher binding to tumour antigen this implies that the valency of HMFG1 epitopes on tumour PEM may be low, resulting in restricted binding at only one site of the ELISA sandwich.

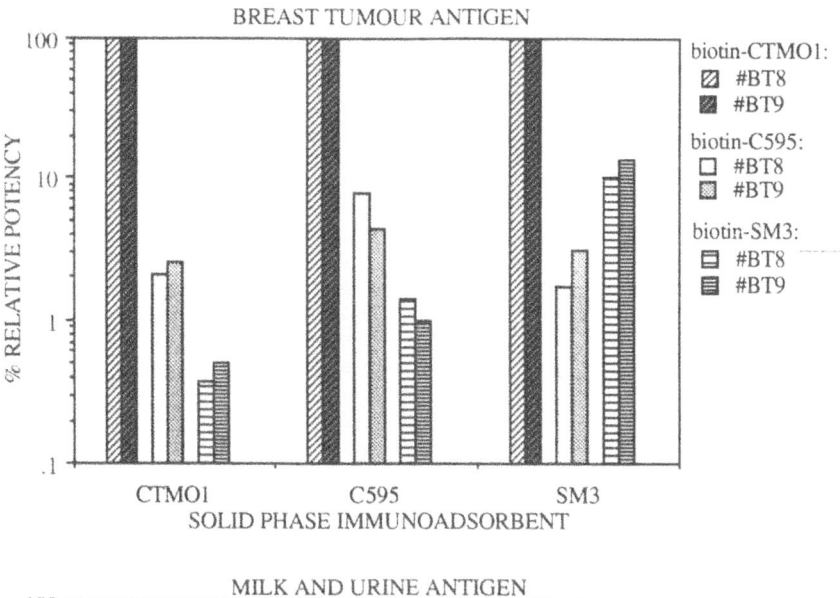

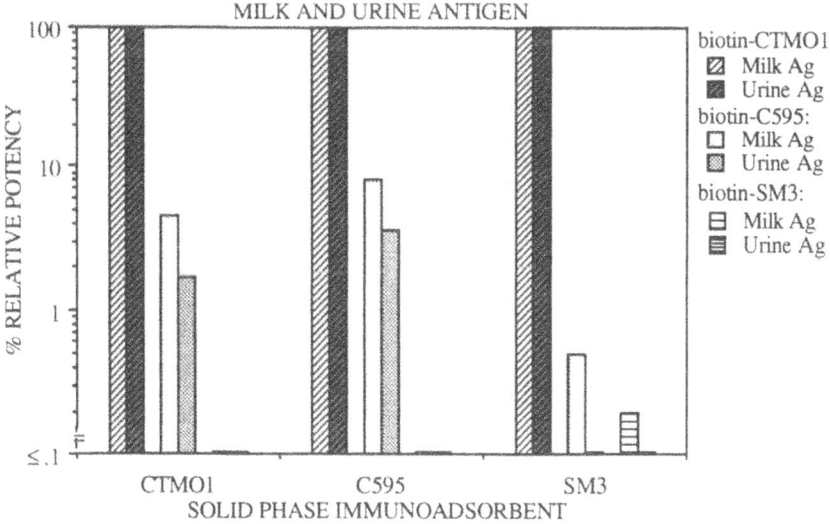

**FIGURE 4** Histogram showing % relative potencies of mCTMO1, C595 and SM3 antibody pairs in a two-site ELISA on antigen sources.

Comparative specificity and affinity of 9 combinations of solid phase/labelled anti-PEM antibody pairs (mCTM01, SM3, C595) has been assessed from titration curves of antigen, where each antibody in turn has been used as solid phase immuno-adsorbent to extract sample antigen in permutations with their biotinylated equivalents to reveal the immuno-adsorbed antigen.

For a given immuno-adsorbent % relative potency was calculated, as the reciprocal sample dilution at 0.5 absorbance units on each titration curve relative to that of the biotinylated mCTM01 titration curve. Results from two different breast tumour homogenates #BT8 and #BT9 (top panel) and human milk and urine antigen (lower panel) are shown.

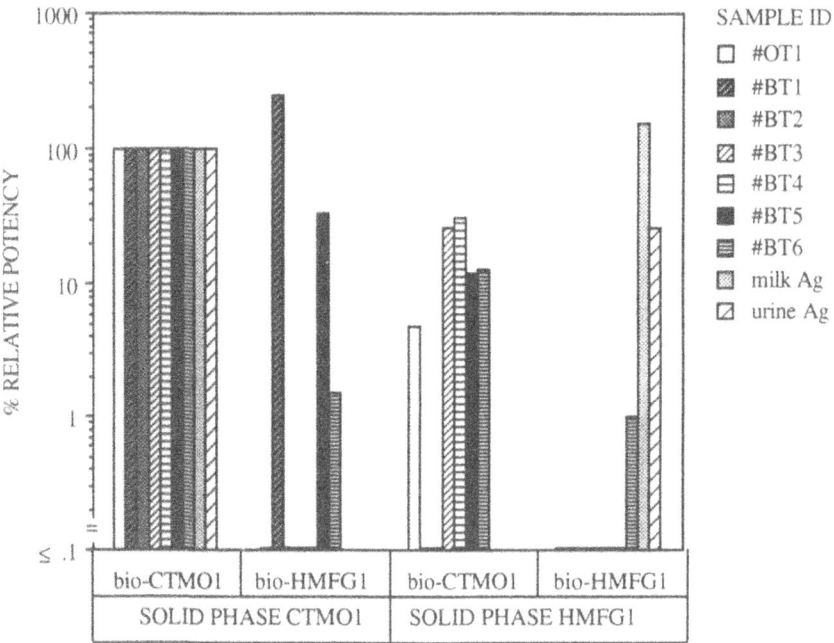

**FIGURE 5** Histogram showing % relative potencies of mCTMO1 and HMFG1 antibody pairs in a two-site ELISA on different tumour samples.

Comparative specificity and binding of 4 combinations of solid phase/labelled HMFG1 and mCTM01 antibody pairs against PEM from one ovarian tumour (#OT1) and six breast tumour (#BT1-6) tissue homogenates. % relative potencies have been determined as for Figure 4, against each biotinylated mCTM01/solid phase mCTM01 pair (100%).Percent relative potency for human milk and urine antigens were determined for the two homologous antibody pairs only.

The relative potency of CTM01 and HMFG1 binding to CTM01 defined epitopes on immuno-adsorbed antigen from different sources, as determined by the two-site ELISA in competition format is shown in Figure 6. A total of seven breast tumour and two ovarian tumour samples, in addition to milk and urine derived antigen, were examined. The PEM was attached to the solid phase by affinity capture with either mCTM01 or murine HMFG1 to define bias due to potential enrichment of sub-populations of PEM. The potencies of HMFG1 are shown relative to unlabelled mCTM01 at 100%. Against milk antigen and in one of the nine tumour samples (#BT1, using mCTM01 extraction) HMFG1 had a similar or greater potency to that of mCTM01. By contrast the relative potency of HMFG1 to urine antigen and to most tumour derived PEMs was much reduced. Relative potency values fell into two groups. In the first, which comprised one ovarian and three breast tumour extracts HMFG1 reactivity was undetectable. In the second group also comprising one ovarian and three breast tumour extracts HMFG1 reactivity was in the range 1.2-8.4% apart from the above exception at 214%. The means of immuno-adsorption of antigen led to a higher estimation of HMFG1 relative potency in 4 cases using an HMFG1 solid phase but gave a lower relative potency in 3 cases compared to using a CTM01 solid phase.

In the case of one ovarian tumour sample (#OT1), serum was available from the same patient. Relative potency of HMFG1 to circulating PEM was 27% but was undetectable against tumour homogenate PEM.

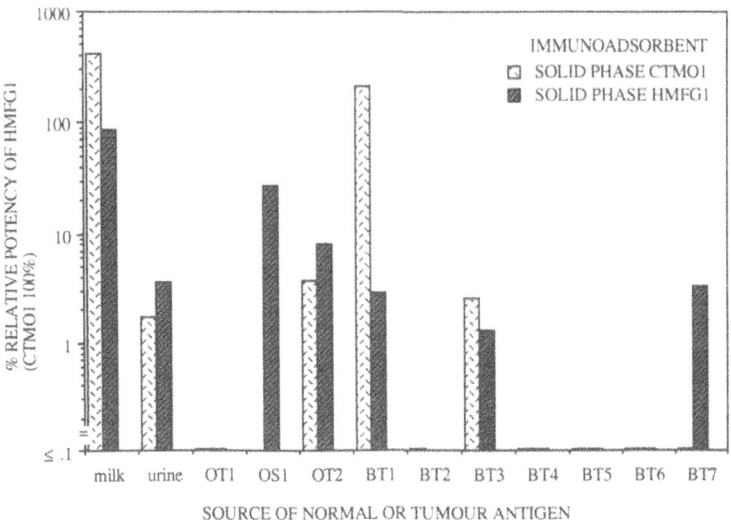

**FIGURE 6** Histogram showing relative potency of HMFG1 compared to mCTMO1 as determined by competition ELISA.

Comparison was made on a total of 7 breast tumour (#BT1-7) and 2 ovarian (#OT1, #OT2) tissue homogenates, one serum sample from patient #OT1 and milk and urine antigens. Immunoadsorption of antigen was carried out by solid phase mCTM01 or HMFG1 prior to the competition stage. Titrations of mCTM01 or HMFG1 were competed against a constant level of biotinylated mCTM01. Relative potencies were calculated from the % relative dose of unlabelled mCTM01 compared to that of HMFG1 at which 50% inhibition of biotinylated mCTM01 binding was observed.

## Construction and analysis of humanized CTM01

Humanized $V_L$ and $V_H$ domains of mCTM01 were designed based on the deduced sequence of CTM01 obtained from cDNA cloning (see Materials and Methods). The human antibody EU was used as the acceptor framework. For each domain the Complementarity Determining Regions (CDRs) (Kabat et al., 1987; Wu and Kabat, 1970) and other residues at locations outside of the CDR's where the murine and human sequences have a different amino acid and are positions predicted to be important for retaining antigen binding (Adair et al., 1991), were substituted into the EU sequence (Kabat et al., 1987). In addition, in hH the generic human residue was used at residues where EU has residues not normally seen in human $V_H$ sequences (see also Queen et al., 1989; Co et al., 1992).

The variable region sequences were assembled from oligonucleotides and cloned into eukaryotic expression vectors to produce genes capable of generating full length IgG4P heavy and kappa light chains, and being transcribed from the human Cytomegalovirus promoter/enhancer.

The humanized genes were expressed in CHO L761h cells (Cockett et al., 1991) in a transient expression experiment to demonstrate that the humanized antibody bound to antigen with affinity similar to that of the mCTM01.This was measured by the competition ELISA (Figure 7), where all supernatant dilutions had been normalized for IgG concentration, by the assembly ELISA. Thus in crude cell culture supernatants hCTM01 showed approximately equivalent relative potencyto mCTMO1. Hybrids were formed by the co-expression in CHO L761h cells of the chimeric CTM01 light chain and the humanized heavy chain, to give cL/hH, or the chimeric CTM01 heavy chain and the humanized light chain, to give hL/cH. Competition binding experiments suggested that hCTMO1 had similar potency to mCTM01 and the cL/hH and hLcH hybrids (Figure 7).

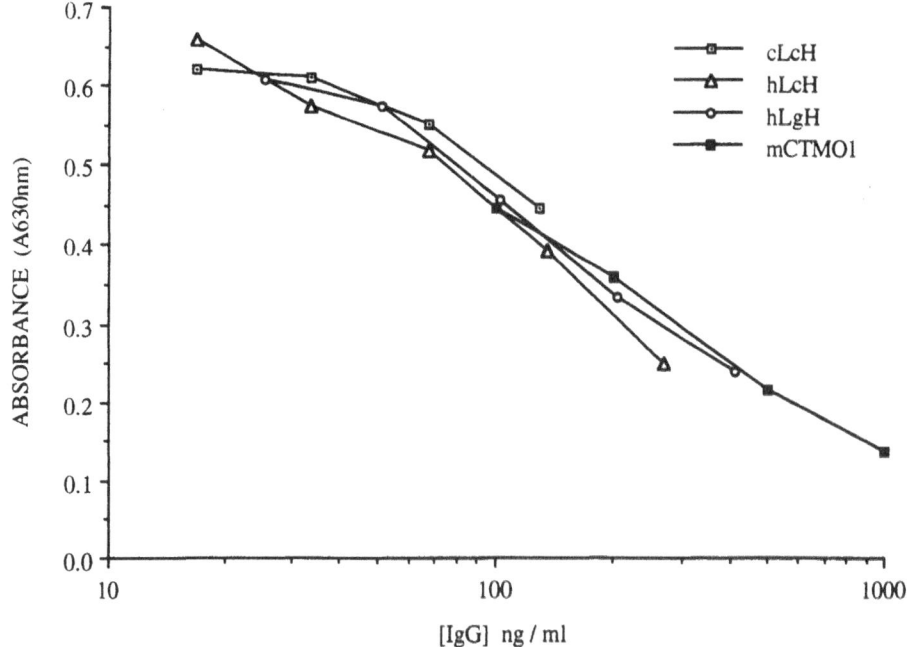

**FIGURE 7** Titration of CHOL761h cell supernatants by competition binding ELISA to monitor the transient expression of various chimeric (c) or humanized (h) IgG4P heavy (H) and kappa light (L) chain gene constructs.

The antibody under test was competed against biotinylated mCTMO1 for binding to solid phase affinity purified milk antigen. Antibody concentration has been normalized following measurement of supernatant human IgG levels using the assembly ELISA. The competition curve of unlabelled mCTMO1 is also shown.

The humanized antibody genes were assembled together on a single expression vector, pAL55 (Figure 1), capable of being transfected into the myeloma cell line NS0 (Bebbington et al., 1992) to form a stable cell line expressing the hCTM01 at high levels. A cell line 18D8 was selected after culture in the presence of 10 μM MSX which produced 700 μg/mL of antibody in small scale shake flask culture and up to 1g/L in larger, air-lift fermentors in serum-free growth medium. Antibody was purified to >95 % purity as determined by SDS-PAGE and HPLC analyses.

**Comparison of relative potency of murine and humanized CTM01**

The relative potency of purified hCTM01 was compared to that of mCTM01 (100%) in the competition ELISA format using either mCTM01 or HMFG1 as immuno-adsorbent and a total of seven breast tumour samples and two ovarian tumour samples along with immuno-purified antigen from milk and urine. A similar pattern of immuno-reactivity was observed for all sources of antigen with the hCTM01 giving a log mean relative potency of 213% (95% confidence interval 199-227%)

Figure 8 shows the competitive binding of unlabelled HMFG1, mCTM01 and hCTM01 against FITC-labelled mCTM01 to breast tumour derived cells where fluorescence intensity measured on single, intact cells has been plotted against unlabelled antibody concentration. HMFG1 competed with <5% relative potency compared to mCTM01 (100%) whereas hCTM01 competed at 176% relative potency.

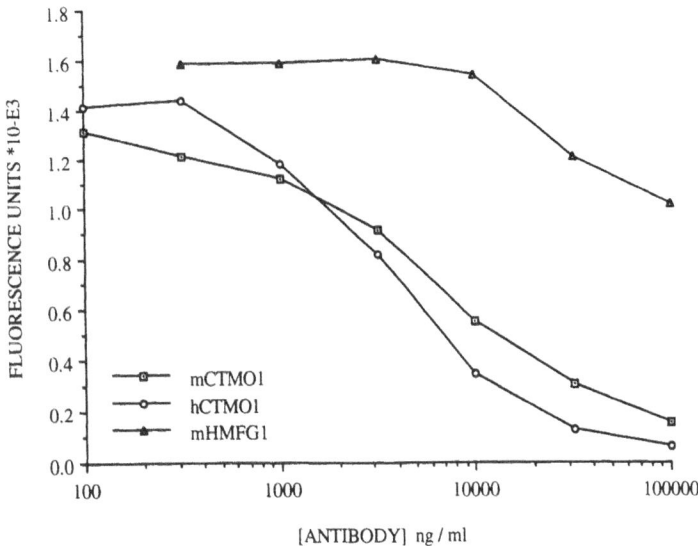

**FIGURE 8**  Competitive inhibition of FITC-mCTMO1 binding to MCF7 cells by murine and humanized CTMO1 and by HMFG1.

Fluorescence intensity was measured on monodisperse, intact cells using flow cytommetry with suitable gating parameters.

## DISCUSSION

### Comparison of CTM01 and other anti-PEMs

Following detailed biochemical studies on the binding of mCTM01 (formerly known as 7F11C7) to and endocytosis within the MCF-7 breast carcinoma cell line, Aboud-Pirak et al., (1988) concluded that this antibody recognized an antigen similar or identical to that recognized by HMFG1 (Burchell et al., 1983) and DF3 (Sekine et al., 1985). In the first part of the present study binding studies were undertaken to confirm this earlier conclusion.

We have shown that mCTM01 reactive antigen, immuno-purified from human milk and urine, is also recognized by HMFG1, HMFG2, C595, SM3 and EMA antibodies which all share closely related epitopes within the VNTR unit of PEM (Price et al., 1990b). Conversely in two-site ELISA experiments HMFG1, C595 and SM3 have been used to immuno-capture antigen from up to seven breast tumour tissue samples and two ovarian tumour tissue samples and in each case mCTM01 was seen to exhibit specific binding to the captured antigens. This suggests either that CTM01 recognizes an epitope which is the same as, or is similar to that seen by the other anti-PEM antibodies, or alternatively recognizes an epitope which co-purifies with and is physically linked to the antigen seen by the other anti-PEM antibodies.

Demonstration that mCTM01 recognizes a similar epitope as anti-PEM antibodies is provided by experiments where mCTM01 was shown to bind, with intensity intermediate to that of C595 or HMFG2 and SM3 or HMFG1, to a 29mer peptide adsorbed to plastic, CTSA<u>PDTRPAPGSTAPPAHGVTSA</u>PDTRP, which contains the VNTR repeat unit (underlined). The latter antibodies are known to bind to a series of overlapping linear peptides within the VNTR unit (Briggs et al., 1991; Dion et al., 1991; Layton et al., 1990) and the similarity in the binding of mCTM01 to this peptide provides suggestive evidence that mCTM01 recognizes an epitope within the protein core of PEM.

Recently a number of groups have cloned the partial or complete cDNA sequence coding for PEM (known as the MUC1 gene) (Gendler et al., 1987; Siddiqui et al., 1988; Wrescher et al., 1990; Ligtenberg et al., 1990). These studies have led to a much clearer understanding of the molecular basis of epithelial mucin polymorphism and have given a better insight into how variant forms may arise in human tumours (Hilkens et al., 1989; Wrescher et al., 1990). MAbs have been described such as SM3, C595, Bre-3 (Blank et al., 1992) and H23 (Keydar et al., 1989), which by immuno-histochemical (Girling et al., 1989), flow cytometry studies (van Dam et al., 1991) and/or xenograft studies have been shown to be relatively tumour specific, the inference being that they react preferentially with sub-populations of PEM which predominate in tumours. Since our ultimate goal was to develop an antibody-drug conjugate for targetted therapy of breast and ovarian cancer a means of, at least semi-quantitatively, comparing its reactivity to tumour tissue PEMs derived from different cancer patients was highly desirable.

We have used the two-site ELISA in a novel manner to investigate the comparative specificity and affinity of two or more antibodies to the heterogeneous antigen, PEM, derived from a number of sources. Our results support the observations of others, in that SM3 appears to recognize a distinct sub-population of PEM present in breast tumour tissue but not present, or present in much reduced amounts in milk or urine derived PEM. In two breast tumour tissues SM3 immuno-adsorption gave a 27 fold enrichment in SM3 reactive antigen (Figure 4) compared to mCTM01 immuno-adsorption. To a lesser degree C595 was also capable of recognizing a tumour sub-population of PEM different from that recognized by SM3, where C595 gave a 2.7 fold enrichment in C595 reactive antigen (Figure 4). In contrast mCTM01 appears to be relatively pan-specific recognizing the SM3 and C595 defined sub-populations better than the homologous antibody.

In the same manner we compared the tumour specificity and affinity of HMFG1 on a larger number of tumour and non-tumour samples. With the exception of milk derived antigen, HMFG1 immuno-adsorption did not result in relative enrichment of HMFG1 reactivity suggesting a similar pan-reactivity to mCTM01. mCTM01 showed higher affinity of binding to antigen in 5/6 tumour samples whether immuno-adsorption was by mCTM01 or by HMFG1.

The competition ELISA format was used to test the relative binding affinity of unlabelled HMFG1 and mCTM01 against breast and ovarian tumour PEM in a manner that was independent of antigen concentration, and would compare binding to mCTM01 defined epitopes. In 4/9 tumour samples using HMFG1 immuno-adsorption HMFG1 could not compete for the mCTM01 epitope (Figure 6), even though HMFG1 epitopes must have been present on the antigen in order for it to be captured. A possible explanation is that HMFG1 epitopes on PEM from some tumours may have limited valency compared to mCTM01 epitopes. In the remaining samples HMFG1 competed for the mCTM01 epitope but with 10-fold lower affinity. A similar pattern was observed using mCTM01 immuno-adsorbed antigen, apart from one tumour sample (#BT1) where HMFG1 had a higher affinity for the mCTM01 epitope. Interestingly where serum and tumour tissue from the same patient was tested a distinctly different pattern of immuno-reactivity was observed between the two sources of PEM (Figure 6, samples #OS1 and #OT1) where HMFG1 reactivity was observed for the serum derived antigen but not for the ovarian tumour derived material. These observations are consistent with the hypothesis that the protein product of the MUC1 gene shows variation due to differential splicing (Wrescher et al., 1991) and post-translational modifications (Hilkens et al., 1989), leading to distinct molecular entities, some of which are predominantly cell membrane members, or cell associated, and some of which are predominantly shed into the extracellular plasma.

From this series of experiments we conclude that HMFG1 and mCTM01 possess a similar degree of pan-reactivity across the tumour tissues studied and with one exception (patient #BT1) HMFG1 has at least a 10-fold lower affinity for antigen. The broad cross reactivity against a range of different tumour antigen sources and its higher relative affinity compared to HMFG1, C595 and SM3 led us to select mCTM01 for humanization.

## Humanization of CTM01

Reconstruction of rodent antibodies to resemble human antibodies has been proposed as a mechanism for avoidance of the immune response which generally occurs when rodent or rodent/human chimeric antibodies are administered to patients (reviewed in Adair, 1992). The process of humanization involves the substitution of the binding site of a human antibody with that of a suitable rodent antibody. In many cases this transfer results in a reduction in the the binding site affinity for antigen. In a small number of cases the net binding affinity of the antibody has been reproduced (Adair et al., 1991; Co et al., 1991) or increased (Carter et al., 1992; Co et al. 1992), although the detail of the binding affinity, measured as differences in enthalpy and entropy of binding may differ between the murine and humanized form (Kelley et al., 1992). The hoped-for reduction in immunogenicity of humanized antibodies remains to be tested in large scale studies, but in primates (Hakimi et al., 1991) and in small Phase I, (Isaacs et al., 1992), and anecdotal studies, (Hale et al., 1989; Mathieson et al., 1990), there does appear to be a benefit in using the humanized form of the antibody.

In this paper we have described a humanized form of the anti-PEM antibody CTM01 in which the binding site affinity for antigen has been reproduced. The humanized form is based on the human antibody EU and incorporates the CDR's from CTM01 and other residues from the framework regions of CTM01 which are believed to be required for the efficient reconstitution of binding affinity (Adair et al., 1991). A cell line expressing hCTM01 has been generated which yields up to 1 g/L of antibody in fermentors in serum-free medium, levels which make the use of antibody-conjugates for cancer therapy a practical proposition. The affinity of hCTM01 for immuno-purified antigen derived from milk, urine and tumour sources appears to be increased compared to that of mCTM01 with a mean relative potency of 213%, while a relative potency of 176% for antigen presented on MCF-7 cells was seen.

The present work has described the humanization of a high affinity anti-PEM antibody to produce an antibody, hCTM01, which displays improved binding affinity to tumour derived PEM. The key question of whether humanization or murine antibodies in general will lead to reduced immunogenicity in patients will ultimately be answered by the clinical testing of this and other humanized antibody therapeutics in the next few years.

## ACKNOWLEDGEMENTS

We wish to acknowledge the contribution of R. Reedman for assistance with cDNA cloning; J. Turner and J. Scothern for oligonucleotide synthesis; H. Brand (Celltech Biologics plc) for Cell Culture Development; G. Renner and S. Fyfe for antibody fermentations of the hCTM01 cell line. We also thank our colleagues at American Cyanamid Inc. for helpful discussions and suggestions.

## REFERENCES

Aboud-Pirak, E., Sergent, T., Otte-Slachmuylder, C., Abarca, J., Trouet, A., and Schneider, Y.-J., 1988, Binding and endocytosis of a monoclonal antibody to a high molecular weight human milk fat globule membrane-associated antigen by cultured MCF-7 breast carcinoma cells, *Cancer Res.*, 48:3188.

Adair, J.R., 1992, Engineering antibodies for therapy, *Immunological Reviews*, 130:1.

Adair, J.R., Athwal, D.S., and Emtage, J.S., 1991, Humanised antibodies, WO91/09967.

Angal, S., King, D.J., Bodmer, M.W., Turner, A., Lawson, A.D.G., Pedley, B., Roberts, G., and Adair, J.R., 1992, A single amino acid substitution abolishes the heterogeneity of a chimeric mouse/human (IgG4) antibody, *Mol. Immunol.*, in press.

Atherton, E., and Sheppard, R.C., 1989, RSolid Phase Synthesis: A practical ApproachS, IRL Press, Oxford.

Baker, T.S., Begent, R.H.J., Dewji, M.R., Conlan, J., and Secher, D.S.,1991, Characterization of the antibody response in patients undergoing radioimmunotherapy with chimeric B72.3, *Antibod. Immunoconj. Radiopharm.*, 4:799.

Bebbington, C.R., 1991, Expression of antibody genes in nonlymphoid mammalian cells, *Methods*, 2:136.

Bebbington, C.R., Renner, G., Thomson, S., King, D., Abrams, D., and Yarranton, G.T., 1992, High-level expression of a recombinant antibody from myeloma cells using a Glutamine synthetase gene as an amplifiable selectable marker, *Bio/Technology*, 10:169.

Begent, R,H,J., Ledermann, J.A., Bagshawe, K.D., Green, A.J., Kelly, A.M.B., Lane, D., Secher, D.S., Dewji, M.R., and Baker, T.S., 1990, PhaseI/II study of chimeric B72.3 antibody in radioimmunotherapy of colorectal carcinoma, *Br. J. Cancer*, 62:487.

Blank, E.W., Pant, K.D., Chan, C.M., Peterson, J.A., and Ceriani, R.L., 1992, A novel anti-breast mucin Mab (Bre-3). Characterization and experimental biodistribution and immunotherapy, *Cancer J.*, 5:38.

Briggs, S., Price, M.R., and Tendler, S.J.B., 1991, Immune recognition of linear peptides in peptide fragments of epithelial mucins, *Immunology*, 73:505.

Burchell, H., Durbin, H., and Taylor-Papadimitriou, J., 1983, Complexity and expression of antigen determinants recognized by monoclonal antibodies HMFG1 and HMFG2 in normal and malignant human mammary epithelial cells, *J. Immunol.*, 131:508.

Burchell, H., Gendler, S., Taylor-Papadimitriou, J.,Girling, A., Lewis, A., Millis, R., and Lamport, D., 1987, Development and characterisation of breast cancer reactive monoclonal antibodies directed to the core protein of the human milk mucin, *Cancer Res.*, 47:5476.

Carter P., Presta, L., Gorman, C.M., Ridgway, J.B.B., Henner, D., Wong, W.L.T., Rowland, A.M., Kotts, C., Carver, M.E., and Shepard, H.M., 1992, Humanization of an anti-p185[HER2] antibody for human cancer therapy, *Proc. Natl. Acad. Sci. USA*, 89:4285.

Catane, R., and Longo, D.L.,1988, Monoclonal antibodies for cancer therapy. *Isr. J. Med. Sci.*, 24:471.

Ceriani, R.L., ed., 1991, RBreast Epithelial Antigens. Molecular Biology to Clinical Applications,S Plenum Press, New York.

Co. M.S., Avdalovic, N.M., Caron, P.C., Avdalovic, M.V., Scheinberg, D.A., and Queen, C. 1992, Chimeric and humanized antibodies with specificity for the CD33 antigen, *J. Immunol.*, 148:1149.

Co, M.S., Deschamps, M., Whitley, R.J., and Queen, C., 1991, Humanized antibodies for antiviral therapy, *Proc. Natl. Acad. Sci. USA*, 88:2869.

Cockett, M.I., Bebbington, C.R., and Yarranton, G.T., 1990, High-level expression of tissue inhibitor of metalloproteinases in Chinese hamster ovary cells using Glutamine synthetase gene amplification, *Bio/Technology*, 8:662.

Cockett, M.I., Bebbington, C.R., and Yarranton, G.T., 1991, The use of engineered E1A genes to transactivate the hCMV-MIE promoter in permanent CHO cell lines, *Nucl. Acids Res.*, 19:319.

Daugherty, B.L., DeMartino, J.A., Law, M.-F., Kawka, D.W., Singer, I.I., and Mark, G.E., 1991, Polymerase chain reaction facilitates the cloning, CDR-grafting and rapid expression of a murine monoclonal antibody directed against the CD18 component of leukocyte integrins. *Nucl. Acids Res.*, 19:2471.

DeNardo, S.J., Warhoe, K.A., OUGrady L.F., DeNardo, G.L., Hellstrom, I., Hellstrom, K.E., and Mills, S.L., 1991a, Radioimmunotherapy with I-131 chimeric L-6 in advanced breast cancer, *in* RBreast Epithelial Antigens. Molecular Biology to Clinical ApplicationsS. Ceriani, R. L., ed., Plenum Press, New York.

DeNardo, S.J., Warhoe, K.A., OUGrady L.F., Gobuty, A.H., Macey, D.J., Hellstrom, I., Hellstrom, K.E., Kroger, L.E., and DeNardo, G.L., 1991b, I-131 Human-chimeric MoAB L6: Bionetics and radioimmunotherapy in patients with metastatic breast cancer, *Antibod. Immunoconj. Immunother.*, 4:34.

Dion, A.S., Smordinsky, N.I., Williams, C.J., Wreschner, D.H., Major, P.P., and Keydov, I., 1991. Recognition of polypeptides by polymorphic epithelial mucin (PEM) specific monoclonal antibodies. *Hybridoma*, 10:595.

Drak, J., Iwasawa, N., Danishefsky, S., and Crothers, D.M., 1991. The carbohydrate domain of calicheamicin $\gamma_1^I$ determines its sequence specificity for DNA cleavage. *Proc. Natl. Acad. Sci. USA*, 88:7464.

Gendler, S.J., Burchell, J.M., Duhig, T., Lamport, D., White, R., Parker, M., and Taylor-Papadimitriou, J., 1987, Cloning of partial cDNA encoding differentiation and tumour associated mucin glycoproteins expressed by human mammary epithelium. *Proc. Natl. Acad. Sci. USA*, 84:6060.

Girling, A., Bartkova, J., Burchell, J., Gendler, S., Gillet, C., and Taylor-Papadimitriou, J., 1989, A core protein epitope of the polymorphic epithelial mucin detected by the monoclonal antibody SM3 is selectively exposed in a range of carcinomas, *Int. J. Cancer*, 43;1072.

Goodman, G., 1991, Phase I trial of chimeric monoclonal antibody L6: Comparisons to murine L6. *6th Annual Conference on Antibody Immunoconjugates and Radiopharmaceuticals. San Diego, USA.*

Hakimi, J., Chizzonite, R., Luke, D.R., Familletti, P.C., Bailon, P., Kondas, J.A., Pilson, R.S., Lin, P., Weber, D.V., Spence, C., Mondini, L.J., Tsien, W.-H., Levin, J.E., Gallati, V.H., Korn, L., Waldmann, T.A., Queen, C., and Benjamin, W.R., 1991, Reduced immunogenicity and improved pharmacokinetics of humanized anti-Tac in cynomolgus monkeys, *J. Immunol.*, 147;1352.

Hale, G., Dyer, M.J., Clark, M.R., Phillips, J.M., Marcus, R., Riechmann, L., Winter, G., and Waldmann, H., 1988, Remission induction in Non-Hodgkin lymphoma with reshaped human monoclonal antibody CAMPATH-1H, *Lancet*, ii:1394.

Hilkens, J., Buijs, F., and Ligtenberg, M., 1989, Complexity of Mam-6, an epithelial sialomucin associated with carcinomas, *Cancer Res.*, 49:786.

Hilkens, J., Ligtenberg, M.J.L., Vos, H.L., and Litvinov, S.V., 1992, Cell membrane-asociated mucins and their adhesion-modulating properties. *Trends in Biochemical Sciences*, 17:359.

Hinman, L.M., Wallace,R.E.,Hamann, P.E., Durr, F.E., and Upeslacis, J. 1991, Calicheamicin immunoconjugates:inluence of analog and linker modification on activity in vivo, *Antibody Immunoconjugates and Radipharmaceuticals, 3:59*.

Isaacs, J.D., Watts, R.A., Hazleman, B.L., Hale, G., Keogan, M.T., Cobbold, S.P., and Waldmann, H., 1992, Humanised antibody therapy for rheumatoid arthritis, *Lancet*, 340:748.

Kelley, R.F., OUConnell, M.P, Carter, P., Presta, L., Eigenbrot, C., Covarrubias, M., Snedcor, B., Bourell, J.H., and Vetterlein, D., 1992, Antigen binding thermodynamics and anti-proliferative effects of chimeric and humanized anti-p185$^{HER2}$ antibody Fab fragments, *Biochemistry*, 31:5434.

Keydar, J., Chou, C.S., Hareuveni, M., Tsarfaty, I., Sahar, E., Selzer, G., Chaitchik, S., and Hizi, A., 1989, Production and characterisation of monoclonal antibodies identifying breast tumour associated antigens, *Proc. Natl. Acad. Sci. USA*, 86:1362.

Khazaeli, M.B., Saleh, M.N., Liu, T.P., Meredith, R.F., Wheeler, R.H., Baker, T.S., King, D., Secher, D., Allen, L., Rogers, K., Colcher, D., Schlom, J., Shochat. T,D., and LoBuglio, A.F., 1991, Pharmacokinetics and immune response of $^{131}$I-chimeric mouse/human B72.3 (human gamma 4) monoclonal antibody in man, *Cancer Res.*, 51:5461.

King, D.J., Adair, J.R., Angal, S., Low, D.C., Proudfoot, K.A., Lloyd, J.C., Bodmer, M., and Yarranton, G.T., 1992, Expression, purification and characterisation of a mouse: human chimeric antibody and chimeric FabU fragment*Biochem. J.*, 281:317.

Knox, S J., Levy, R., Hodgkinson, S., Bell, R., Brown, S., Wood, G.S., Hoppe, R., Abel, E.A., Steinman, L., Berger, R.G., Gaiser, C., Young, G., Bindl, J., Hanham, A., and Reichert, T., 1991, Observations on the effect of chimeric anti-CD4 monoclonal antibody in patients with Mycosis Fungoides, *Blood*, 77:20.

Kabat, E.A., Wu, T.T., Reid-Miller, M., Perry, H.M. and Gottesman, K.S., 1987, Sequences of Proteins of Immunological Interest, 4th edition. United States Department of Health and Human Services, Washington DC.

Layton, G.T., Devine, P.L., Warren, J.A., Birrell, G., Xing, P.-X., Ward, B.G., and McKenzie, I.F.C., 1990, Monoclonal antibodies reactive with the breast carcinoma-associated mucin core repeat sequence peptide also recognise the ovarian carcinoma-associated sebaceous gland-antigen, *Tumor Biol.*, 11:274.

Lee, M.D., Dunne, T.S., Siegel, M.M., Chang, C.C., Morton, G.O. and Borders, D.B., 1987a, Calicheamicins, a novel family of antitumor antibiotics. 1. Chemistry and partial structure of calicheamicin $\gamma_1^I$, *J. Am. Chem. Soc.*, 109:3464.

Lee, M.D., Dunne, T.S., Chang, C.C., Ellestad, G.A., Siegel, M.M., Morton, G.O., McGahren, W.J. and Borders, D.B., 1987b, Calicheamicins, a novel family of antitumor antibiotics. 2. Chemistry and solution structure of calicheamicin $\gamma_1^I$, *J. Am. Chem. Soc.*, 109:3466.

Lewis, A.P., and Crowe, J.S., 1991, Immunoglobulin complementarity determining region grafting by recombinant polymerase chain reaction to generate humanised monoclonal antibodies, *Gene*, 101:297.

Ligtenberg, M.J., Vos, H.L., Gennissen, A.M., and Hilkens, J., 1990. Episialin, a carcinoma associated mucin, is generated by a polymorphic gene encoding splice variants with alternative amino termini, *J. Biol. Chem.*, 265:5573.

LoBuglio, A.F., Wheeler, R.H., Trang, J., Haynes, A., Rogers, K., Harvey, E.B., Sun, L. Ghrayeb, J., and Khazaeli, M.B.,1989. Mouse/human chimeric monoclonal antibody in man: Kinetics and immune response, *Proc. Natl. Acad. Sci. USA*, 86:4220.

LoBuglio, A.F., Meredith, R., Wheeler, R.H., Rogers, K.J., Liu, T., Allen, L., Polansky, A., Plott, G., and Khazaeli, M.B., 1991, Chimeric monoclonal antibody studies in colo-rectal cancer. *in* RMonoclonal Antibodies Applications in Clinical OncologyS Epenetos, A. A., ed., Chapman and Hall Medical, London.

Mathieson, P.W., Cobbold, S.D., Hale, G., Clark, M.R., Oliveira, D.B., Lockwood, C.M., and Waldmann, H., 1990. Monoclonal antibody therapy in systemic vasculitis. *New Engl. J. Med.*, 323:250.

Meredith, R.F., Khazaeli, M.B., Plott, W.E., Saleh, M.N., Liu, T., Allen, L.F., Russell, C.D., Orr, R.A., Colcher, D., Schlom, J., Shochat, D., Wheeler, R.W., and LoBuglio, A.F., 1992b, Phase I trial of Iodine-131-chimeric B72.3 (human IgG4) in metastatic colorectal cancer, *J. Nucl. Med.*, 33:23.

Meredith, R.F., LoBuglio, A.F., Plott, W.E., Orr, R.A., Brezovich, I.A., Russell, C.D., Harvey, E.B., Yester, M.V., Wagner, A.J., Spencer, S.A., Wheeler, R.H., Saleh, M.N., Rogers, K.J., Polansky, A., Salter, M.M., and Khazaeli, M.B., 1991, Pharmacokinetics, immune response, and biodistribution of Iodine-131-labeled chimeric mouse/human IgG1,κ 17-1A monoclonal antibody, *J. Nucl. Med.*, 32:1162.

Meredith, R.F., Khazaeli, M.B., Plott, W.E., Brezovich, I.A., Russell, C.D., Wheeler, R.H., Spencer, S.A., and LoBuglio, A.F., 1992a, Comparison of two mouse/human chimeric antibodies in patients with metastatic colon cancer, *Antibod. Immunoconj. Radiopharm.*, 5:75.

Morrison, S.L., Johnson, M.J., Herzenberg, L.A., and Oi, V.T., 1984, Chimeric human antibody molecules: Mouse antigen-binding domains with human constant region domains. *Proc. Natl. Acad. Sci. USA.*, 81:6851.

Nicolaou, K.C., Dai, W.-M., Tsav, S.-C., Estevez, V.A., and Wrasidlo, W., 1992, Designed enedienes: a new class of DNA-cleaving molecules with potent and selective anticancer activity, *Science*, 256:1172.

Price, M.R., Clarke, A.J., Robertson, J.F.R., OUSullivan, C., Baldwin, R.W, and Blamey, R.W., 1990a, Detection of polymorphic epithelial mucins in the presence in the serum of systemic breast cancer patients using the monoclonal antibody NCRC-11, *Cancer Immunol. Immunother.*, 31:269.

Price, M.R., Crocker, G., Edwards, S., Nagra, C.S., Robins, R.A., Williams, M., Blamey, R.W., Swalow, D.M., and Baldwin, R.W., 1987, Identification of a monoclonal antibody-defined breast carcinoma antigen in body fluids, *Eur. J. Cancer Clin. Oncol.*, 23:1169.

Price, M.R., Hudecz, F., OUSullivan, C., Baldwin, R.W, Edwards, P.M., and Tendler, S.J.B., 1990b, Immunological and structural features of the protein core of human polymorphic epithelial mucin, *Mol. Immunol.*, 27:795.

Price, M.R., Pugh, J.A., Hudecz, F., Griffiths, W., Jacobs, E., Symonds, I.M., Clarke, A.J., Chan, W.C., and Baldwin, R.W., 1990c, C595- a monoclonal antibody against the protein core of human urinary epithelial mucin commonly expressed in breast carcinomas, *Br. J. Cancer*, 61:681.

Queen, C., Schneider, W.P., Selick, H.E., Payne, P.W., Landolfi, N.F., Duncan, J.F., Avdalovic, N.M., Levitt, M., Junghans, R.P., and Waldmann, T.A., 1989, A humanized antibody that binds to the interleukin 2 receptor, *Proc. Natl. Acad. Sci. USA.*, 86:10029.

Saiki, R.K., Gelfand, D.H., Stoffel, S., Scharf, S.F., Higuchi, R., Horn, R.T., Mullis, K.B., and Ehrlich, H.A., 1988, Primer-directed enzymatic amplification of DNA with a thermostable DNA polymerase, *Science*, 239:487.

Saleh, M.N., Khazaeli, M.B., Wheeler, R.H., Allen, L., Tilden, A.B., Grizzle, W., Reisfeld, R.A., Yu, A.L., Gillies, S.D., and LoBuglio, A.F., 1992, Phase I trial of the chimeric anti-GD2 monoclonal antibody ch14.18 in patients with malignant melanoma, *Hum. Antibod. Hybridomas*, 3:19.

Sekine, H., Ohno, T., and Kufe, D.W., 1985, Purification and characterization of high molecular weight glycoprotein detected in human milk and human carcinoma, *J. Immunol.*, 135:3610.

Soule, H.D., Albert, S., Brennan, M., Vazquez, J., and Long, A., 1973. A human cell line froma pleural effusion derived from a breats carcinoma *J. Natl. Cancer Inst.*, 51:1409.

Stephens, P.E., and Cockett, M.I., 1989, The construction of a highly efficient and versatile set of mammalian expression vectors, *Nucl. Acids Res.*, 17:7110.

Taylor-Papadimitriou, J., Peterson, J.A., Arklie, J., Burchell, J., Ceriani, R.L., and Bodmer, W.F., 1981, Monoclonal antibodies to epithelium specific components of human milkfat globule membrane:productin and reaction with cells in culture,*Int. J. Cancer*, 28:17.

Toneguzzo, F., Hayday, A.C., and Keating, A., 1986, Electric field mediated DNA transfer: transient and stable gene expression in human and mouse lymphoid cells, *Mol. Cell Biol.*, 6:703.

Trang, J.M., LoBuglio, A.F., Wheeler, R.H., Harvey, E.B., Sun, L., Ghrayeb, J., and Khazaeli, M.B., 1990, Pharmacokinetics of a mouse/human chimeric monoclonal antibody (C-17-1A) in metastatic adenocarcinoma patients. *Pharmacol. Res.*, 7: 587.

Van Dam, P.A., Lowe, D.G., Watson, J.V., Jobling, T.W., Chard, T., and Shepard, J.H., 1991. Multi-parameter flow cytometric quantitation of the expression of the tumour associated antigen SM3 in normal and neoplastic ovarian tissue. *Cancer*, 68:169.

Wreschner, D.H., Hareuveni, M., Tsarfaty, I., Smorodinsky, N., Horev, J., Zaretsky, J., Kotkes, P., Weiss, M., Lathe, R., Dion, A and Keydar, I., 1990. Human epithelial tumour antigen cDNA sequences. *Eur. J. Biochem.*, 189:463.

Wreschner, D.H., Tsarfaty, I., Hareuveni, M., Zaretsky, J., Smorodinsky, N., Weiss, M., Zrihan, S., Burstein, M., Horev, J., Kotkes, P., Lathe, R., Hart, C.A., McCarthy, K., Williams, C., Dion, A., and Keydar, I., 1991, Molecular analysis of H23 epithelial antigen-differentially spliced full length cDNAs and gene, *in* RBreast Epithelial Antigens. Molecular Biology to Clinical ApplicationsS Ceriani, R.L., ed., Plenum Press, New York.

Wu, T.T., and Kabat, E.A., 1970, An analysis of the sequences of the variable regions of Bence Jones proteins and myeloma light chains and their implications for antibody complementarity, *J. Exp. Med.*, 132:211.

# TOWARDS AN IMMUNOTHERAPY FOR p185[HER2] OVEREXPRESSING TUMORS

Paul Carter[1], Maria L. Rodrigues[1], Gail D. Lewis[2], Irene Figari[3]
and M. Refaat Shalaby[4]

Departments of Protein Engineering[1], Cell Biology[2], Endocrinology[3]
and Medicinal and Analytical Chemistry[4]
Genentech Inc, 460 Point San Bruno Boulevard
South San Francisco, CA 94080

## INTRODUCTION

The protooncogene, *HER2* (also known as c-*erb*B-2, *neu*, and HER-2 / *neu*) encodes a receptor tyrosine kinase, p185[HER2] which is homologous to the EGF receptor (EGFr). *HER2* was found to be amplified from 2 to 20-fold in up to ~ 30% of primary human breast cancers[1]. Furthermore, *HER2* amplification was shown to be a strong prognosticator of decreased overall survival and overall time to relapse[1] *HER2* amplification and/or overexpression has subsequently been correlated with poor clinical prognosis in several additional malignant human diseases including: ovarian cancer[2, 3], endometrial cancer[4, 5], gastric cancer[6] and adenocarcinoma of the lung[7].

Monoclonal antibodies (MAb) have proved to be very powerful tools for probing the role of p185[HER2] and its rat homolog, p185[*neu*], in neoplastic cell growth (reviewed in Ref. 8). Further advances will surely follow in the wake of the recent identification and cloning of ligands for p185[HER2] (Ref. 9-11) and p185[*neu*] (Ref. 12, 13). Here we focus on the evolution of potential antibody-based therapeutics for human cancers in which *HER2* is amplified and/or overexpressed.

*Antigen and Antibody Molecular Engineering in Breast Cancer Diagnosis and Treatment*, Edited by R.L. Ceriani, Plenum Press, New York, 1994

83

## MURINE MAb 4D5 IS POTENTIALLY USEFUL FOR IMMUNOTHERAPY OF p185[HER2] OVEREXPRESSING TUMORS

A panel of murine MAb was generated which are reactive with the extracellular domain of p185[HER2], but not the homologous EGFr[14]. The anti-p185[HER2] MAb known as 4D5 was selected for further study since it was found to be the most effective in retarding the growth of a variety of human tumor cell lines overexpressing p185[HER2] in monolayer culture. MAb 4D5 has a number of additional properties (reviewed in Ref. 15, 16) which suggest that it might be potentially useful for immunotherapy of p185[HER2] overexpressing tumors. MAb 4D5 down regulates p185[HER2] from the surface of cells[17] and inhibits colony formation in soft agar suggesting that it may be reversing the transformed phenotype[18.] MAb 4D5 localizes to p185[HER2] overexpressing tumor xenografts in nude mice[16] and furthermore inhibits their growth[15]. In addition, MAb 4D5 reverses the TNF-α resistant phenotype which appears to be characteristic of breast tumor cells overexpressing p185[HER2] (Ref. 18).

## *HUMANIZATION* OF MURINE MAb 4D5 TO ENHANCE ITS CLINICAL POTENTIAL

A major limitation in the clinical use of rodent MAb is an anti-globulin response during therapy[19, 20]. A partial solution to this problem is to construct chimeric antibodies by coupling the rodent antigen-binding variable domains to human constant domains[21, 22]. The isotype of the human constant domains may be varied to tailor the chimeric antibody for participation in antibody-dependent cellular cytotoxicity (ADCC) and complement-dependent cytotoxicity (CDC)[23]. Such chimeric antibody molecules are still ~30% rodent in sequence and are capable of eliciting a significant anti-globulin response. This potential immunogenicitiy problem of chimeric antibodies may be minimized by *humanization* as pioneered by Winter and colleagues[24-26]. Rodent antibodies are humanized by grafting the six antigen-binding complimentarity determining region loops from their variable domains into a human antibody. Thus the rest of the variable domains, known as framework regions, and the constant domains are human in origin. Several different variations on the basic humanization strategy have been devised (reviewed in Ref. 27). In some cases it has been necessary to install one[26] or several[28] murine framework region residues into the humanized antibody to obtain comparable antigen binding affinity to the murine parent antibody. It seems likely that antibody humanization may soon be superseded by direct routes to human antibodies. For example, the advent of antibody display phage[29] has enabled the isolation of human antibodies from antibody phage libraries[30].

We chose to humanize the well characterized 4D5 MAb (see above) as a step towards developing an immunotherapeutic for therapy of p185[HER2] overexpressing tumors, rather than attempt to directly isolate a human antibody with a similar set of properties. The most potent humanized version of the antibody, known as huMAb4D5−8, binds the extracellular

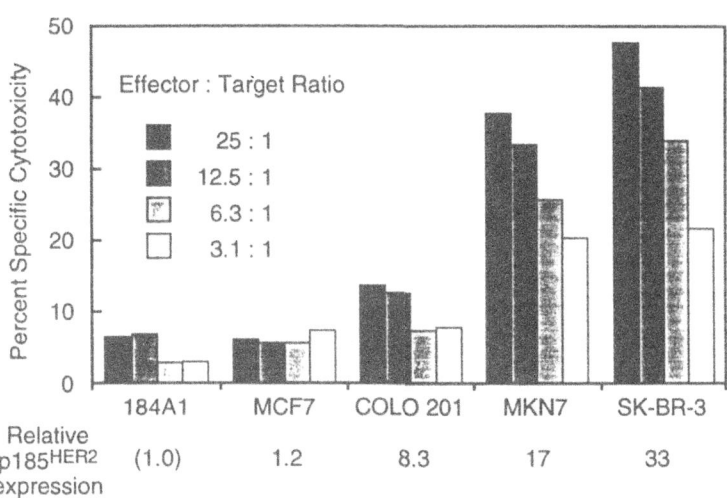

**Figure 1.** ADCC of human peripheral blood mononuclear effector cells mediated by humAb4D5-8 against the cells lines: 184A1 (normal breast epithelium), MCF7 (breast tumor), COLO201 (colo-rectal tumor), MKN7 (gastric tumor) and SK-BR-3 (breast tumor)[32]. Percent specific cytotoxicity was calculated from the difference in $^{51}Cr$ released from the target cells in a 4 hr assay in the presence or absence of antibody. The level of surface p185$^{HER2}$ was determined by FACS® analysis[32] and is expressed relative to that on the 184A1 cell line.

domain of p185[HER2] about 3-fold more tightly than the murine parent antibody and is almost as potent in inhibiting the proliferation of SK-BR-3 breast tumor cells[31].

## SECONDARY IMMUNE FUNCTIONS OF huMAb4D5-8

The human IgG1 isotype is the preferred one for supporting ADCC and CDC as judged by using matched sets of chimeric[23] or humanized[26] antibodies and was therefore chosen for humAb4D5-8. As anticipated, huMAb4D5-8 supports ADCC against tumor cells overexpressing p185[HER2] in the presence of human effector cells[31] whereas the parent antibody (murine IgG1) does not. Importantly, the efficiency of ADCC correlates with the extent of p185[HER2] overexpression[32] (Figure 1). For the cell lines: SK-BR-3, MKN7, MCF7, COLO201 and 184A1 the relative expression levels of p185[HER2] are 33, 17, 8.3, 1.2 and 1.0, respectively, as judged by FACS® analysis[32]. SK-BR-3 and MKN7 cells are efficiently killed by ADCC, COLO201 cells slightly less so, whereas MCF7 and 184A1 cells are not readily susceptible to ADCC. These data are consistent with the correlation between antigen density and the tumor susceptibility to secondary immune functions of antibodies previously observed by others[33]. The enhanced susceptibility to ADCC of tumor cell lines which overexpress p185[HER2] at high levels bodes well for the on-going clinical trial using humAb4D5-8 since the highest level of p185[HER2] overexpression correlates with the poorest clinical prognosis[1,2]. The minimal cytotoxicity observed against normal cell lines (WI-38, Ref. 31; 184A1, Ref. 32) is also encouraging since low levels of p185[HER2] are observed on a variety of normal epithelial cells[34]. Antibody specificity for tumor compared to normal tissue expressing the same (or similar) antigen at lower levels is one of the fundamental issues that must be addressed in using antibodies for anti-cancer therapy (reviewed in Ref. 35).

## BEYOND *NAKED* ANTIBODIES FOR IMMUNOTHERAPY OF p185[HER2] OVEREXPRESSING TUMORS

Studies from several different groups have suggested a number of promising strategies to augment naked antibodies for potential immunotherapy of p185[HER2] overexpressing tumors (Table 1). The feasibility of retargeting effector cells to specifically lyse tumor cells using bispecific antibodies (BsAb) has been well demonstrated *in vitro* and in animal tumor models *in vivo* (reviewed in Ref. 45 and 46). Furthermore a bispecific F(ab')$_2$ fragment (anti-glioma associated antigen / anti-CD3) was found to have clinical efficacy in glioma patients[47]. Lysis of tumor cells appears to be mediated by the release of cytolytic granules from T cells bound to their surface *via* the bispecific antibody. In addition, release of the cytokines TNF-α and IFN-γ by recruited T cells may block the growth of bystander tumor cells[46].

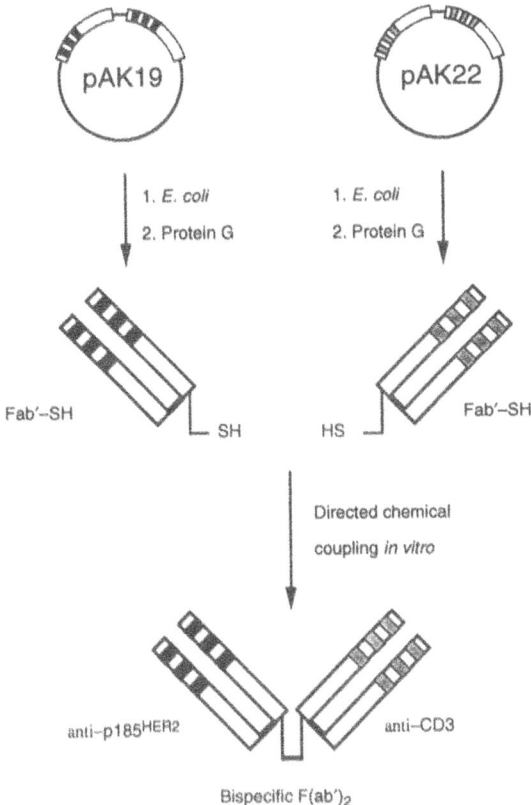

**Figure 2.** Construction of humanized bispecific (anti-p185[HER2] / anti-CD3) F(ab′)$_2$. Humanized anti-p185[HER2] and anti-CD3 Fab′ fragments were separately expressed in *E. coli* from plasmids pAK19 (Ref. 48) and pAK22 (Ref. 37), respectively. The Fab′ fragments were purified using Streptococcal protein G and the bispecific F(ab′)$_2$ then constructed by directed chemical coupling[37].

**Table 1.** Strategies for augmenting the anti-tumor activity of anti-p185[HER2] and anti-p185[neu] MAb

---

Bispecific antibodies for effector cell retargeting

        anti-p185[HER2] / anti-CD3 for retargeting T cell[36-39]

        anti-p185[HER2] / anti-FcγRIII for retargeting large granular lymphocytes[40]

Synergistically acting combinations of MAb

        2 x anti-p185[neu] (Ref. 41)

        2 x anti-p185[HER2] (Ref. 42)

        anti-p185[HER2] + anti-EGFr[54]

MAb with synergistically acting chemotherapeutic

        anti-p185[HER2] + CDDP[15, 43]

Immunotoxins

        anti-p185[HER2] - *Pseudomonas* exotoxin[44]

---

We[36, 37] and others[38, 39] have constructed BsF(ab' )$_2$ fragments with specificities for p185[HER2] and CD3 which were found to be highly effective in retargeting the cytotoxic activity of T cells against p185[HER2] overexpressing tumor cells. We developed a facile route to the construction of a humanized anti-p185[HER2] / anti-CD3 BsF(ab' )$_2$ fragment which may encourage the more widespread clinical use of such bifunctional molecules (Figure 2). Our strategy relies upon an *E. coli* expression system which secretes functional humanized Fab' fragments at gram per liter titers[48]. Traditional directed chemical coupling of Fab' fragments is then used to efficiently form BsF(ab' )$_2$ *in vitro*[49, 50].

Large granular lymphocytes represent an alternative population of effector cells to T cells whose cytotoxic activity may be unleashed upon tumor cells using appropriately designed BsAb. For example, a bispecific antibody with specificites against p185[HER2] and FcγRIII (CD16) was purified from an appropriate hybrid hybridoma[40]. This BsAb directed efficient lysis of several different breast tumor cell lines overexpressing p185[HER2] by human large granular lymphocytes, including MDA-MB-175 which overexpresses p185[HER2] by only a few fold.

In addition to BsAb, combinations of MAb also appear to be promising strategies for the development of potential therapies for p185[HER2] overexpressing tumors. For example, two MAb directed against different epitopes on the rat p185[neu] protein were found to have synergistic anti-tumor effects *in vivo* in a nude mouse xenograft model[41]. An apparently similar pair of MAb has been identified for the human protein, p185[HER2], and found to inhibit the growth of human tumor cell lines growing as xenografts in nude mice and even reduce established tumors[42]. Formation of highly constrained lattices of p185[HER2] on cell surfaces induced by the MAb combinations may be important to this anti-tumor activity since combinations of the corresponding Fab fragments did not show the pronounced anti-tumor effect.

It may be possible to enhance the clinical efficacy of anti-p185[HER2] MAb by combined treatment with anti-tumor drugs. The cytotoxic effect of the chemotherapeutic *cis*-diamminedichloroplatinum (CDDP) against human tumor cells overexpressing p185[HER2] is enhanced both *in vitro* and *in vivo* by anti-p185[HER2] MAb[43] including 4D5 (Ref. 15). The molecular basis of this enhancement remains to be elucidated but one plausible explanation is that the anti-p185[HER2] MAb impair DNA repair since CDDP is known to alkylate DNA. The anti-tumor activity of CDDP has also been observed *in vivo* for EGFr overexpressing tumors in the presence of anti-EGFr MAb[51].

The development of potential anti-p185[HER2] therapies may be complicated by interaction between p185[HER2] and EGFr. -Binding of EGF to EGFr induces heterodimerization with p185[HER2] (Ref. 52, 53). However the functional significance of the p185[HER2] / EGFr heterodimers in normal and neoplastic cell growth remains to be determined. Intriguingly, a combination of MAb directed against rat p185*neu* and human EGFr were found to have synergistic anti-tumor activity in nude mice implanted with rodent fibroblasts transformed with genes for both of these receptors[54].

## CONCLUSIONS AND PERSPECTIVES

Two principal factors have driven the recent proliferation of different approaches to the development of potential immunotherapies for p185[HER2] overexpressing human tumors. Firstly, much progress has been made towards understanding the role of *HER2* amplification and overexpression in neoplastic cell growth (reviewed in Ref. 55). Secondly, rapid advances have been made in technologies which enhance the clinical utility of antibodies (reviewed in Ref. 56) including direct routes to human antibodies through antibody-phage (reviewed in Ref. 57). One engineered molecule - our humanized anti-p185[HER2] antibody[31] - is currently being evaluated in a phase II clinical trial for the treatment of p185[HER2]-overexpressing breast cancer. Another engineered molecule - our humanized BsF(ab')₂ (anti-p185[HER2] / anti-CD3)[36, 37]- is highly effective in retargeting T cells to lyse tumor cells overexpressing p185[HER2] *in vitro* making it a strong candidate for a potential immunotherapy.

## REFERENCES

1. Slamon, D. J., Clark, G. M., Wong, S. G., Levin, W. J., Ullrich, A. and McGuire, W. L. Human breast cancer: correlation of relapse and survival with amplification of the HER-2/*neu* oncogene. *Science* 235:177 (1987).

2. Slamon, D. J., Godolphin, W., Jones, L. A., Holt, J. A., Wong, S. G., Keith, D. E., Levin, W. J., Stuart, S. G., Udove, J., Ullrich, A. and Press, M. F. Studies of the HER-2/*neu* proto-oncogene in human breast and ovarian cancer. *Science* 244:707 (1989).

3.  Berchuck, A., Kamel, A., Whitaker, R., Kerns, B., Olt, G., Kinney, R., Soper, J. T., Dodge, R., Clarke-Pearson, D. L., Marks, P., McKenzie, S., Yin, S. and Bast, R. C. Overexpression of *HER-2 / neu* is associated with poor survival in advanced epithelial ovarian cancer. *Cancer Res.* 50:4087 (1990).

4.  Borst, M. P., Baker, V. V., Dixon, D., Hatch, K. D., Shingleton, H. M. and Miller, D. M. Oncogene alterations in endometrial carcinoma. *Gynecol. Oncol.* 38:364 (1990).

5.  Berchuck, A., Rodriguez, G., Kinney, R. B., Soper, J. T., Dodge, R. K., Clarke-Pearson, D. L. and Bast, R. C. Overexpression of HER-2 / *neu* in endometrial cancer is associated with advanced stage disease. *Am. J. Obstet. Gynecol.* 164:15 (1991).

6.  Yonemura, Y. Ninomiya, I., Yamaguchi, A., Fushida, S., Kimura, H., Ohoyama, S., Miyazaki, I., Endou, Y., Tanaka, M. and Sasaki, T. Evaluation of immunoreactivity for erbB-2 protein as a marker of poor short term prognosis in gastric cancer. *Cancer Res.* 51:1034 (1991).

7.  Kern, J. A., Schwartz, D. A., Nordberg, J. E., Weiner, D. B., Greene, M. I., Torney, L. and Robinson, R. A. p185$^{neu}$ expression in human lung adenocarcinomas predicts shortened survival. *Cancer Res.* 50:5184 (1990).

8.  Myers, J. N., Drebin, J. A., Wada, T. and Greene, M. I. Biological effects of monoclonal antireceptor antibodies reactive with *neu* oncogene product, p185$^{neu}$. *Methods Enzymol.* 198:277 (1991).

9.  Lupu, R., Colomer, R., Zugmaier, G., Sarup, J., Shepard, M., Slamon, D. and Lippman, M. E. Direct interaction of a ligand for the *erb*B2 oncogene product with EGF receptor and p185$^{erbB2}$. *Science* 249:1552 (1990).

10. Lupu, R., Colomer, R., Kannan, B. and Lippman, M. E. Characterization of a growth factor that binds exclusively to the *erbB-2* receptor and induces cellular responses. *Proc. Natl. Acad. Sci. USA* 89:2287 (1992).

11. Holmes, W. E., Sliwkowski, M. X., Akita, R. W., Henzel, W. J., Lee, J., Park, J. W., Yansura, D., Abadi, N., Raab, H., Lewis, G. D., Shepard, H. M., Kuang, W.-J., Wood, W. I., Goeddel, D. V. and Vandlen, R. L. Identification of heregulin, a specific activator or p185$^{erbB2}$. *Science* 256:1205 (1992).

12. Wen, D., Peles, E., Cupples, R., Suggs, S. V., Bacus, S. S., Luo, Y., Trail, G., Hu, S., Silbiger, S. M., Ben Levy, R., Koski, R. A., Lu, H. S. and Yarden, Y. Neu differentiation factor: a transmembrane glycoprotein containing an EGF domain and an immunoglobulin homology unit. *Cell* 69:559 (1992).

13. Peles, E., Bacus, S. S., Koski, R. A., Lu, H. S., Wen, D., Ogden, S. G., Ben Levy, R. and Yarden, Y. Isolation of the Neu/HER-2 stimulatory ligand: a 44 kd glycoprotein that induces differentiation of mammary tumor cells. *Cell* 69:205 (1992).

14. Fendly, B. M., Winget, M., Hudziak, R. M., Lipari, M. T., Napier, M. A. and Ullrich, A. Characterization of murine monoclonal antibodies reactive to either the

human epidermal growth factor receptor or HER2/*neu* gene product. *Cancer Res.* 50:1550 (1990).

15. Shepard, H. M., Lewis, G. D., Sarup, J. C., Fendly, B. M., Maneval, D., Mordenti, J., Figari, I., Kotts, C. E., Palladino Jr., M. A., Ullrich, A. and Slamon, D. Monoclonal antibody therapy of human cancer: taking the HER2 protooncogene to the clinic. *J. Clin. Immunol.* 11:117 (1991).

16. Park, J. W., Stagg, R., Lewis, G. D., Carter, P., Maneval, D., Slamon, D. J., Jaffe, H. and Shepard, H. M. Anti-p185[HER2] monoclonal antibodies: biological properties and potential for immunotherapy. *In* "Breast Cancer: Cellular and Molecular Biology", Lippman, M. E. and Dickson, R. B., eds., Kluwer Academic Publishers, Boston, pp 193-211 (1991).

17. Sarup, J. C., Johnson, R. M., King, K. L., Fendly, B. M., Lipari, M. T., Napier, M. A., Ullrich, A. and Shepard, H. M. Characterization of an anti-p185[HER2] monoclonal antibody that stimulates receptor function and inhibits tumor cell growth. *Growth Reg.* 1:72 (1991).

18. Hudziak, R. M., Lewis, G. D., Winget, M., Fendly, B. M., Shepard, H. M., and Ullrich, A. p185[HER2] monoclonal antibody has antiproliferative effects *in vitro* and sensitizes human breast tumor cells to tumor necrosis factor. *Mol. Cell. Biol.* 9:1165 (1989).

19. Miller, R. A., Oseroff, A. R., Stratte, P. T. and Levy, R. Monoclonal antibody therapeutic trials in seven patients with T-cell lymphoma. *Blood* 62:988 (1983).

20. Schroff, R. W., Foon, K. A., Beatty, S. M., Oldham, R. K. and Morgan Jr. , A. C. Human anti-murine immunoglobulin responses in patients receiving monoclonal antibody therapy. *Cancer Res.* 45:879 (1985).

21. Morrison, S. L., Johnson, M. J., Herzenberg, L. A. and Oi, V. T. *Proc. Natl. Acad. Sci. USA* 81:6851 (1984).

22. Boulianne, G. L., Hozumi, N. and Shulman, M. J. Production of functional chimaeric mouse/human antibody. *Nature* 312:643 (1984).

23. Brüggemann, M., Williams, G. T., Bindon, C. I., Clark, M. R., Walker, M. R., Jefferis, R., Waldmann, H. and Neuberger, M. S. Comparison of the effector functions of human immunoglobulins using a matched set of chimeric antibodies. *J. Exp. Med.* 166:1351 (1987).

24. Jones, P. T., Dear, P. H., Foote, J., Neuberger, M. S., and Winter, G. Replacing the complementarity-determining regions in a human antibody with those from a mouse. *Nature* 321:522 (1986).

25. Verhoeyen, M., Milstein, C. and Winter, G. Reshaping human antibodies: grafting an antilysozyme activity. *Science* 239:1534 (1988).

26. Riechmann, L., Clark, M., Waldmann, H., and Winter, G. Reshaping human antibodies for therapy. *Nature* 332:323 (1988).

27. Presta, L. G. Antibody engineering. *Current Opinion Str. Biol.* 2:593 (1992).

28. Queen, C., Schneider, W. P., Selick, H. E., Payne, P. W., Landolfi, N. F., Duncan, J. F., Avdalovic, N. M., Levitt, M., Junghans, R. P. and Waldmann, T. A. A humanized antibody that binds to the interleukin 2 receptor *Proc. Natl. Acad. Sci. USA* 86:10029 (1989).

29. McCafferty, J., Griffiths, A. D., Winter, G. and Chiswell, D. J. Phage antibodies: filamentous phage displaying antibody variable domains. *Nature* 348:552 (1990).

30. Marks, J. D., Hoogenboom, H. R., Bonnert, T. P., McCafferty, J., Griffiths, A. D. and Winter, G. By-passing immunization. Human antibodies from V-gene libraries displayed on phage. *J. Mol. Biol.* 222:581 (1991).

31. Carter, P., Presta, L., Gorman, C. M., Ridgway, J. B. B., Henner, D., Wong, W. L. T., Rowland, A. M., Kotts, C., Carver, M. E. and Shepard, H. M. Humanization of an anti-p185$^{HER2}$ antibody for human cancer therapy. *Proc. Natl. Acad. Sci. USA* 89:4285 (1992).

32. Lewis, G. D., Figari, I., Fendly, B., Wong, W. L., Carter, P., Gorman, C. and Shepard, H. M. Differential responses of human tumor cells lines to anti-p185$^{HER2}$ monoclonal antibodies *Cancer Immunol. Immunother.* 37:255 (1993).

33. Herlyn, D., Powe, J., Ross, A. H., Herlyn, M. and Koprowski, H. Inhibition of human tumor growth by IgG2a monoclonal antibodies correlates with antibody density on tumor cells. *J. Immunol.* 134:1300 (1985).

34. Press, M. F., Cordon-Cardo, C. and Slamon, D. J. Expression of the HER-2/*neu* proto-oncogene in normal human adult and fetal tissues. *Oncogene* 5:953 (1990).

35. Schlom, J. Antibodies in cancer therapy: basic principles of monoclonal antibodies, basic principles and applications. *In* "Biologic Therapy of Cancer", DeVita Jr., V. T., Hellman, S. and Rosenberg, S. A., eds., J. B. Lippincott Company, Philadelphia, pp 464-481 (1991).

36. Shalaby, M. R., Shepard, H. M., Presta, L., Rodrigues, M. L., Beverley, P. C. L., Feldmann, M. and Carter, P. Development of humanized bispecific antibodies reactive with cytotoxic lymphocytes and tumor cells overexpressing the *HER2* protooncogene. *J. Exp. Med.*175:217 (1992).

37. Rodrigues, M. L., Shalaby, M. R., Werther, W., Presta, L. and Carter, P. Engineering a humanized bispecific F(ab' )$_2$ fragment for improved binding to T cells. *Internat. J. Cancer Suppl.* 7:45 (1992).

38. Nishimura, T., Nakamura, Y., Tsukamoto, H., Takeuchi, Y., Tokuda, Y., Iwasawa, M., Yamamoto, T., Masuko, T., Hashimoto, Y. and Habu, S. Human c-*erbB*-2 proto-oncogene product as a target for bispecific-antibody-directed adoptive tumor immunotherapy. *Int. J. Cancer* 50:800 (1992).

39. Sugiyama, Y., Aihara, M., Shibamori, M., Deguchi, K., Imagawa, K., Kikuchi, M., Momota, H., Azuma, T., Okada, H., Alper, O., Hitomi, J. and Yamaguchi, K.

*In vitro* anti-tumor activity of anti-c-*erb*B-2 x anti-CD3ε bifunctional monoclonal antibody. *Jpn. J. Cancer Res.* 83:563 (1992).

40. Ring, D. B., Shi, T., Hsieh-Ma, S. T., Reeder, J., Eaton, A. and Flatgaard, J. Targeted lysis of human breast cancer cells by human effector cells armed with bispecific antibody 2B1 (anti-c-erbB-2 / anti-Fcγ receptor III). *In* "Breast Epithelial Antigens", Ceriani, R. L., ed., Plenum Press, New York, pp 91-104 (1991).

41. Drebin, J. A., Link, V. C. and Greene, M. I. Monoclonal antibodies reactive with distinct domains of the *neu* oncogene-encoded p185 molecule exert synergistic anti-tumor effects *in vivo*. *Oncogene* 2:273 (1988).

42. Kasprzyk, P. G., Song, S. U., Di Fiore, P. P. and King, C. R. Therapy of an animal model of human gastric cancer using a combination of anti-*erb*B-2 monoclonal antibodies. *Cancer Res.* 52:2771 (1992).

43. Hancock, M. C., Langton, B. C., Chan, T., Toy, P., Monahan, J. J., Mischak, R. P. and Shawver, L. K. A monoclonal antibody against the c-*erbB*-2 protein enhances the cytotoxicity of *cis*-diamminedichloroplatinum against human breast and ovarian tumor cell lines. *Cancer Res.* 51:4575 (1991).

44. Batra J. K., Kasprzyk, P. G., Bird, R. E., Pastan, I. and King, C. R. Recombinant anti-erbB2 immunotoxins containing *Pseudomonas* exotoxin. *Proc. Natl. Acad. Sci. USA* 89:5867 (1992).

45. Nelson, H. Targeted cellular immunotherapy with bifunctional antibodies. *Cancer Cells* 3:163 (1991).

46. Segal, D. M., Qian, J.-H., Mezzanzanica, D., Garrido, M. A., Titus, J. A., Andrew, S. M., George, A. J. T., Jost, C. R., Perez, P. and Wunderlich, J. R. Targeting of anti-tumor responses with bispecific antibodies. *Immunobiol.* 185:390 (1992).

47. Nitta, T., Sato, K., Yagita, H., Okumura, K. and Ishii, S. Preliminary trial of specific targeting therapy against malignant glioma. *Lancet* 335:368 (1990).

48. Carter, P., Kelley, R. F., Rodrigues, M. L., Snedecor, B., Covarrubias, M., Velligan, M. D., Wong, W. L. T., Rowland, A. M., Kotts, C. E., Carver, M. E., Yang, M., Bourell, J. H., Shepard, H. M. and Henner, D. High level *Escherichia coli* expression and production of a bivalent humanized antibody fragment. *Bio/Tech.* 10:163 (1992).

49. Brennan, M., Davison, P. F. and Paulus, H. Preparation of bispecific antibodies by chemical recombination of monoclonal immunoglobulin G₁ fragments. *Science* 229:81 (1985).

50. Glennie, M. J., McBride, H. M., Worth, A. T. and Stevenson, G. T. Preparation and performance of bispecific F(ab'γ)2 antibody containing thioether-linked Fab'γ fragments. *J. Immunol.* 139:2367 (1987).

51. Aboud-Pirak, E., Hurwitz, E., Pirak, M. E., Bellot, F., Schlessinger, J. and Sela, M. Efficacy of antibodies to epidermal growth factor receptor against KB carcinoma *in vitro* and in nude mice. *J. Natl. Cancer Inst.* 21:1605 (1988).

52. Goldman, R., Ben Levy, R., Peles, E. and Yarden Y. Heterodimerization of the erbB-1 and erbB-2 receptors in human breast carcinoma cells: a mechanism for receptor transregulation. *Biochem.* 29:11024 (1990).

53. Spivak-Kroizman, T., Rotin, D., Pinchasi, D., Ullrich, A., Schlessinger, J. and Lax, I. Heterodimerization of c-erbB2 with different epidermal growth factor receptor mutants elicits simulatory or inhibitory responses. *J. Biol. Chem.* 267:8056 (1992).

54. Wada, T., Myers, J. N., Kokai, Y., Brown, V. I., Hamuro, J., LeVea, C. M. and Greene, M. I. Anti-receptor antibodies reverse the phenotype of cells transformed by two interacting proto-oncogene encoded receptor proteins. *Oncogene* 5:489 (1990).

55. Allred, D. C., Tandon, A. K., Clark, G. M. and McGuire, W. L. Expression and prognostic significance of the HER-2/*NEU* oncogene during the evolutionary progression of human breast cancer. *In* "Breast Epithelial Antigens", Ceriani, R. L., ed., Plenum Press, New York, pp 69-82 (1991).

56. Waldmann, T. A. Monoclonal antibodies in diagnosis and therapy. *Science* 252: 1657 (1991).

57. Marks, J. D., Hoogenboom, H. R., Griffiths, A. D. and Winter, G. Molecular evolution of proteins on filamentous phage. Mimicking the strategy of the immune system. *J. Biol. Chem.* 267:16007 (1992).

# BRANCHING N-LINKED OLIGOSACCHARIDES IN BREAST CANCER

Bozena Korczak[1,2], Paul Goss[3], Bernard Fernandez[1], Michael Baker[3], and James W. Dennis[1]

[1]Samuel Lunenfeld Research Institute
Mount Sinai Hospital
600 University Avenue
Toronto, Ontario
M5G 1X5
Canada

[2]Allelix Inc.
Goreway Dr.
Mississauga, Ontario

[3]Toronto General Hospital
Department of Medicine
University of Toronto

## SUMMARY

Tumor progression in rodent and human tumors is commonly associated with changes in glycoprotein glycosylation, in particular increased $\beta$1-6GlcNAc-branching, a regulatory step in expression of polylactosamine and extended-chain Lewis antigens. Loss of the branched oligosaccharides in murine tumor cells either due to somatic mutation, or treatment of the cells with the oligosaccharide processing inhibitor swainsonine, blocks tumor cells invasion in vitro and reduces solid tumor growth in vivo. Swainsonine and other inhibitors of N-linked oligosaccharide processing may be useful anti-cancer drugs, a premise which has begun to be tested in humans.

**Glycoprotein glycosylation in transformed cells.** Malignant transformation is generally accompanied by the expression of larger oligosaccharide structures on cellular glycoproteins[1]. This phenomena has been observed in rodent tumor cells

*Antigen and Antibody Molecular Engineering in Breast Cancer Diagnosis and Treatment*, Edited by R.L. Ceriani, Plenum Press, New York, 1994

95

transformed by activated oncogenes (i.e., H-ras, v-fps, v-src), by DNA tumor viruses, and by chemical carcinogenesis (reviewed in[2]). A fraction of N-linked oligosaccharides in transformed fibroblasts cells are generally more branched at the trimannosyl core (i.e., -GlcNAc$\underline{\beta 1\text{-}6}$Manα1-6Manβ-). Consistent with the presence of these structures, UDP-GlcNAc:α6Man β6-N-acetylglucosaminyltransferase V (i.e., GlcNAc-TV) activity, the enzyme that initiates the β1-6 linked antenna was found to be elevated 3-10 fold, while other glycosyltransferase activities remained unchanged[3,4]. In mammalian cells there are at least six distinct branching GlcNAc-Ts which substitute the trimannosyl core of N-linked oligosaccharides, a process that is completed in the median Golgi before further addition of galactose (Gal), sialic acid (SA) and fucose (Fuc) occurs in the trans Golgi[5]. The GlcNAc-Ts utilize UDP-GlcNAc as sugar donor and add GlcNAc to the trimannosyl core (bold) in the positions and linkages shown below.

GlcNAc-TVI    GlcNAcβ1-4

GlcNAc TV     GlcNAc$\underline{\beta 1\text{-}6}$

GlcNAc TII    GlcNAcβ1-2**Man**α1-6

GlcNAc-T-III               GlcNAcβ1-4**Man**β1-4GlcNAcβ1-4GlcNAcβ1-Asn

GlcNAc-TI     GlcNAcβ1-2**Man**α1-3

GlcNAc-TIV    GlcNAcβ1-4

GlcNAc-TIII has been shown to be elevated in rat and human hepatomas[6]. Structural analysis of oligosaccharides in choriocarcinoma[7], and in HepG2 hepatoma cells[8] suggests that GlcNAc-TIV and TIV may also be elevated in tumors of the liver. However, upregulation of β1-6 branched structures and GlcNAc-TV activity have been observed in wide variety of rodent tumors (reviewed in[2]). Although antibodies to GlcNAc-branched sequences in glycoproteins and glycolipids have been developed[9], none of these reagents react specifically to the -GlcNAc$\underline{\beta 1\text{-}6}$Manα1-6Manβ- portion of complex-type N-linked oligosaccharides. The plant lectin leukoagglutinin (L-PHA) is a more specific probe, and binds to a portion of the oligosaccharide which includes -GlcNAc$\underline{\beta 1\text{-}6}$Manα1-6Manβ- as shown in bold below[10].

**Galβ1-4GlcNAc$\underline{\beta 1\text{-}6}$**

**Galβ1-4GlcNAcβ1-2Manα1-6**

Manβ1-4GlcNAcβ1-4GlcNAcβ1-Asn

Galβ1-4GlcNAcβ1-2Manα1-3

Galβ1-4GlcNAcβ1-4

Further substitutions of α2-3 linked sialic acid or polylactosamine (i.e., repeats of Galβ1-4GlcNAcβ1-3) onto the terminal Gal of the structure shown above does not inhibit L-PHA binding, and these are common termini found on tetra-antennary oligosaccharides[10]. However, L-PHA binding to β1-6 branched oligosaccharides is reduced by substitution of the antenna with α2-6 linked sialic acid or α1-3 linked fucose[11].

**β1-6 Branching in human tumors.** Increased β1-6 branching of N-linked oligosaccharides has been detected in human carcinomas of breast, colon and in melanomas[2,12,13]. In a study of 60 breast cases, carcinomas and fibroadenomas which were designated atypical had significantly increased L-PHA staining compared to benign hyperplasia. Similar results were observed for colon carcinoma where Duke's stage C colon carcinomas showed significantly greater L-PHA reactivity than stage A tumors. These observations suggest that increased expression of L-PHA reactive oligosaccharides is associated with tumor progression in the breast and colon, and with metastatic disease in the colon. Using L-PHA histology, essentially all high grade malignancies of colon, breast and melanoma showed increased L-PHA reactivity compared to benign and normal tissues. L-PHA does not react with normal epithelium, brain, liver, or muscle, but does bind to vascular endothelial cells, some interstitial fibroblasts and monocytes.

Polylactosamine or type 2 chains (i.e., repeating Gal$\beta$1-4GlcNAc$\beta$1-3) are the backbone for substitution with fucose and sialic acid to produce Le$^x$, Le$^y$, sialyl Le$^x$ and polymeric forms of these antigens. The type 2 based Lewis sequences are neo-expressed or over-expressed in a majority of human carcinomas of the colon[14], bladder[15], breast[16], and lung[17]. Type 2-based Lewis antigens in colon cancer were found to be significantly elevated in glycoproteins, and their detection in the serum of colon carcinoma patients has been correlated with the severity of the disease (i.e., Duke's stage), and with recurrence[14]. Notably, the expression of extended chain Le$^x$, sialy Le$^x$ and Le$^y$ antigens appear to be more cancer specific than the short chain forms of these antigens which are also expressed in a high proportion of benign polyps[18-20]. The synthesis of type 2 chain requires $\beta$1-4Gal-T and $\beta$1-3GlcNAc-T(i), the latter appears to be rate limiting, and substitution of the chains by fucosyltransferases. However, $\beta$1-3GlcNAc-T(i) has been shown to preferentially substitute the Gal$\beta$1-4GlcNAc$\beta$1-2(Gal$\beta$1-4GlcNAc$\underline{\beta 1-6}$)Man portion of N-linked oligosaccharides in vitro[21]. This suggests that cooperative action of $\beta$1-3GlcNAc-T(i) and $\beta$1-6GlcNAcTV is an important consideration in the regulation of polylactosamine and extended-chain Lewis antigens expression. This appears to be the case for SP1 mammary carcinoma cells and H-ras transformed rat2 fibroblasts, where GlcNAc-T(i) activity is not limiting and up-regulation of GlcNAc-TV activity in the metastatic sublines is associated with increased type 2 chain content in N-linked oligosaccharides[4]. In parallel, type 2 chains associated with O-linked oligosaccharides also appeared to increase due to the O-linked-specific ß1-6 branching enzyme UDP-GlcNAc:Gal$\beta$1-3GalNAc$\alpha$-R (GlcNAc to GalNAc) $\beta$1-6GlcNAc-T (i.e., core 2 GlcNAc-T) activity. Like the N-linked enzyme GlcNAc-TV, core 2 GlcNAc-T appears to be a key regulatory step for extension of O-linked structures with polylactosamine and related extended-chain Lewis antigens[4].

**Murine mammary carcinoma.** The murine mammary carcinoma cell lines SP1[22] and MTI CI.5/7[23] become metastatic following transfection with activated H-ras and provide a model for the study of molecular events associated with tumor progression. SP1 cells express very little -GlcNAc$\underline{\beta 1-6}$Man$\alpha$1-6Manß- branched oligosaccharide but following transfection with activated H-ras, the tumor cells show enhanced GlcNAc-TV activity and -GlcNAc$\underline{\beta 1-6}$Man$\alpha$1-6Manß- branching of oligosaccharides as well as metastatic potential in mice[4,24].

Metastatic sublines have also been generated by treating SP1 cells *in vitro* with the calcium ionophore A23187, phorbol ester or both reagents, then injecting the cells into mice and isolating tumor cells from spontaneous lung metastases[25]. Cell lines derived from individual lung nodules were shown to be clonal in their origin, derived from different progenitor cells and the lines retained metastatic potential when re-injected subcutaneously into mice. Acquisition of the metastatic phenotype is accompanied by increased GlcNAc-TV activity and $\beta$1-6 branched oligosaccharides as indicated by L-PHA reactivity of membrane glycoproteins (figure 1).

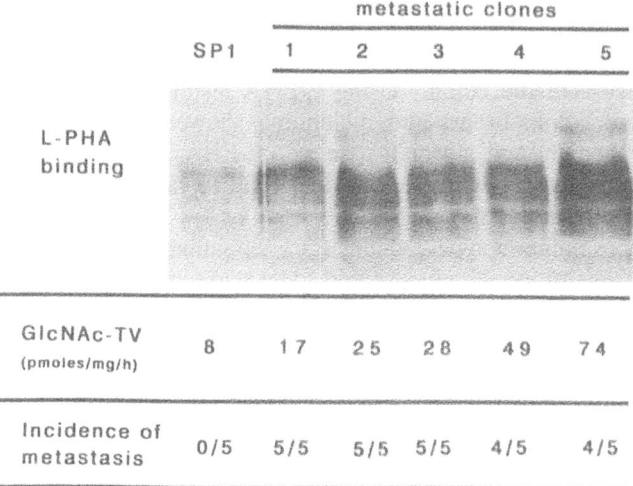

metastatic clones

|  | SP1 | 1 | 2 | 3 | 4 | 5 |
|---|---|---|---|---|---|---|
| L-PHA binding | | | | | | |
| GlcNAc-TV (pmoles/mg/h) | 8 | 17 | 25 | 28 | 49 | 74 |
| Incidence of metastasis | 0/5 | 5/5 | 5/5 | 5/5 | 4/5 | 4/5 |

**Figure 1** Comparison of L-PHA reactivity, GlcNAc-TV and incidence of metastasis in SP1 and metastatic sublines. The sublines 2-6 were generated by treating SP1 cells *in vitro* with the calcium ionophore A23187, phorbol ester or both reagents, then injecting the cells into mice and establishing tumor cell lines from spontaneous lung metastases as previously described[25]. 1), A1a; 2), A3a were from A23187-treated SP1 cells, 3), P1b from phorbol ester, 4), M1a; 5), M2a from treatment with both reagents. L-PHA reactivity of membrane glycoproteins in the 80-160 Kd size range is shown and was preformed as described[24]. Ratio in the bottom row is the number of mice with spontaneous lung metastasis per number of mice injected subcutaneously with $10^5$ tumor cells 28 days earlier. Tumor take at the subcutaneous site was 100%.

Cell surface glycosylation in SP1 cells is only one of many changes that occur with progression to the metastatic phenotype. Metastatic sublines of SP1 secreted more protease activity into the culture medium capable of degrading extracellular matrix. For example, steady state levels of transin mRNA were 15-20 fold greater than in SP1 cells, while tissue inhibitor of metalloproteinase (TIMP) mRNA was decreased 3-5 fold[26]. TIMP binds to, and inhibits metalloproteinases and has been shown to inhibit tumor cell invasion in vitro and metastasis in vivo[27,28]. A qualitatively similar shift in expression of these genes was rapidly induced in nonmetastatic SP1 cells following the addition of conditioned medium from metastatic cells[29]. The gene-regulating activity in the conditioned medium from metastatic cells was heat-labile suggesting that it was protein in nature. Furthermore, responsiveness to the factor(s) secreted by metastatic sublines was blocked by the protein synthesis inhibitor cycloheximide. The addition of basic fibroblast growth factor to cultures of SP1 cells mimicked the effect of the conditioned medium from metastatic cells as an inducer of transin expression in SP1 cells[29]. These observations suggest that enhanced production of autocrine growth factors by metastatic tumor cells can not only facilitate tumor cell proliferation, but also promote invasion by altering the expression of genes coding for proteases and their inhibitors.

**Inhibition of oligosaccharide processing blocks metastasis.** Transformation-related changes in glycosylation appear at different times during tumor progression[20], and include a variety of structures other than those mentioned above. Therefore, if specific oligosaccharide sequences contribute to malignant tumor growth, then experimental manipulation designed to inhibit their expression on metastatic tumor cells would be expected to reduce tumor growth and metastasis. Indeed, glycosylation mutants of highly metastatic tumor cell lines have been studied (reviewed in[2]). The effect of specific glycosylation mutations on tumor cell metastasis is quite striking[24,30-32], and suggests that loss of sialic acid, or $\beta$1-6 branching reduces metastatic potential with little or no effect on tumorigenicity (i.e., the ability to form a tumor at the site of tumor cell injection).

**Swainsonine.** Swainsonine is a plant alkaloid and potent inhibitor of Golgi $\alpha$-mannosidase II[33], a processing enzyme required to remove the mannose residues shown in bold below. As such, swainsonine blocks expression of the transformation-associated $\beta$1-6 branched N-linked oligosaccharides, diverting the pathway into "hybrid-type" structures as shown below.

**Man$\alpha$1-6**
    Man$\alpha$1-6
**Man$\alpha$1-3**        Man$\beta$1-4GlcNAcß1-4GlcNAc$\beta$1-AsnSA$\alpha$2-
3(6)Galß1-4GlcNAcß1-2Man$\alpha$1-3

Swainsonine-treated murine MDAY-D2 and B16F10 tumor cells are less metastatic in mice[34,35], and the anti-colonization effect of swainsonine is enhanced by administering the drug to mice in their drinking water at 2.5 ug/ml[34]. The growth rate of SP1T24Hras1 tumors in syngeneic mice was inhibited by constant infusion of swainsonine using Alzet mini osmotic pumps implanted subcutaneously into the mice (figure 2). Similarly, human MeWo melanoma and HT29m colon carcinoma tumor xenografts in athymic nude mice is reduced by treating the mice with swainsonine[36,37]. Swainsonine at 4 mg/kg/day administered to mice by miniosmotic pump reduced the growth rate of MeWo melanoma tumors by 50-60% and blocked expression of complex-type oligosaccharide in tumors and intestine of the mice by 85%[37]. Kino et al.[38] found that intraperitoneal injection of 100 mg/kg/day of swainsonine eliminated ascited tumor growth in mice. DeSantis et al.[39] have shown that T24H-ras-transfected NIH 3T3 cells lose their ability to grow in an anchorage-independent manner when cultured in the presence of swainsonine. The alkaloid blocked invasion by metastatic SP1 sublines into human amnion basement membranes while increasing tumor cell adhesion *in vitro*[40]. Similarly, swainsonine and deoxymannojirimycin have been shown to inhibit human melanoma cell invasion into reconstituted basement membranes, and this effect was readily reversed when the drugs were removed[41]. Swainsonine also inhibits invasion of amnion membranes by human trophoblasts, an invasive but non-transformed cell that expresses high levels of $\beta$1-6 branched oligosaccharides[42].

Loss or truncation of $\beta$1-6 branched oligosaccharides in metastatic tumor cells has pleiotropic effects on cellular phenotype, including increased adhesion to extracellular matrix (ECM) proteins[43], decreased adhesion to microvascular endothelial cells[44], reduced cell motility and invasion into ECM in vitro[40-42], and reduced cellular response to autocrine growth stimulation[37,45]. These observations suggest that simplification of the complex-type oligosaccharides in tumor cells may affect the malignant or differentiated phenotype, in a pleiotropic manner, possibly at the level of gene expression.

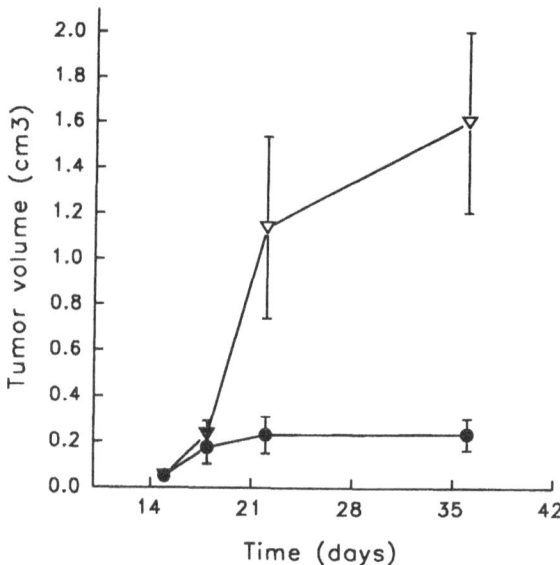

**Figure 2** Growth of SP1 tumors in syngeneic CBA/J mice treated with either saline,▽; or 4 mg/kg/day of swainsonine,○; by mini osmotic pump. Mice were injected subcutaneously with $10^5$ SP1T24Hras1 cells, a metastatic subline of SP1[24]. Alzet mini-osmotic pumps were installed subcutaneously on the opposite flank. The tumor volume was calculated from an average of minimum and maximum diameters measurements for groups of five mice as previously described[37].

In this regard, metastatic sublines of the SP1 mammary carcinoma cultured in the presence of swainsonine for 48 h showed approximately 3 fold enhancement of TIMP and c-jun mRNA levels while urokinase (uPA) transcripts remained unchanged (figure 3). Somatic mutations which blocked completion of $\beta$1-6 branched complex-type oligosaccharides in CHO cells, MDAY-D2 lymphoma cells and MeWo human melanoma cells were also associated with increased TIMP and c-jun gene transcription[46]. Nuclear-run-on assays showed that transcription of the TIMP gene was increased in cells where N-linked oligosaccharide processing was inhibited. In a study by Seftor et al.[41], swainsonine treatment of human melanoma cells also inhibited invasion in vitro and was associated with decreased type IV collagenase mRNA levels[41]. These observations suggest that transformation-associated changes in glycoprotein glycosylation in human, murine and hamster cell lines may affect the transcription of select genes, including TIMP and metalloproteinases which may influence the invasive phenotype. Furthermore, cell-specific patterns of glycoprotein glycosylation may be an integral element of cellular phenotype controlling expression of select genes.

Swainsonine also has positive effects on the immune system of the host (reviewed in[47]). In particular, the alkaloid has been shown to alleviate both chemically-induced and tumor-associated immune suppression, increase NK cell activity and increase IL-2 production by lymphocytes. These effects be may related to enhanced responsiveness of lymphoid cells to oligomannose-binding lymphokines such as IL-1, IL-2 and TNF[48]. Therefore, the therapeutic or anti-tumor effects of swainsonine in vivo may be a combination of host-dependent immune modulation and, at the tumor level, loss of N-linked oligosaccharides which facilitate tumor growth and metastasis.

These observations suggest that swainsonine or other inhibitors of N-linked oligosaccharide processing may be useful anti-cancer drugs, a premise which has begun to be tested in humans. We are currently conducting a phase I trial of swainsonine at the Toronto General Hospital.

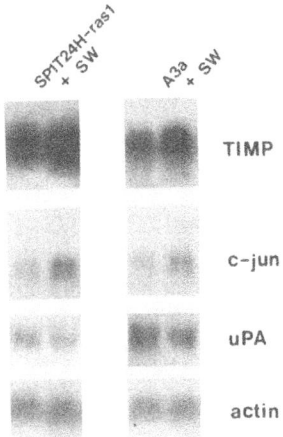

**Figure 3** Effects of swainsonine on TIMP, c-jun, uPA and actin mRNA levels in metastatic sublines of SP1 murine mammary carcinoma cell lines, SP1.T24Hras1 and A3a. Tumor cells were cultured in the absence or presence of 1 ug/ml of swainsonine for 48 h, and RNA was prepared and analyzed by Northern analysis.

## REFERENCES

1. L. Warren, C.A. Buck, and G.P. Tuszynski. Glycopeptide changes and malignant transformation: a possible role for carbohydrate in malignant behavior. *Biochim. Biophys. Acta* 516:97-127 (1978).
2. J.W. Dennis. Changes in glycosylation with malignant transformation and tumor progression. In: M. Fukuda (ed.), Cell Surface Carbohydrates and Cell Development, pp. 161-194, CRC Press. 1991.
3. K. Yamashita, Y. Tachibana, T. Ohkura, and A. Kobata, A. Enzymatic basis for the structural changes of asparagine-linked sugar chains of membrane glycoproteins of baby hamster kidney cells induced by polyoma transformation. *J. Biol. Chem.* 260:3963-3969 (1985).
4. S. Yousefi, E. Higgins, Z. Doaling, O. Hindsgaul, A. Pollex-Kruger, and J.W. Dennis. Increased UDP-GlcNAc:Gal $\beta$1-3GalNAc-R (GlcNAc to GalNAc) $\beta$1-6 N-acetylglucosaminyltransferase activity in transformed and metastatic murine tumor cell lines: control of polylactosamine-synthesis. *J. Biol. Chem.* 266:1772-1783 (1991).
5. H. Schachter. Biosynthetic controls that determine the branching and microheterogeneity of protein-bound oligosaccharides. *Biochem. Cell Biol.* 64:163-181 (1986).

6. S. Narasimhan, H. Schachter, and S. Rajalakshmi. Expression of N-acetylglucosaminyltransferase III in hepatic nodules during rat liver carcinogenesis promoted by orotic acid. *J. Cell Biol.* 263:1273-1281 (1988).

7. A. Kobata. Structural changes induced in the sugar chains of glycoproteins by malignant transformation of producing cells and their clinical application. *Biochimie* 70:1575-1585 (1988).

8. B. Campion, D. Leger, J.-M. Wieruszeski, J. Montreuil, and G. Spik. Presence of fucosylated triantennary, tetraantennary and pentaantennary glycans in transferrin synthesized by the human hepatocarcinoma cell line Hep G2. *Eur. J. Biochem.* 184:405-413 (1989).

9. B.A. Fenderson, E.J. Nichols, H. Clausen, and S.-I. Hakomori. A monoclonal antibody defining a binary N-acetyllactosaminyl structure in lactoisooctasylceramide (IV$^6$Gal$\beta$1 --> 4GlcNAcnLc$_6$): a useful probe for determining differential glycosylation patterns between normal and transformed human fibroblasts. *Mol. Immunol.* 23:747-754 (1986).

10. R.D. Cummings, and S. Kornfeld. Characterization of the structural determinants required for the high affinity interaction of asparagine-linked oligosaccharides with immobilized Phaseolus vulgaris leukoagglutinating and erthroagglutinating lectins. *J. Biol. Chem.* 257:11230-11234 (1982).

11. M. Bierhuizen, H. Edzes, W. Schiphorst, D. Van Den Eijinden, and W. Van Dij k. Effects of $\alpha$2-6 linked sialic acid and $\alpha$1-3 linked fucose on the interaction of N-linked glycopeptides and related oligosaccharides with immobilized phaseolus vulgaris leukoagglutinating lectin (L-PHA). *Glycoconjugate J.* 5:85-97 (1988).

12. J.W. Dennis, and S. Laferte. Oncodevelopmental expression of -GlcNAc $\beta$1-6M an $\alpha$1-6Man $\beta$1-6 branching of Asn-linked oligosaccharides in human breast carcinomas. *Cancer Res.* 49:945-950 (1989).

13. B. Fernandes, U. Sagman, M. Auger, M. Demetrio, and J.W. Dennis. $\beta$1-6 branched oligosaccharides as a marker of tumor progression in human breast and colon neoplasia. *Cancer Res.* 51:718-723 (1991).

14. A.K. Singhal, T.F. Orntoft, E. Nudelman, S. Nance, L. Schibig, M.R. Stroud, H. Clausen, and S. Hakomori. Profiles of Lewis$^x$-containing glycoproteins and glycolipids in sera of patients with adenocarcinoma. *Cancer Res.* 50:1375-1380 (1990).

15. C. Cordon-Cardo, V.E. Reuter, K.O. Lloyd, J. Sheinfeld, W.R. Fair, L.J. Old, and M.R. Melamed. Blood group-related antigens in human urothelium: enhanced expression of precursor, Le$^x$, and Le$^y$ determinants in urothelial carcinoma. *Cancer Res.* 48:4113-4120 (1988).

16. A. Brown, T. Feizi, H.C.Gool, M.J. Embleton, J.K. Picard, and R.W. Baldwin. A monoclonal antibody against human colonic adenoma recognizes difucosylate type-2-blood-group chains. *Bioscience Reports* 3:163-170 (1983).

17. K. Zenita, Y. Kirhata, A. Kitahara, K. Shigeta, K. Higuchi, K. Hirashima, T. Murachi, T., Takeda, and R. Kannagi. Fucosylated type-2 chain polylactosamine antigens in human lung cancer. *Int. J. Cancer* 41:344-349 (1988).

18. Y.S. Kim, M. Yuan, S.H. Itzkowitz, Q. Sun, T. Kaizu, A. Palekar, B.F. Trump, and S. Hakomori. Expression of Le$^Y$ and extended Le$^Y$ blood group-related antigens in human malignant, premalignant, and nonmalignant colonic tissues. *Cancer Res.* 46:5985-5992 (1986).

19. S.H. Itzkowitz, M. Yuan, Y. Fukushi, A. Palekar, P.C. Phelphs, A.M. Shamsuddin, B.F. Trump, S. Hakomori, and Y.S. Kim. Lewis[X] and sialylated Lewis[X]-related antigen expression in human malignant and non-malignant colonic tissue. *Cancer Res.* 46:2627-2632 (1986).
20. S.-I. Hakomori. Aberrant glycosylation in tumors and tumor-associated carbohydrate antigens. *Adv. Cancer Res.* 52:257-331 (1989).
21. D.H. van den Eijnden, A.H.L. Koenderman, and W.E.C.M. Schiphorst. Biosynthesis of blood group i-active polylactosaminoglycans. *J. Biol. Chem.* 263:12461-12465 (1988).
22. C. Waghorne, R.S. Kerbel, and M.L. Breitman. Metastatic potential of SP1 mouse mammary adenocarcinoma cells is differentially induced by activated and normal forms of c-H-ras. *Oncogene* 1:149-155 (1987).
23. K. H. Vousden, S.A. Eccles, H. Purvies, and C.J. Marshall. Enhanced spontaneous metastasis of mouse carcinoma cells transfected with an activated c-Ha-ras-1 gene. *Int. J. Cancer* 37:425-433 (1986).
24. J.W. Dennis, S. Laferte, C. Waghorne, M.L. Breitman, and R.S. Kerbel., $\beta$ 1-6 branching of Asn-linked oligosaccharides is directly associated with metastasis. *Science* 236:582-585 (1987).
25. B. Korczak, C. Whale, and R.S. Kerbel. Possible involvement of Ca2+ mobilization and protein kinase C activation in the induction of spontaneous metastasis by mouse mammary adenocarcinoma cells. *Cancer Res.* 49: 2597-2602 (1989).
26. B. Korczak, R.S. Kerbel, and J.W. Dennis. Constitutive expression and secretion of proteases in non-metastatic SP1 mammary carcinoma cells and its metastatic sublines. *Int. J. Cancer* 48:557-561 (1991).
27. P. Mignatti, E. Robbins, and D.B. Rifkin. Tumor invasion through the human amniotic membrane: requirement for a proteinase cascade. *Cell* 47:487-498 (1986).
28. R. Khokha, P. Waterhouse, S. Yagel, P.K. Lala, C.M. Overall, G. Norton, and D.T. Denhardt. Antisense RNA-induced reduction in murine TIMP levels confers oncogenicity on Swiss 3T3 cells. *Science* 243: 947-950 (1989).
29. B. Korczak, R.S. Kerbel, and J.W. Dennis. Autocrine and paracrine regulation of tissue inhibitor of metalloproteinases (TIMP), transin and urokinase gene expression in metastatic and nonmetastatic mammary carcinoma cells. *Cell Growth & Differentiation* 2:335-343 (1991).
30. J. Finne, M.M. Burger, and J.P. Prieels. Enzymatic basis for a lectin resistant phenotype: increase in a fucosyltransferase in mouse melanoma cells. *J. Cell Biol.* 92:277-282 (1982).
31. C.L. Reading, P.N. Belloni, and G.L. Nicolson. Selection of lectin attachment variants of malignant murine lymphosarcoma cell lines. *JNCI* 64:1241-1249 (1980).
32. J.W. Dennis. Different metastatic phenotypes in two genetic classes of WGA-resistant tumor cell mutants. *Cancer Res.* 46:4594-4600 (1986).
33. D.R. Tulsiani, T.M. Harris, and O. Touster. Swainsonine inhibits the biosynthesis of complex glycoproteins by inhibition of Golgi mannosidase II. *J. Biol. Chem.* 257:7936-7939 (1982).
34. J.W. Dennis. Effects of swainsonine and polyinosinic-polycytidylic acid on murine tumor cell growth and metastasis. *Cancer Res.* 46:5131-5136 (1986).

35. M.J. Humphries, K. Matsumoto, S.L. White, and K. Olden. Oligosaccharide modification by swainsonine treatment inhibits pulmonary colonization by B16-F10 murine melanoma cells. *Proc. Natl. Acad. Sci. USA* 83:1752-1756 (1986).

36. J.W. Dennis, K. Koch, and D. Beckner. Inhibition of human HT29 colon carcinoma growth in vitro and in vivo by swainsonine and human interferon-α2. *JNCI* 81:1028-1033 (1989).

37. J.W. Dennis, K. Koch, S.Yousefi, and I. VanderElst. Growth inhibition of human melanoma tumor xenografts in athymic nude mice by swainsonine. *Cancer Res.* 50:1867-1872 (1990).

38. T. Kino, N. Inamura, K. Nakahara, S. Kiyoto, T. Goto, H. Terano, M. Kohsaka, H. Oaki, and H. Imanaka. Effect of swainsonine on mouse immunodeficient system and experimental murine tumor. *Journal Antibiotics* 38:936-940 (1985).

39. R. DeSantis, U.V. Santer, and M.C. Glick. NIH 3T3 cells transfected with human tumor DNA lose the transformed phenotype when treated with swainsonine. *Biochem. Biophys. Res. Commun.* 142:348-353 (1987).

40. S. Yagel, R. Feinmesser, C. Waghorne, P.K. Lala, M.L. Breitman, and J.W. Dennis. Evidence that β 1-6 branched Asn-linked oligosaccharides on metastatic tumor cells facilitate invasion of basement membranes. *Int. J. Cancer* 44:685-690 (1989).

41. R.E.B. Seftor, E.A. Seftor, W.J. Grimes, L.A. Liotta, W.G. Stetler-Stevenson, D.R. Welch, and M.J.C. Hendrix. Human melanoma cell invasion is inhibited in vitro by swainsonine and deoxymannojirimycin with a concomitant decrease in collagenase IV expression. *Melanoma Research* 1: 43-54 (1991).

42. S. Yagel, R.S. Kerbel, T. Eldar-Gera, and J.W. Dennis. Basement membrane invasion by first trimester human trophoblast: requirement for branched complex-type Asn-linked oligosaccharides. *Clin. Exp. Metastasis* 8: 305-318 (1990).

43. J.W. Dennis, C. Waller, R. Timpl, and V. Schirrmacher. Sialic acid on metastatic tumor cells reduces cell attachment to fibronectin and collagen type IV. *Nature* 300:274-276 (1982).

44. I. Cornil, R.S. Kerbel, and J.W. Dennis. Tumor cell surface β1-4 linked galactose binds to lectin(s) on microvascular endothelial cells and contributes to organ colonization. *J. Cell Biol.* 111:773-782 (1990).

45. I. VanderElst, and J.W. Dennis. N-linked oligosaccharide processing and autocrine-stimulation of tumor cell proliferation. *Exp. Cell Res.* 192:612-613 (1991).

46. B. Korczak, and J.W. Dennis. Inhibition of N-linked oligosaccharide processing in tumor cells is associated with enhanced tissue inhibitor of metalloproteinases (TIMP) gene expression. *Int. J. Cancer* (in press: 1992).

47. M.J. Humphries, and K. Olden. Asparagine-linked oligosaccharides and tumor metastasis. *Pharm. & Therap.* 44:85-105 (1989).

48. A. Muchmore, J. Decker, A. Shaw, and P. Wingfield. Evidence that high mannose glycopeptides are able to functionally interact with recombinant tumor necrosis factor and recombinant interleukin 1. *Cancer Res.* 50: 6285-6290 (1990).

# SPECIFICITY OF THE IgG RESPONSE IN MICE AND HUMAN BREAST CANCER PATIENTS FOLLOWING IMMUNIZATION AGAINST SYNTHETIC SIALYL-Tn, AN EPITOPE WITH POSSIBLE FUNCTIONAL SIGNIFICANCE IN METASTASIS

B. Michael Longenecker[1,2,4], Mark Reddish[1], Rao Koganty[1], and Grant D. MacLean[3,4]

[1]Immunotherapeutics Division, Biomira Inc.
2011 - 94 Street, Edmonton, Alberta T6N 1H1
[2]Department of Immunology, University of Alberta
Edmonton, Alberta T6N 2H7
[3]Department of Medicine, University of Alberta
Edmonton, Alberta T6N 2R7
[4]Cross Cancer Institute, 11560 University Avenue
Edmonton, Alberta T6G 1Z2

## SUMMARY

Several investigators have shown that the expression of the sialyl-Tn (STn) epitope on cancer associated mucins is associated with a poor prognosis in several human cancers suggesting that STn may have functional significance in metastasis. We postulate that antibodies against the STn-epitope can inhibit metastasis. We generated a synthetic "mimic", NANA$\alpha$(2$\rightarrow$6)GalNAc$\alpha$-O-Crotyl (STn-crotyl), of the natural O-linked epitope on mucins, NANA$\alpha$(2$\rightarrow$6)GalNAc$\alpha$-O-Serine (STn-serine). STn-crotyl was conjugated to the carrier protein KLH through the crotyl linker arm and a "vaccine" containing STn-KLH plus Detox™ adjuvant was formulated. The immunogenicity of the vaccine was evaluated in BALB/c mice and in metastatic breast cancer patients. The specificity and titres of IgG antibodies were evaluated by ELISA on ovine submaxillary mucin (OSM) solid phases. OSM is a convenient source of repeating, natural O-linked STn-serine structures. Mice immunized three times with as little as 0.25 µg of STn-KLH produced a median IgG titre of over 1:5000 on solid phase OSM. Anti-OSM IgG monoclonal antibodies generated from these mice were completely inhibited in their binding to solid phase OSM equally well by STn-serine and STn-crotyl synthetic haptens but not by several other closely related synthetic haptens.

*Antigen and Antibody Molecular Engineering in Breast Cancer Diagnosis and Treatment*, Edited by R.L. Ceriani, Plenum Press, New York, 1994

105

Breast cancer patients immunized 2-8 times with 25 or 100 µg of the same vaccine produced median peak IgG titres 1:1280 measured on STn-HSA and 1:80 on OSM. Once again, hapten inhibition experiments with the human sera demonstrated the specificities of the IgG antibodies for STn-crotyl and STn-serine, but not against several other related synthetic haptens. We found little or no evidence that the artificial linker arm (crotyl linker) contributed significantly to either the titre or affinity of the antibodies generated in either mice or human breast cancer patients. This suggests that the antibodies recognized the cancer-associated disaccharide NANA$\alpha$(2$\rightarrow$6)GalNAc. Evidence of a clinical response was noted in several of the immunized breast cancer patients with other patients showing prolonged disease stability.

## INTRODUCTION

Our program developing Active Specific Immunotherapy (ASI) for cancers is focussed on the use of synthetic cancer associated antigens as immunogens attempting to generate immune responses against defined epitopes on cell surface mucin molecules which are integral membrane glycoproteins on carcinoma cells. The rationale for targeting mucin epitopes is that: (a) mucins mask or inhibit immune effector mechanisms directed against other cell surface antigens[1,2]; (b) cell surface mucins exist as flexible rods which protrude relatively great distances from the cell membrane surface and hence, are the first points of contact by immune effector cells and antibodies[3]; and (c) certain carbohydrate epitopes on cell surface mucins may have functional significance in the metastatic process[4] and are associated with a poor prognosis[5,6].

### Rationale of Multiepitopic Anti-Mucin Approach to ASI

The development of formulations for clinically effective ASI will probably have to reflect the antigenic heterogeneity of human cancers. For example, the cancer-associated epitope STn shows marked heterogeneity in its expression on some breast cancers[7]. In our preliminary studies[8], testing an STn ASI formulation in women with metastatic breast cancer , we have observed several "mixed responses" where at least one metastatic lesion has decreased in size while others have progressed. Such mixed responses could relate to the heterogeneous expression of STn, and could thus reflect the need for multiepitopic ASI formulations for control of metastatic cancers.

### Targeting Peptide Epitopes on Mucin Molecules

For the development of ASI, our group has focussed on antigenetic determinants found on cancer cell surface mucins. It is now well recognized that cell surface mucins may have important functions in cell communication and signal transduction[9,10]. MUC1 is the first mucin gene to be cloned and mapped[11]. It is expressed on the cell surface of breast cancer cells where it is under-glycosylated[12] and hence antigenically different from normal cell mucins exposing normally cryptic carbohydrate[13] and peptide[14] epitopes.

The core peptide encoded by the MUC1 gene contains a tandem repeat of the 20-amino acid sequence PDTRPAPGSTAPPAHGVTSA. The PDTRP region of the core peptide is of particular interest to immunologists because: (a) It is an immunodominant B-cell epitope in mice[14]. Many monoclonal antibodies (MAbs) generated following immunization of mice with the MUC1 mucin bind to, or near, this epitope. (b) Human CTL cell lines have been derived from human cancer patients which only lyse tumor cells which express cell surface MUC1 and this lysis is specifically blocked by MAbs against the PDTRP epitope, suggesting that PDTRP is also a T-cell epitope in humans[15]. (c) We have shown that PDTRP containing synthetic peptides function as DTH (T-cell) epitopes in mice, inducing DTH reactions against tumor cells expressing human MUC1[16]. (d) It has been shown that vaccinia virus constructs containing the human MUC1 gene can be used to protect mice against growth of murine tumors transfected with and expressing the human MUC1 cell surface mucin[17]. (e) We have shown that immunogenic synthetic peptides containing MUC1 PDTRP sequences can be used for effective ASI in mice bearing mouse mammary carcinoma cells transfected with and expressing the human MUC1 cell surface mucin[16]. It is noteworthy that MUC1 synthetic peptides which induce only DTH and not antibody appeared to induce better anti-tumor activity than peptides which induced both antibody plus DTH, suggesting the importance of cellular immunity in anti-MUC1 peptide ASI[16].

**Targeting Carbohydrate Epitopes on Mucin Molecules**

The Thomsen-Friedenreich (TF) antigen is a human pan-carcinoma carbohydrate determinant expressed on cancer-associated mucins having the structure $\beta Gal1 \rightarrow 3\alpha GalNAc$[18]. TA3-Ha is a murine mammary adenocarcinoma which expresses a mucin (epiglycanin) which also expresses multiple TF epitopes[1,2]. We have used the TA3-Ha animal model to demonstrate that synthetic TF conjugated to KLH plus Detox™ adjuvant can be used for effective ASI against TA3-Ha tumors provided that low dose cyclophosphamide is first given to inhibit T-suppressor cell functions[19]. Based on these encouraging results in the animal model, we conducted a Phase I clinical trial in ovarian cancer patients with widespread disease and showed that TF-KLH plus Detox™ (following a single low dose of cyclophosphamide prior to the first ASI treatment) was non-toxic and induced a specific humoral immune response directed against the TF epitope[20]. Encouraged by these results, we turned our attention toward the use of synthetic STn-KLH conjugates plus Detox™ adjuvant in metastatic breast cancer patients[8] to determine the specificity of the humoral immune response to this important epitope.

**Sialyl-Tn, A Carbohydrate Epitope on Mucin Molecules Is An Independent Predictor Of Poor Prognosis**

Itzkowitz and co-workers[5] were the first to suggest that the expression of the STn epitope on colon cancer is associated with a poorer prognosis than patients whose colon cancers were STn negative. Recently, a paper by Kobayashi and co-workers demonstrated that the presence of the STn epitope on circulating mucins was a strong and independent predictor of poor prognosis in ovarian cancer patients, independent of tumor grade, stage, or histologic subtype[6]. These workers found that STn serum negative ovarian cancer patients had a 5-year survival of approximately 85% vs. approximately 10% for STn positive patients. Such a strong association of STn with prognosis suggest that the STn epitope may have functional significance in the metastatic cascade[4,5].

## Both Humoral and Cell-Mediated Immunity May Be Important For Effective ASI

Evidence from many animal models suggests that cell-mediated immunity (CMI) is the most important immune response associated with tumor regression seen following biomodulation. Indeed, when considering peptide epitopes like PDTRP as targets for immunotherapy as mentioned above, the evidence supports the importance of CMI. It is reasonable to suggest that CMI directed against cell surface MUC1 peptide on carcinoma cells might be expected to attack already established metastases and reduce the size of or eliminate these lesions[16,17]. We have provided evidence that anti-MUC1 DTH reactions may lead to "bystander killing" of even antigen negative tumor cell variants[16].

However, antibodies induced against carbohydrate epitopes like STn may inhibit tumor cell invasion or metastasis[4,5,6], and may also possibly trigger antibody mediated cytotoxicity and inflammatory reactions. Of relevance, it has been shown that specific anti SLe[a] and SLe[x] antibodies can inhibit tumor cells binding to the E-Selectin on activated endothelial cells[21] whereby it would presumably block metastasis by blocking this key step. In this paper, we examine the generation and specificity of an IgG response to a synthetic STn vaccine in mice and human metastatic breast carcinoma patients.

## MATERIALS AND METHODS

### Antigens and Haptens

All haptens and immunoconjugates were provided by Biomira, Inc. (Edmonton, AB, Canada): $\alpha$DGalNAc-OR = Tn; $\beta$DGal(1$\rightarrow$3)$\alpha$DGalNAc-OR = TF$\alpha$; $\alpha$DNeuNAc(2$\rightarrow$6)$\alpha$DGalNAc-OR = sialyl-Tn; $\alpha$DNeuNAc(2$\rightarrow$6)$\beta$DGalNAc-OR = $\beta$sialyl-Tn. R is the crotyl linker arm that can be used for covalent attachment of the hapten to a protein carrier. Sialyl-Tn-Serine hapten was also synthesized = $\alpha$DNeuNAc(2$\rightarrow$6)$\alpha$DGalNAc-O-Serine.

### ASI Formulation Preparation For Human Use

Sialyl-Tn-KLH was provided as a sterile, pyrogen-free pharmaceutically acceptable formulation by Biomira, Inc. Detox™ (RIBI ImmunoChem Research, Inc., Hamilton, MT, U.S.A.) is a sterile, pyrogen-free preparation[22] and is formulated as a lyophilized oil droplet emulsion containing monophosphoryl lipid A and cell wall skeleton from <u>Mycobacterium phlei</u>. Immediately prior to injection, the STn-KLH was reconstituted with phosphate-buffered saline (PBS) and added to the lyophilized Detox™ to give a final volume of approximately 1.0 mL at a final concentration of STn-KLH of 25, 100 or 500 µg. The final mixture was administered as one-half volume (~0.5 mL) of each dose injected subcutaneously into each of two sites, alternating each treatment between upper arms (deltoid region) and anterolateral thighs.

## Mouse Immunizations

Mice were immmunized (10 per group) subcutaneously on days 0, 14 and 28 with STn-KLH emulsified in Ribi Adjuvant System (RAS). Doses ranged between 0.25 µg and 100 µg all delivered in a total volume of of 0.2 mL split into two injection sites. Immune sera were obtained on days 12, 26 and 40.

## ELISA for Anti-STn Antibodies

Microtitre 96-well plates were coated with ovine submaxillary mucin (OSM) or with hapten-HSA conjugates. Control wells were coated with HSA only. Coated plates were blocked with 0.8% gelatin. Serial dilutions of sera were incubated on the antigen-coated plates at room temperature for 1 hour, after which the wells were thoroughly washed. Alkaline phosphatase-labeled specific anti-mouse or anti-human IgG, or IgM, (Kirkegaard and Perry Laboratories, Inc., Gaithersburg, MD, U.S.A.) antibodies were added to appropriate wells and incubated at room temperature for 1 hour. Each plate was then thoroughly washed and $p$-nitrophenyl phosphate substrate was added to each well. After 30 min. at room temperature, 1 $\underline{M}$ HCl was added to each well to stop the enzyme reaction and the absorbance was read on an enzyme-linked immunosorbent assay (ELISA) reader. Positive control high-titre patient sera were used on each plate to ensure reproducibility of results among plates and assays. Background optical density (OD) readings on HSA-coated wells were subtracted from readings obtained on STn-HSA-coated wells. The results of the titration are reported as the reciprocal of the highest serum dilution at which the optical density was greater than 0.12[20].

## Hapten Inhibition of the Anti-STn ELISA

An appropriate dilution of immune serum calculated to give an OD of approximately 1.0 when tested with an ELISA with STn-HSA or OSM on the solid phase was mixed with the appropriate dilution of hapten in microtitre plates. All dilutions were made in PBS, pH 7.4. The hapten-serum mixtures were incubated overnight at 2-6°C and the next morning transferred to ELISA plates containing solid-phase STn-HSA or OSM. The covered ELISA plate was then incubated at room temperature for 1 hour and the ELISA was developed as described above. For other hapten inhibition studies, reactions were performed essentially the same except that a kinetic read method was performed using the Vmax plate reader (Molecular Devices). A total of 30 readings were taken and a rate kinetic determined by regression that is expressed as milli O.D./minute.

## Complement-Mediated Lysis

DU4475 cells[23] were labelled with $^{51}$Cr as previously described[20]. Fifty μL of diluted sera were mixed with 50 μL of $10^4$ of labelled DU4475 target cells. Plates were incubated at 4°C for 1 hour and then washed using 100 μL of PBS and 1% BSA. One hundred microlitres of 10% complement in PBS (Lo Tox H Rabbit Complement, Cedarlane Labs. Ltd., Hornby, ON, Canada) were added to all wells and incubated for 1 hour at 37°C. The reaction was stopped by adding 75 μL of cold PBS and the plates were centrifuged at 1,000 rpm for 10 min. A fraction of the supernatant was collected and counted in a gamma counter. Control wells containing target cells in PBS alone, complement alone, and TritonX-100 (total release) were included in each plate.

The percent specific $^{51}$Cr release was calculated as follows:

$$\frac{[\text{cpm (experimental)} - \text{cpm (spontaneous release in complement alone)}]}{[\text{cpm (maximum release)} - \text{cpm (spontaneous release in complement alone)}]} \times 100$$

## Clinical Trial Design

The first study of STn-KLH plus Detox™ involved 12 patients with previously histologically proven breast cancer with clinical or radiological evidence of metastatic disease. There were two doses of immunoconjugate tested, the first 100 μg, and the second 25 μg. Patients number 1 to 6 inclusive received 100 μg each treatment, and patients 7 to 12 have received 25 μg per treatment. All patients gave valid written informed consent and were aware of the Phase I nature of this program.

Three days prior to the first ASI, each patient was treated with a single intravenous bolus treatment of Cyclophosphamide (Cy), 300 mg/$m^2$, (with an antiemetic and 1000 mL of normal saline intravenously for hydration).

For each patient, the first four ASI treatments were scheduled at two weekly intervals. Eligibility for a further four ASI treatments depended upon subsequent evaluation, including acceptable toxicity, evidence of disease stability or even clinical response, and evidence of an immune response to the STn epitope. The four "booster" immunizations were to be given at four weekly intervals.

## RESULTS

### Anti-OSM IgG Response of CAF$_1$ Mice Following Immunization With STn-KLH Plus Detox™ Adjuvant

Three groups of ten mice each were immunized three times with 0.25 μg, 0.5 μg and 1.0 μg of STn-KLH, respectively. Serum samples were collected 12 days after each immunization and the IgG titre of each mouse was determined by ELISA on both ovine submaxillary mucin (OSM) and synthetic STn-crotyl-HSA conjugate solid phases. OSM was chosen because it is a convenient natural source of repeating sialyl-Tn determinants, which are O-linked on the mucin molecule[24].

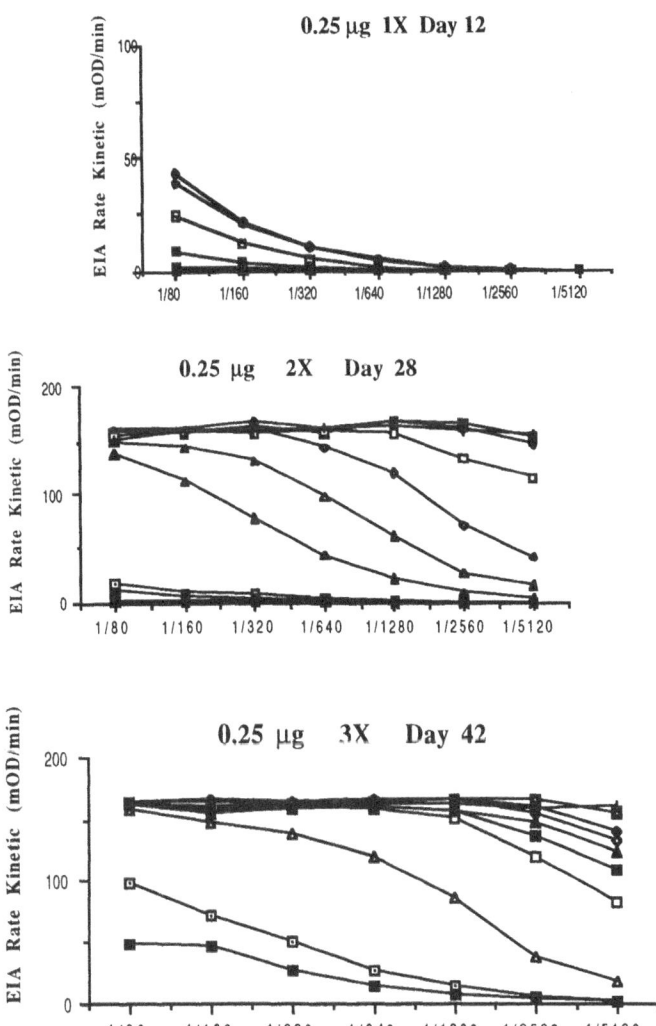

**Figure 1.** The effects of multiple boostings with low doses, 0.25μg, of STn-KLH is analyzed by a kinetic ELISA method specific for murine anti-OSM IgG.

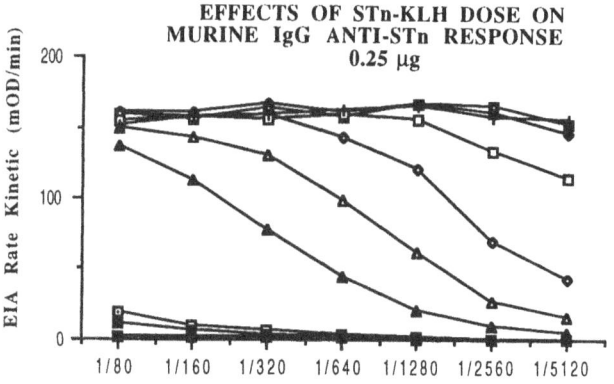

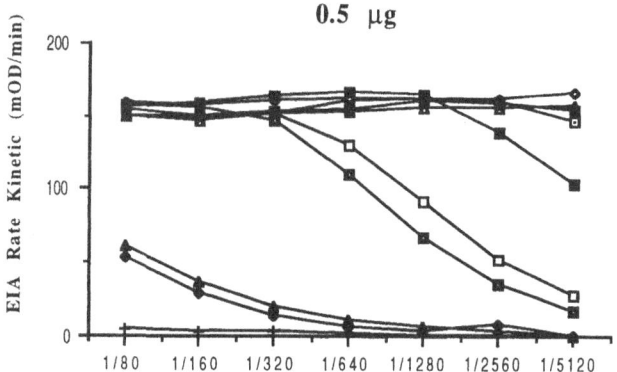

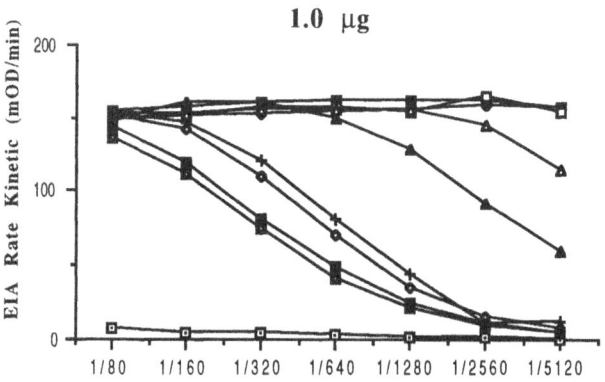

**Figure 2.** The effect STn-KLH dose on the murine IgG response is analyzed by kinetic ELISA. CAF1 mice (n=10) were immunized twice on days 0 and 14 and immune serum obtained on day 26. Doses of 0.25μg, 0.5 μg and 1.0 μg are shown. All doses in excess of 1 μg showed titres greater than 1/5120 in this analysis.

Preimmune sera showed no significant anti-OSM IgG binding. All mice in all three dosage groups developed significant IgG titres following the third immunization and most of the mice given even the lowest dose (0.25 µg) of STn-KLH developed anti-OSM titres in excess of 1:5000 (Figs. 1 and 2). Groups of mice immunized with 10, 20, 50 and 100 µg of STn-KLH produce comparable titres (data not shown).

## Specificity of Murine Anti-OSM IgG MAbs Induced Following Immunization With STn-KLH Plus Detox™

In order to ascertain the specificity on a clonal level, we generated anti-OSM IgG producing B-cell hybridomas from the spleen cells of mice immunized with STn-KLH plus Detox™. Several clones were analysed with virtually identical results. Hapten inhibition studies demonstrated that only synthetic STn, but not related synthetic structures like TF and Tn haptens inhibited specific anti-OSM MAb binding (data not shown). In further hapten inhibition studies, we compared three different forms of synthetic sialyl-Tn for hapten inhibition (see Fig. 3).

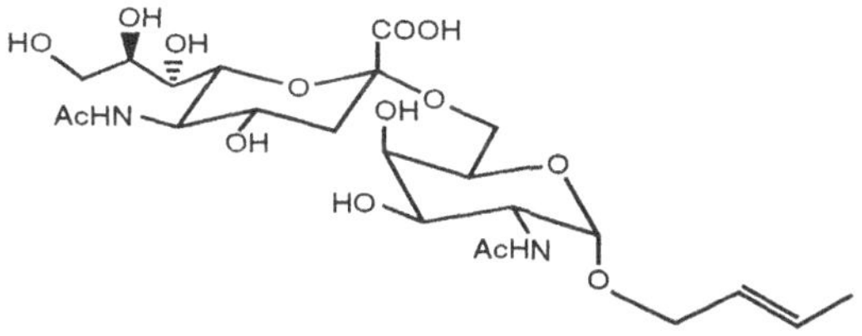

NANA α(2-6) GalNAc α-O-Crotyl
($ST_N$ - CROTYL)

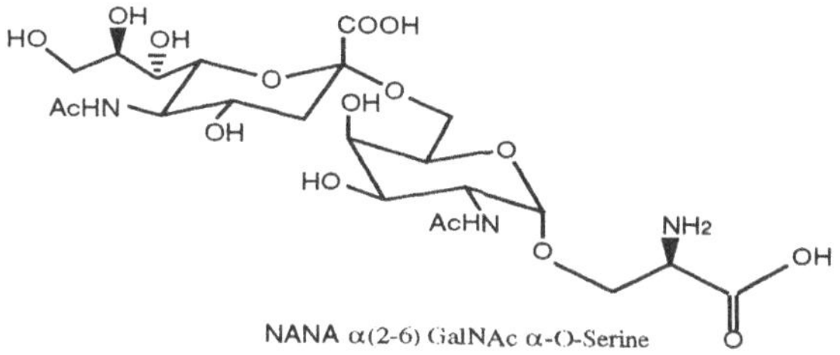

NANA α(2-6) GalNAc α-O-Serine
($ST_N$ - O - SERINE)

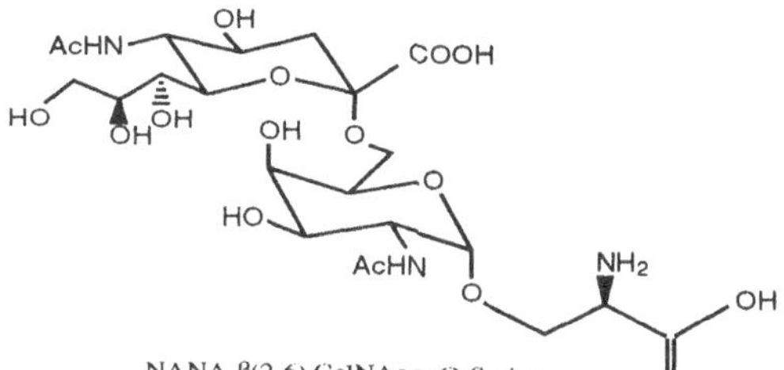

NANA β(2-6) GalNAc α-O-Serine
(β(2-6) $ST_N$ - O - SERINE)

Figure 3.

α2→6 STn-crotyl is the hapten that was used for conjugation to KLH by way of the crotyl linker arm to generate the STn-KLH immunogen used in all the studies reported in this paper. In Fig. 3, a comparison is made between the structures of α2→6 STn-crotyl; β2→6 STn-serine and α2→6 STn-serine. The STn-O-serine is the "natural" hapten as STn is naturally O-linked on mucins through serine (see Fig. 3).

The β2→6 STn-O-serine is the unnatural β anomer of sialyl-Tn. Fig. 4 demonstrates that both STn-crotyl and STn-O-serine (alpha) produce equivalent and complete inhibition of binding of one of the anti-OSM MAbs, which is representative of several other MAbs, but the unnatural β anomer of STn does not significantly inhibit the binding to OSM. These MAbs were also shown to bind to tumor cells bearing the STn epitope (data not shown). The binding on tumor cells is equivalent to results obtained with anti-STn MAbs B72.3 and TKH2. Hapten inhibition of polyclonal IgG antibodies from STn-KLH immunized mice show similar results (see Fig. 5).

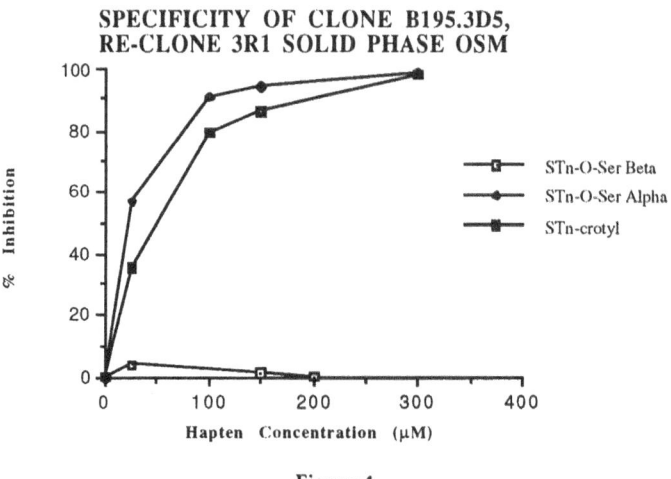

Figure 4.

## Immunization of Breast Cancer Patients Using STn-KLH Plus Detox™

The same lot (#10) of STn-KLH studied in the mouse experiments described above was used with Detox™ adjuvant to immunize metastatic breast cancer patients. Using STn-HSA in a solid phase ELISA, it was shown that all patients developed IgM and IgG specific for the synthetic STn hapten (data not shown). Following immunization, most patients were shown to develop increased titres of complement mediated cytotoxic antibodies, partially inhibited by synthetic STn hapten, but not by the related TF hapten (Table 1). We also detected IgG antibodies reactive with synthetic STn-HSA as well as natural STn determinants expressed on OSM – the STn specificity of this reactivity being confirmed by synthetic hapten inhibition (see Table 2 and Figs. 6 and 7).

**Table 1.** Hapten inhibition of complement mediated cytotoxicity.

| SERUM [1] FROM PATIENT # | PBS | INHIBITING HAPTEN (4 mM) | | | |
| | | STn | % INHIBITION | TF | % INHIBITION |
| --- | --- | --- | --- | --- | --- |
| 1 | $31 \pm 4$ [2] | $12 \pm 2$ [3] | 61% | $27 \pm 2$ [5] | 13% |
| 3 | $38 \pm 5$ | $28 \pm 5$ [4] | 26% | $38 \pm 2$ [5] | 0% |
| 6 | $29 \pm 2$ | $5 \pm 1$ [3] | 83% | $32 \pm 5$ [5] | 0% |
| 7 | $40 \pm 3$ | $28 \pm 3$ [3] | 30% | $38 \pm 2$ [5] | 5% |

[1]Serum taken after 3 or 4th immunization. Pre-immunization cytotoxicity was less than 10%
[2]Mean % $^{51}$Cr release $\pm$ S.D. using the DU4475 human breast cancer cell line.
[3]p<0.001 compared to PBS control.
[4]p<0.005 compared to PBS control.
[5]Not significantly different from PBS control.

**Table 2.** Hapten inhibition of anti-STn IgG from a breast cancer patient following immunization with STn-KLH plus Detox™ adjuvant tested on OSM solid phase.

| INHIBITING HAPTEN[1] | 4 WEEKS AFTER 6th IMMUNIZATION | 5 WEEKS AFTER 8th IMMUNIZATION |
| --- | --- | --- |
| TF-crotyl | 0 | 8 |
| Tn-crotyl | 17 | 0 |
| ßSTn-serine | 19 | 20 |
| STn-serine | 88 [3] | 91 |
| STn-crotyl | 90 | 91 |

[1]Tested at 0.25 mM hapten.
[2]Serum sample tested at a 1:5 dilution: IgG anti-OSM titre of the sample was 1:80.
[3]% Inhibition of binding in an ELISA.

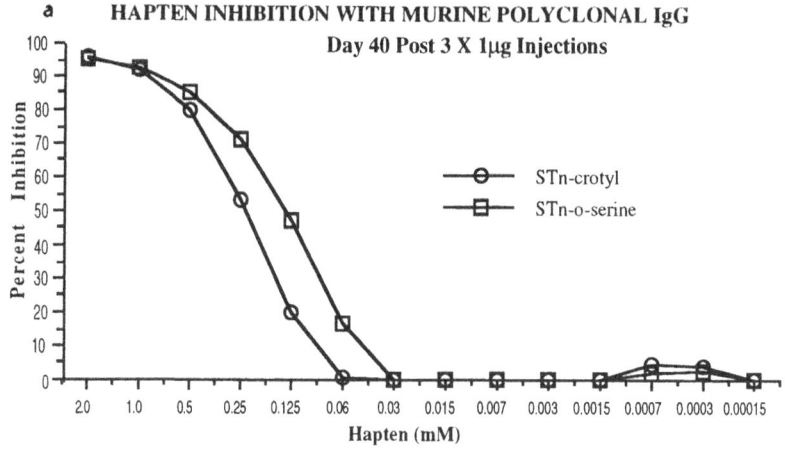

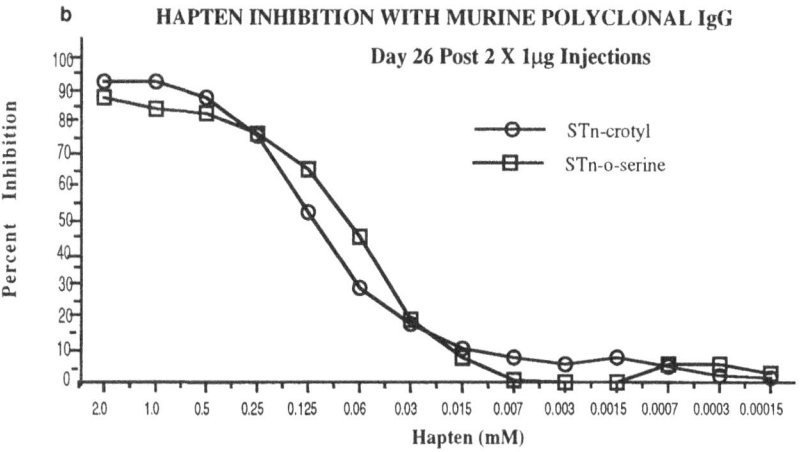

**Figure 5.** The hapten specificity of the murine polyclonal IgG response to STn-KLH is examined by inhibition of binding to an STn-HSA solid phase. In Fig. 5a, the post 3 injections (1µg dose) IgG response is tested with both STn-crotyl and STn-O-serine haptens. In Fig. 5b, the post 2 injections IgG response is tested similarly.

In all patients, IgG antibodies to STn-HSA developed more rapidly and reached higher titres than those to OSM (data not shown). Nevertheless, significant IgG binding to OSM developed in all patients with maximum titres ranging from 1:10 – 1:640 with a median titre of 1:80. The specificities of the anti-OSM antibodies were determined by hapten inhibition of their binding to OSM. Table 2 illustrates inhibition of serum IgG binding to OSM by 0.25 mM of Tn, TF or the three forms of the STn hapten shown in Fig. 3. Once again, the specificity of the sera was directed primarily to STn-O-serine and STn-crotyl.

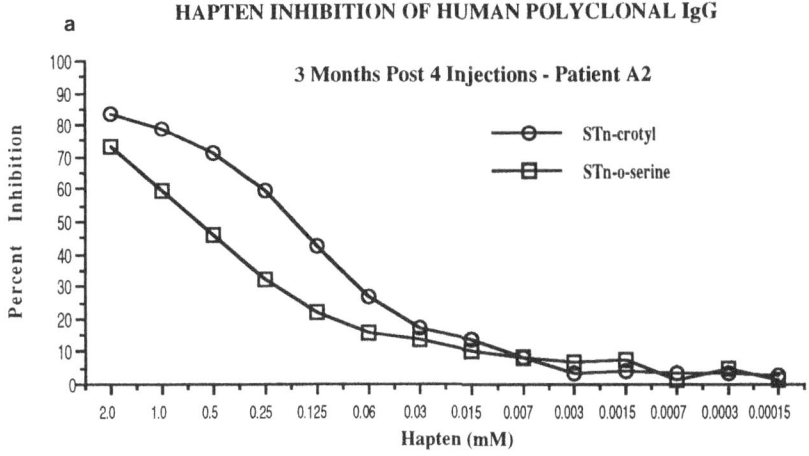

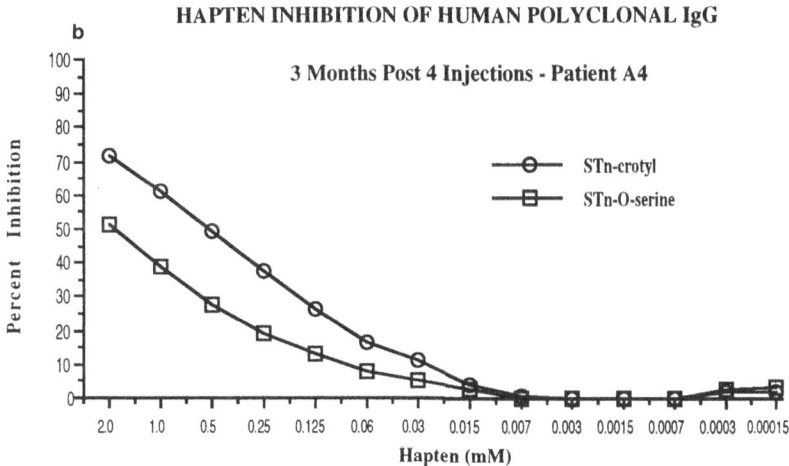

**Figure 6.** The hapten specificity of human IgG anti-STn antibody is analyzed by inhibition of binding to an STn-HSA solid phase using STn-crotyl and STn-O-serine haptens. In Fig. 6a, the 3 months post 4 injection serum from patient A2 is tested. In Fig. 6b, the 3 months post 4 injection serum from patient A4 is tested.

Fig. 6 shows the hapten inhibition of binding of the human IgG antibodies to an STn-HSA solid phase and Fig. 7 shows hapten inhibition of binding of the same serum samples to an OSM solid phase. In contrast to serum samples taken during the first course of four immunizations, several samples taken after monthly boosters were inhibited in their OSM binding by much lower concentrations of STn hapten, approximately 50% inhibition by 2 mM STn hapten (see Fig. 7) versus approximately 50% inhibition by 500 µM of STn hapten in serum samples taken after the first course (data not shown), suggesting a higher affinity of binding for the later serum samples. In addition, much lower hapten concentrations are required to inhibit the binding of the human IgG antibodies to OSM than to STn-HSA (compare Figs. 6 and 7). The fact that STn-serine hapten inhibits as well or better than STn-crotyl hapten indicates that the crotyl linker arm does not contribute significantly to the affinity of the antibody response. The specificity of the IgG antibodies for the STn determinant was further confirmed by the observation that neuraminidase treatment of OSM and STn-HSA eliminated the binding of the antibodies (data not shown).

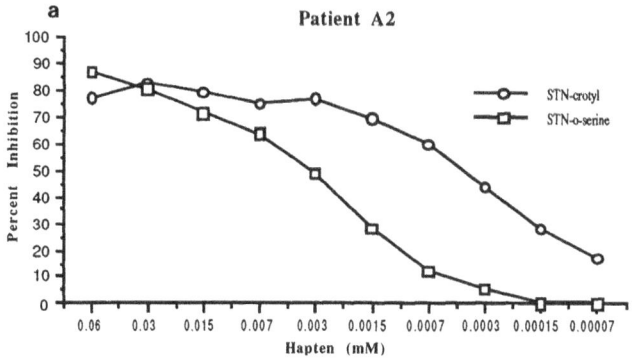

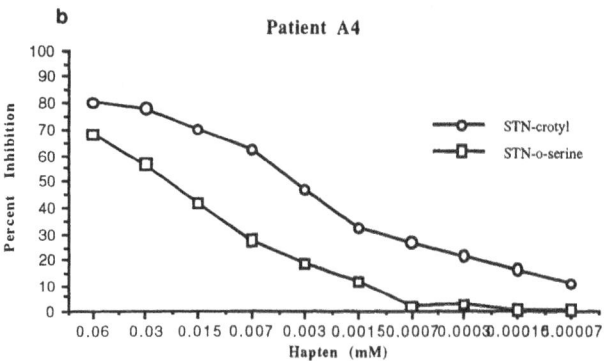

**Figure 7.** The hapten specificity of human IgG anti-STn antibody is analysed by inhibition of binding to an ovine submaxillary mucin coated solid phase using STn-crotyl and STn-O-serine haptens. In Fig. 7a, the 3 months post 4 injections serum from patient A2 is tested. In Fig. 7b, the 3 months post injections serum from patient A4 is tested.

Evaluation of clinical efficacy in a small pilot study is difficult. Five patients are alive twelve or more months after entry, and another four patients are alive six or more months after entry into the study. All three patients with known widespread bulky disease progressed despite ASI, two having died from widespread cancer. Two patients had partial responses, each lasting six months. While several patients had disease stability for three to 13.5 months, one patient with pulmonary metastases remains stable fifteen months after entry into the program (see Table 3).

## DISCUSSION

The use of synthetic antigens as immunogens for active specific immunotherapy (ASI) always raises the question of the relevance of the synthetic antigen as a proper mimic of the natural epitope. In the case of the sialyl-Tn epitope, both the natural and synthetic disaccharide, $NANA\alpha(2\rightarrow6)GalNAc\alpha$-O are exactly the same based on $^{13}C$ and $^{1}H$ NMR spectral studies of both natural disaccharide cleaved from OSM[25,26], the disaccharide serine structures synthesized by Ogawa[27] and by us, and our disaccharide with the crotyl linker arm. In addition, both well characterized anti-STn MAbs B72.3[28] and TKH2[29] react specifically with our synthetic STn-crotyl epitope. Furthermore, the anti-STn MAb described here binds to tumor cells in an equivalent manner to these well characterized anti-STn MAbs (unpublished data).

**Table 3.** Summary of clinical outcome in breast cancer patients immunized with STn-KLH plus Detox™ adjuvant.

| RESPONSE STATUS | # PATIENTS | TIME TO PROGRESSION (months) |
|---|---|---|
| Partial Response | 2 | 6, 7 |
| Stable | 5 [1] | 4.5, 7, 10.5 |
| Mixed Response | 2 | 2, 4 |
| Progressive Disease | 3 [2] | PD |

[1]Two patients still stable at 13.5 and 15 months.
[2]These patients entered the study with bulky disease.

We have employed a two carbon crotyl linker arm in our synthetic hapten STn-crotyl for conjugation to KLH to generate our STn-KLH ASI vaccine. Fig. 8a shows the structure of the STn-crotyl-KLH immunogen illustrating the conjugation to epsilon amino groups on lysines on the KLH. In contrast, Fig. 8b shows the natural O-linked STn structure as part of a hypothetical mucin core structure. The crotyl linker is slightly different from the natural "linker" which attaches the disaccharide to mucins through an O-linked serine (see Figures 3 and 8). In the present study, we have attempted to analyse whether the specificities of the IgG antibodies generated using the STn-crotyl structure recognized the "unnatural" crotyl linker arm versus the "natural" O-linked serine on mucins. The antibody specificity analysis presented here indicates that the crotyl linker arm does not contribute significantly to the antibody specificities and affinities despite the structural differences between the two glycoconjugates.

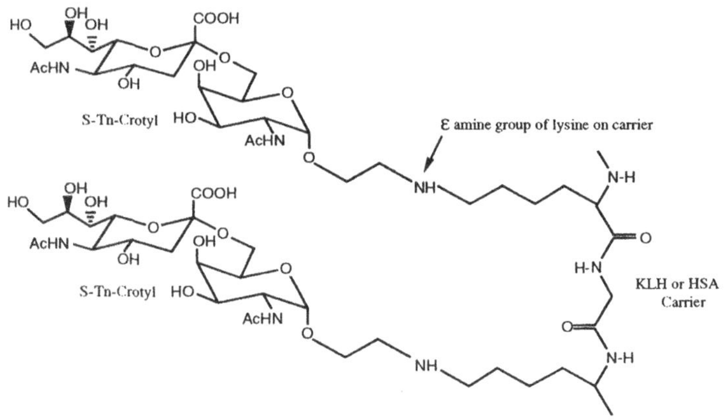

**Figure 8a.** The crotyl linker provides a two carbon spacer between the epsilon-amino group of lysine on KLH and the STn-disaccharide. The two carbon crotyl spacer is exactly the same length as the "natural" serine spacer.

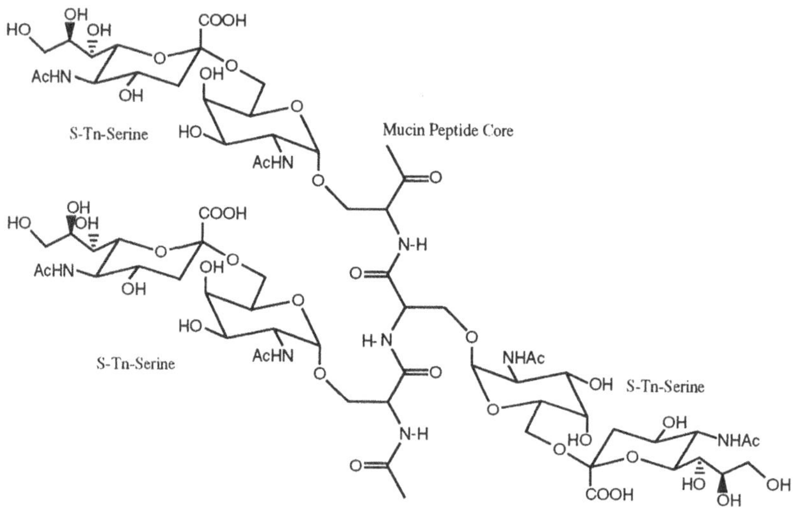

**Figure 8b.** A "cluster" of three sialyl-Tn disaccharides O-linked on serine molecules which are part of a hypothetical peptide core of a mucin molecule.

Nevertheless, we examined whether there were significant differences in antibody elicited following immunization with STn-crotyl-KLH in its binding to the two structures, STn-crotyl and STn-serine. In the mouse studies, high titres (>1:5000) of IgG binding to the natural O-linked STn determinants on OSM were generated following the third immunization with even the lowest dose of STn-KLH vaccine employed (0.25 µg per injection). Only slightly higher IgG titres were noted when tested on STn-crotyl-HSA. IgG monoclonal antibodies generated from these mice showed excellent binding to OSM as well as to tumor cells expressing STn. Both STn crotyl and STn-serine haptens produced equivalent complete inhibitions of binding of these MAbs to OSM, demonstrating the specificity of the MAbs against the disaccharide sugars of STn but not the crotyl or serine "linker arms". Furthermore, the mouse IgG polyclonal antibodies generated using the STn-crotyl-KLH immunogen which bind to STn-crotyl-HSA were also equally inhibited by STn-crotyl and STn-serine haptens. Thus, the evidence strongly suggests that the murine IgG response to STn-crotyl-KLH does not involve significant recognition of the crotyl linker arm and results in the generation of high titres of IgG antibodies recognizing the natural STn determinant on mucin molecules.

In breast cancer patients immunized with the STn-KLH vaccine, the anti-STn titres generated were lower than in the mice immunized with the same vaccine. For example, the median IgG titre tested on an STn-HSA solid phase was 1:1280 and 1:80 on an OSM solid phase. The higher titres in the mice could reflect an altered state of immune regulation due to the use of inbred mice or the lower titres in the patients could also be due to an altered state of immune regulation due to the presence of breast cancer, or it could reflect the *in vivo* absorption of the antibodies by STn structures on the tumor mass or secreted mucin molecules. This is being investigated. Once again, however, little or no contribution of the crotyl linker arm was noted (see Table 2 and Fig. 6).

Nevertheless, it may be important that STn epitope specific antibodies can be induced by ASI in patients with breast cancer. While STn specific cell mediated immunity may be important for tumor cell lysis, it is possible that anti-STn IgG antibodies could have an important functional role in inhibiting metastasis and achieving disease stability.

From our small pilot studies to date, it could be misleading or erroneous to reach conclusions about any clinical efficacy of the STn-KLH plus Detox™ formulation for ASI of breast cancers. However, the two partial responses and the apparent prolonged disease stability in some of the other patients are encouraging. The two mixed responses challenge us to continue to develop multiepitopic formulations to induce polyvalent responses against heterogeneous cancers.

One point that is still not clear is whether cyclophosphamide pretreatment enhances the immune response to our ASI formulation in humans. The previous results from our murine studies suggested that cyclophosphamide was important to inhibit or abrogate the T-suppressor activity believed induced by the cancer secreted mucins[2]. Current studies are investigating different strategies of utilizing cyclophosphamide, as well as comparisons with and without cyclophosphamide. There may also be better methods to modulate the T-suppressor cell activity induced by cancer-associated mucins.

Using synthetic mimics of cancer mucin epitopes in ASI both in mice and in humans with cancers to study the specific IgG responses may lead to a clearer understanding of the role of mucins in the biomodulation of cancers. It is our intention to develop multiepitopic formulations targeting carbohydrate, peptide and glycopeptide mucin epitopes which we believe could be clinically effective for the control of common antigenically heterogeneous human cancers.

# REFERENCES

1.  J.F. Codington, D.M. Frim. Cell-surface macromolecular and morphological changes related to allotransplantability in the TA3 tumor. In: Manson LA (ed) Biomembranes, Vol. 2, Plenum, New York, p. 207.

2.  P.S. Fung, B.M. Longenecker. Specific immunosuppressive activity of epiglycanin, a mucin-like glycoprotein secreted by a murine mammary adenocarcinoma (TA3-Ha). *Cancer Res*, 50: 4308 (1990).

3.  N. Jentoff. Why are proteins O-glycosylated? *Trends Biochem Sci*, 15: 291 (1990).

4.  H. Ogawa, M. Inoue, O. Tanizawa, M. Miyamoto and M. Sakurai. Altered expression of sialyl-Tn, Lewis antigens and carcinoembryonic antigen between primary and metastatic lesions of uterine cervical cancers. *Histochemistry*, 97: 311 (1992).

5.  S.H. Itzkowitz, E.J. Bloom, W.A. Kokal, G. Modin, S.-I. Hakomori, and Y.S. Kim. Sialosyl-Tn: a novel mucin antigen associated with prognosis in colorectal cancer patients. *Cancer*, 66: 1960 (1990).

6.  H. Kobayashi, Terao, Toshihiko and Y.Kawashima. Serum sialyl Tn as an independent predictor of poor prognosis in patients with epithelial ovarian cancer. *Journal of Clinical Oncology*, 10(1): 95 (1992).

7.  A. Thor, N. Ohuchi, C.A. Szpak, W.W. Johnston, and J. Schlom. Distribution of oncofetal antigen tumor-associated glycoprotein-72 defined by monoclonal antibody B72.3. *Cancer Research*, 46: 3118 (1986).

8.  G.D. MacLean, M. Reddish, R.R. Koganty, T. Wong, S. Gandhi, M. Smolenski, J. Samuel, J.M. Nabholtz and B.M. Longenecker. Immunization of breast cancer patients using a synthetic sialyl-Tn glycoconjugate plus Detox™ adjuvant. *Cancer Immunol Immunother*, 36: 215 (1993).

9.  G. Parry, J.C. Beck, L. Moss, J. Bartley, G.K. Ojakian. Determination of apical membrane polarity in mammary epithelial cell cultures. The role of cell-cell, cell-substrate and membrane-cytoskeletal interaction. *Exp Cell Res*, 188: 302 (1990).

10. N. Peat, S.J. Gendler, E.-N. Lalani, T. Duhig, J. Taylor-Papadimitriou. Tissue specific expression of a human polymorphic epithelial mucin (MUC1) in transgenic mice. *Cancer Res.*, 52: 1954 (1992).

11. S.J. Gendler, C.A. Lancaster, J. Taylor-Papadimitriou, T. Duhig, N. Peat, J. Burchell, L. Pemberton, E.-N. Lalani, and D. Wilson. Molecular cloning and expression of the human tumor-associated polymorphic epithelial mucin, PEM. *J. Biol Chem*, 265: 15286 (1990).

12. S.R. Hull, A. Bright, K.L. Carraway, M. Abe, D.F. Hayes, D. Kufe. Oligosaccharide differences in the DF3 sialomucin antigen from normal human milk and the BT-20 human breast carcinoma cell line. *Cancer Commun*,1: 261 (1989).

13. F. Torben, N.H. Orntoft, N.C. Langkilde. O-linked mucin-type glycoproteins in normal and malignant colon mucosa: lack of T-antigen expression and accumulation of Tn and sialosyl-Tn antigens in carcinomas. *Int J Cancer*, 45: 666 (1990).

14. J. Burchell, S. Gendler, J. Taylor-Papadimitriou, A. Girling, A. Lewis, R. Millis, D. Lamport. Development and characterization of breast cancer reactive monoclonal antibodies directed to the core protein of the human milk mucin. *Cancer Res*, 47: 5476 (1987).

15. D.L. Barnd, M.S. Lan, R.S. Metzgar, O.J. Finn. Specific, major histocompatibility complex-unrestricted recognition of tumor-associated mucins by human cytotoxic T cells. *Proc Natl Acad Sci USA*, 86: 7159 (1989).

16. L. Ding, E.-N. Lalani, M. Reddish, R. Koganty, T. Wong, J. Samuel, M.B. Yacyshyn, A. Meikle, P.Y.S. Fung, J. Taylor-Papadimitriou, and B.M. Longenecker. Immunogenicity of synthetic peptides related to the core peptide sequence encoded by the human MUC1 mucin gene: effect of immunization on the growth of murine mammary adenocarcinoma cells transfected with the human MUC1 gene. *Cancer Immunol Immunother*, 36: 9 (1992).

17. M. Hareuveni, C. Gautier, M.-P. Kieny, D. Wreschner, P. Chambon, R. Lathe. Vaccination against tumor cells expressing breast cancer epithelial tumor antigen. *Proc Natl Acad Sci USA*, 87: 9498 (1990).

18. G.F. Springer. T and Tn, general carcinoma autoantigens. *Science*, 224: 1198 (1984).

19. P.Y.S. Fung, R. Koganty, B.M. Longenecker. Active specific immunotherapy of a murine mammary adenocarcinoma using a synthetic tumor-associated glycoconjugate. *Cancer Res*, 50: 4308 (1990).

20. G.D. MacLean, M. B. Bowen-Yacyshyn, J. Samuel, A. Meikle, G. Stuart, J. Nation, S. Poppema, M. Jerry, R. Koganty, T. Wong and B.M. Longenecker. Active immunization of human ovarian cancer patients against a common carcinoma (Thomsen-Friedenreich) determinant using a synthetic carbohydrate antigen. *Journal of Immunotherapy*, 11: 292 (1992).

21. J.L. Magnani. The tumor markers, Sialyl Le[a] and Sialyl Le[x] bind ELAM-1. *Glycobiology*, 1: 318 (1991).

22. M.S. Mitchell, J. Kan-Mitchell, R.A. Kempf, W. Harle, H. Shau and S. Lind. Active specific immunotherapy for melanoma: phase I trial of allogeneic lysates and a novel adjuvant. *Cancer Res*, 48: 5883 (1988).

23. A.J. Langlois, W.D. Holder Jr., J.D. Iglehart, W.A. Nelson-Rees, S.A. Wells Jr. and D.P. Bolognesi. Morphological and biochemical properties of a new human breast cell line. *Cancer Res*, 39: 2604 (1979).

24. D.H. Hill, M. Schwyzer, H.M. Steinman, and R.L. Hill. Ovine submaxillary mucin. Primary structure and peptide substatus of UDP-N-Acetylgalactosamine: mucin transferase. *J. Biol. Chem*, 252: 3799 (1977).

25. T.A. Gerken. The solution structure of mucin glycoproteins: proton NMR studies of native and modified submaxillary mucin. *Arch. Biochem. Biophys*, 247: 239 (1986).

26. T. Tsuji and T. Osawa. Carbohydrate structures of bovine submaxillary mucin. *Carbohydrate Research*, 151: 391 (1986).

27. H. Iijima and T. Ogawa. Total synthesis of 3-0-[-2-Acetamide-6-0-(N-Acetyl-a-D Neuraminyl-2-deoxy-a-D-galactopyronosyl]-L-serine and a stereo isomer. *Carbohydrate Research*, 172: 183 (1988).

28. F.G. Hanisch, G. Uhlenbruek, H. Egge and J. Peter-Katalinic. A B72.3 second-generation monoclonal antibody (CC49) defines the mucin-carried carbohydrate epitope Galß(1Æ3)[NeuAca(2Æ6)] GalNAc. *J. Biol. Chem*, 370: 21 (1989).

29. T. Kjeldsen, H. Clausen, S. Hirohashi, T. Ogawa, H. Iijima and S. Hakomori. Preparation and characterization of monoclonal antibodies directed to the tumor-associated O-linked sialosyl 2-6-a-N-acetylgalactosaminyl (sialosyl Tn) epitope. *Cancer Res*, 48: 2214 (1988).

# VACCINATION AGAINST BREAST CANCER - STUDIES IN AN ANIMAL MODEL

Nechama I. Smorodinsky[1], Ronit Yarden[1], Lior Carmon[1],
Mara Hareuveni[2], Daniel H. Wreschner[1] and Iafa Keydar[1]

[1]Department of Cell Research and Immunology
George S. Wise Faculty of Life Sciences
Tel Aviv University, Tel Aviv 69978
and [2]Sourasky Medical Center
Tel Aviv, Israel

## INTRODUCTION

One of the main mortality causes around the world are malignant diseases. In spite of the development of new cytotoxic drugs and new therapeutic protocols the death rate is still high due to failure of the response to treatment in metastatic cases[1]. Numerous factors set one tumor apart from another. Tumor specific markers are invaluable for diagnostic, prognostic and therapeutic purposes and enable the clinician to decide on treatment regimes.

New approaches for the prevention and treatment of metastatic spread should be designed. The approach that we would like to suggest is immunotherapy, namely to encourage the potential of the patient's immune system to fight the disease. Tumor cells differ from normal cells in their antigenic repertoire. The tumor associated antigens might elicit immunological responses in the patient that would eliminate tumor cells. Attempts were made in the past few decades to identify, characterize and isolate possible candidates for tumor associated antigens (TAAs). It was found that cellular tumor-associated antigens are often differentiation antigens, that are expressed at trace levels in normal cells and overexpressed in tumor cells[2,3]. These antigens have considerable promise as targets for active or passive immunotherapy.

An antigen of epithelial origin that is aberrantly expressed in breast tumor tissue, has been identified in our lab with a monoclonal antibody (MoAb) H23, raised against particulate antigens released by T47D cells, a human breast cancer cell line[4]. MoAb H23 detects an epithelial tumor antigen.

This epithelial tumor antigen is the product of the recently named MUC1 locus, and although a normal epithelial cell protein, it is expressed at exceptionally high levels in human breast cancer tissue. Furthermore, sera of metastatic breast cancer patients contain elevated amounts of MUC1-H23 Ag[5]. This feature may be used as a prognostic factor in evaluating the status of breast cancer patients. In addition to its detection in body fluids, MUC1-H23 Ag can be detected by immunohistochemical staining of malignant breast tissue. Its cellular localization has been variously referred to as apical, membranous, intracytoplasmic or focal. It therefore appears that

*Antigen and Antibody Molecular Engineering in Breast Cancer Diagnosis and Treatment*, Edited by R.L. Ceriani, Plenum Press, New York, 1994

125

besides qualitative changes in the level of antigen expression in malignant tissue, varying protein forms that localize to different cellular and extracellular compartments probably exist. Viable intact breast tumor cells can be immunofluorescently stained with H23 MoAb indicating that one of the MUC1-H23 Ag forms is a membrane associated protein[6].

As MUC1-H23 Ag is markedly overexpressed in breast tumor tissue and has documented clinical significance in monitoring breast cancer patients, the relevance of MUC1-H23 to the malignant phenotype is of prime importance.

Initial protein studies indicated that the antigen is polymorphic, of high molecular weight and extensively post-translationally modified by the addition of complex sugar residues[7-9]. Molecular studies revealed that the MUC1-H23 Ag protein is unique in that it contains an array of between 20 and 80 highly conserved tandem repeating 20 amino acid units (coded for by tandem repeating 60 base pair units), that constitute greater than 50% of the total protein. Amino acid sequences of differenct MUC1-H23 Ag forms were deduced from the nucleotide sequence of isolated non repeat cDNAs. The diversity of protein forms is generated by a series of alternative splicing events.

One form lacking the transmembrane domain is likely to be secreted from the cell, whereas the second form is probably bound to the cell membrane[6,10]. These results correlate well with the known cell surface localization of MUC1-H23 Ag as well as with the secretion of MUC1-H23 Ag into body fluids.

MUC1-H23 Ag is over-expressed in breast cancer and can therefore be considered a member of the TAA family. In addition, evidence that some specific cellular cytotoxic immunity against this antigen exists in breast cancer patients was recently reported in a study conducted by O. Finn and her colleagues[11,12]. These findings suggest that MUC1-H23 Ag has considerable potential as a target for active immunotherapy.

The application of modern biotechnology to the identification and production of protective antigens has generated many molecularly designed vaccine candidates that have the potential to prevent a wide variety of diseases. Such vaccine candidates may be purified extracts of the organism, genetically engineered recombinant proteins, small synthetic peptides or anti-idiotypic antibodies (anti-Id). The use of defined products in vaccines, as opposed to whole crude extracts, has the advantage of excluding extraneous and toxic cellular or nuclear components.

The increased understanding of the roles played by Id and anti-Id in the regulation of the immune response led to several practical applications in vaccine research. In animal models, these observations were used in the enhancement and induction of antibody response to parasites, bacterial and viral pathogens[13-15]. These studies confirmed that when appropriately manipulated, anti-Id can serve as effective inducers of T and B cell immunity to pathogens. In several other studies anti-tumor reaction could be observed[16-19]. Mice, which were immunized either with purified anti-Id antibody (Ab2ß), or with hybridoma cells which produce Ab2ß, showed specific immune responses, humoral or cellular [delayed-type hypersensitivity (DHT) reaction], against a challenge with the original tumor (against which Ab1 was raised). Moreover, Raychaudhuri et al.[17] showed that in some cases anti-Id immunization resulted in inhibition of tumor growth. Robins et al.[22] using a human mAb anti-Id antibody (105AD7) obtained anti-tumor immune responses in 6 patients with advanced colorectal cancer. The potential of antibodies of type Ab2ß to modulate the immune response of cancer patients to their tumor[19-21] opens new aspects in cancer control.

In our previous studies[23] we have reported the production of two rabbit anti-Id antibodies against human MoAb B11 and 4.6/6. These anti-Id antibodies reacted with the antigen-binding site of B11 and 4.6/6. Immunization with anti-idiotypic antibodies bearing the internal image of the antigen provided immunization against human breast cancer antigen HuMTV without the exposure to the initial antigen. Anti-Id vaccines opens up novel avenues with new therapeutic potential.

## METHODS

### Monoclonal antibodies (MoAb)

H23 MoAb - The details of the production of this mouse MoAb were reported elsewhere[4]. H23 MoAb reacted with human breast epithelial tumor antigen. H23 MoAb was purified from ascites of BALB/c mice.

### Preparation of antiidiotypic (anti-Id) antibodies to MoAb H23

Two-month-old rabbits were used to generate the anti-Id antibodies. Two rabbits were s.c. immunized with 50 $\mu$g per injection of purified H23 antibody at an interval of three weeks. The first three injections were carried out with complete Freund's adjuvant (CFA; Difco, Detroit, MI) and subsequently once with incomplete adjuvant (ICFA). Sera were obtained and precipitated at 40% saturation of ammonium sulfate, dialyzed against phosphate-buffered saline (PBS) and extensively adsorbed on Sepharose column conjugated to pooled mouse IgG. To obtain specific anti-Id antibodies, the effluent from the above Sepharose column was affinity purified on a column consisting of polyacrylhydrazide-agarose, to which H23 antibodies were conjugated. Elution of anti-H23 antibodies was performed with 0.1 N acetic acid in 0.9% NaCl (pH 3.3). The eluates were immediately titrated to pH 5.0 with phosphate buffer (0.1 M, pH 8.0) and then dialyzed against PBS.

### Direct binding of anti-Id antibodies to their Id

Enzyme-linked immunosorbent assay (ELISA) was employed: 96-well polystyrene microtiter plates (Nunc, Roskilde, Denmark; Immunolon II) were coated with 10$\mu$g/ml of myeloma MOPC-P3 IgG or with purified MoAb H23. Blocking of unbound sites was performed with 0.5% gelatin in PBS. Wells were washed with 0.1% gelatin in PBS (washing buffer). Dilutions of rabbit anti-Id antibody were incubated for 4 h at room temperature and their binding to the respective immunoglobulins was quantitated by adding goat anti-rabbit Ig conjugated to alkaline phosphatase, for 18 h at 4°C. After several washes with washing buffer, the substrate p-nitrophenyl phosphate, 0.6 mg/ml in substrate buffer, pH 9.8 (Sigma, St. Louis, MO) was added. All liquid volumes added in ELISA were 50$\mu$l except the substrate which was 200$\mu$l. The plates were read at 405 nm in an automatic microtiter reader MR-600 (Dynatech, Alexandria, VA).

### Cell and antigens

Mouse mammary cell line Mm5mt, the transfected cell line Mm5-35 expressing secreted form of MUC1-H23Ag and the human breast carcinoma cell line T47D were grown in Dulbecco's modified Eagle's medium supplemented with 10% FBS. H23-antigen was isolated from the media of T47D cells as detailed elsewhere[24].

### Transfection experiments

10 $\mu$g of DNA of one of the expression plasmids were mixed with 1 $\mu$g of plasmid, pAG60, encoding the neomycin resistant selection marker and diluted with 420$\mu$l of TE (Tris HCl 10mM, EDTA 0.1mM, pH7.5); 60$\mu$l of 2M CaCl$_2$ solution were added to the DNA by gentle mixing. The obtained solution was transferred

dropwise to 480μl HBSx2 (280mM NaCl, 50mM HEPES, 1.5mM Na$_2$HPO$_4$ x 2H$_2$O, pH 7.12). The precipitate was formed for 30 minutes at room temperature and added dropwise on top of 10$^6$ cells, covered by 10ml complete medium. Twenty four hours later the cells were washed 3 times with PBS before adding fresh medium containing 750μg/ml G418 for selection of transfected clones. G418-resistant foci were subcultured and tested for reaction with mAb H23. Single-cell lines were established by limiting dilution from positive clones. Flow cytometry was used to confirm that all cells expressed the antigen. Mm5mt-neo (Mm5-24) and Mm5mt-S form (Mm5-35) were propagated in Dulbecco's modified Eagle's medium supplemented with 10% FBS, penicillin (100u/ml) and streptomycin (100μg/ml).

**Detection of H23 antigen on the surface of T47D and Mm5-35 cells by flow cytometry**

T47D and Mm5-35 cells were grown in culture flasks and harvested with 0.05% EDTA-PBS. A single cell suspension of 10$^6$ washed cells was incubated in tubes with either 1μg of MoAb H23, MoAb anti MMTV-gp52 (kindly supplemented by Dr. A. Tax), or P3-mouse myeloma IgG. The binding of the antibodies was determined with fluorescein isothiocyanate (FITC)-goat anti mouse (F(ab')2 antibodies incubated for 45 min at 4°C. Following repeated washings the cell suspension was examined by a fluoresceine activated cell sorter (FACS) analyzer (Becton-Dickinson, Mountain View, CA).

**Immunization of mice with anti-Id antibodies**

Four groups of female C3Heb mice, raised at the animal quarters of Tel Aviv University (20 mice in each group), were immunized according to the following protocol: group 1 with PBS only; group 2 with rabbit anti-H23Id; group 3 with 10$^6$ irradiated T47D cells; and group 4 with 10$^6$ irradiated Mm5mt cells. Each mouse was injected three times with either 100μg/50μl per injection of antibody or PBS. The first injection was given with CFA and subsequent two with ICFA. Mice were bled one week following the last injection. Sera of the immunized mice were examined for the presence of antibodies against MUC1-H23Ag by ELISA.

**Detection of antibodies against MUC1-H23Ag in immunized mice**

Polystyrene plates with 96 flat-bottom wells were coated with 20μg/ml of MUC1-H23Ag in carbonate buffer (0.05 M, pH 9.6), overnight at 4°C. The coated wells were subjected to serial dilutions of the individual sera (in duplicates) and incubated for 4 hours at room temperature. Following three washes, goat anti-mouse IgG conjugated to alkaline phosphatase (Sigma) was added and incubated for 18 hours at 4°C. Bound alkaline phosphatase conjugate was measured by adding p-nitrophenyl phosphate (0.6 mg/ml in substrate buffer, pH 9.8, Sigma). Absorbance was read at 405 nm.

**Detection of cell mediated immunity against tumor cells bearing MUC1-H23Ag in mice immunized with anti Id antibodies**

The cell mediated immunity elicited in mice immunized with anti H23Id against T47D and Mm5-35 cells (expressing the H23Ag) was studied. MLT response (Proliferative response of the spleen cells stimulated with the tumor cells) was performed in triplicate. T47D, Mm5mt or Mm5-35 cells were exposed to X-ray radiation. 5x10$^4$ cells/well were distributed in 96 well plates in 10% FBS containing DMEM for 24 hours. Twenty four hours later splenocytes from the tested mice, $2 \times 10^5$/well were added for 72 hours in enriched RPMI-1640 medium supplemented with 1% Normal Mouse Sera (from C3Heb mice). Subsequently, $1 \mu Ci$/well $^3$H-thymidine was added for overnight incubation. Counts per minute (cpm) were determined following harvesting of the cells onto glass microfiber and addition of scintillation fluid.

## RESULTS

The identification of genes and their protein products that are abnormally expressed in breast cancer may lead to new therapeutic means for this neoplasia. One of the therapeutic protocols to be used in the future may be immunization of patients. The efficacy of molecular mimics of human gene products to protect a diseased patient will be tested in this study. To this end, a mouse model system was generated using mouse mammary cells Mm5mt transfected with the human gene H23Ag.

### STRUCTURE OF THE H23-MUC1 GENE AND cDNA CLONES

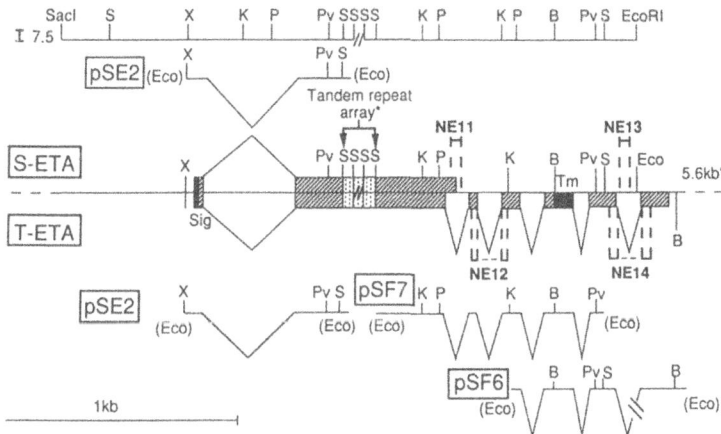

**Figure 1.** S-ETA and T-ETA represent the structure of the mRNA species encoding the S and Tm forms of H23-MUC1. Boxed, coding sequence; solid boxes are major hydrophobic zones within the encoded polypeptides; Sig, N-terminal signal sequence; Tm, putative transmembrane anchor region. I7.5 (above) gives the restriction map of the genomic H23-MUC1; the tandem repeat array in this clone contains 37 copies of the repeat unit (not shown). pSE2, pSF7 and pSF6 are cDNA clones used for assembly of the full length H23-MUC1 coding sequences. NE11-14 show the locations of oligonucleotide probes designed to detect S and Tm coding sequences. Restriction site abbreviations are: B, BalI; Eco, EcoRI; K, KpnI; P, Psvt1; Pv, PvuII; S, SmaI; X, XmnI.

### Tumor cells expressing H23Ag

Full length cDNAs encoding the S and T forms of H23-MUC1 (Fig. 1) were constructed by reassembly of partial cDNA clones with the help of a vector ppolyII, reexcised from its polylinker and inserted between BamHI and SalI sites (Sec form) or BamHI and EcoRV (Tm form) of pHMG, a plasmid comprising the promoter region, the untranslated first exon, and the first intron of the mouse housekeeping gene encoding 3-hydroxy-3-methylglutaryl-CoA reductase[25]. The polylinker of pHMG plasmid is followed by a 123-base-pair fragment containing a polyadenylation signal from simian virus 40 (SV40). Mm5mt - a mouse mammary carcinoma cell line was cotransfected with pAG60 (a plasmid determining G418 resistance) and either pHMG-ETA-S or the expression plasmid vector pHMG, by a modification of the calcium phosphate precipitation method[26]. In this study we present the transfection with the H23-MUC1 secreted form only.

In order to determine if Mm5-35 cells express the MUC1-H23Ag, both Mm5-35 and Mm5-24 were grown as monolayers on chamber slides (Lab-tek), fixed in cold acetone and incubated with either H23 MoAb or with MOPC-P3 myeloma IgG (control). Fig. 2 shows the cytoplasmic staining in Mm5-35 cells with MoAb H23. No fluorescence was obtained in the control cells Mm5-24 with MoAb H23 or in Mm5-35 cells with the MOPC-P3 IgG (data not shown).

## IMMUNOFLUORESCENCE ANALYSIS OF MOUSE MAMMARY TUMOR CELLS EXPRESSING MUC1-H23

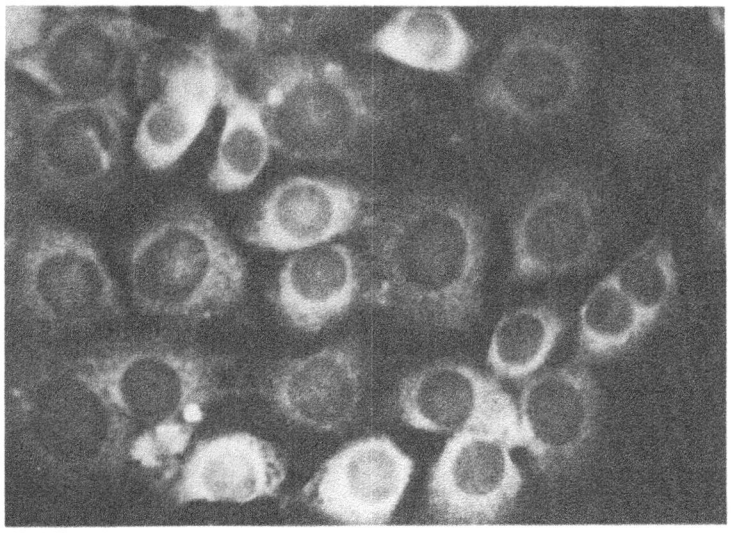

**Figure 2**. Immobilized Mm5-35 cells were stained with 10μg/ml H23 MoAb, followed by incubation with FITC-goat anti mouse Ig and counterstained with Evans blue. Total fluorescence under UV illumination was photographed on black and white film to reveal specific MUC1-H23 fluorescence. (x50).

The transfectants Mm5-35 and the Mm5-24 (control) were also assayed by FACS for the expression of MUC1-H23Ag. Since the transfectants were derived from the mouse mammary Mm5mt cells producing MMTV, the FACS was performed in addition to the H23 MoAb with the MoAb against the MMTV-gp52. As control to the mouse MoAb the MOPC-P3 IgG was used. Fig. 3 shows that both the control transfectant Mm5-24 as well as the Mm5-35 express the viral antigen gp52. On the other hand MUC1-H23 antigen was expressed only by the Mm5-35 cells. No reaction was observed with the control MOPC-P3 IgG. The expression of

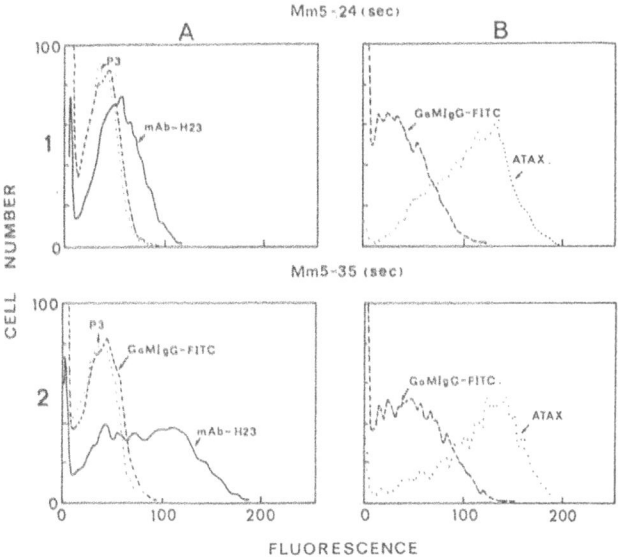

**Figure 3**. (1) Control Mm5-24 cells labeled with MoAb H23 (A) and with anti-MMTV gp52 MoAb (ATAX) (B). (2) Mm5-35 cells labeled with MoAb H23 (A) and with anti-MMTV gp52 (B). P3 IgG secreted by the MOPC-P3 Plasmacytoma was used as control mouse immunoglobulin for both cells (A and B).

the MUC1-H23Ag by the Mm5/35/sec cells was demonstrated also by Western blot analysis of the cell extracts (data not shown).

**Tumorigenicity of Mm5-35**

Does the transfection of Mm5mt cells with the human gene affect the ability of these cells to cause tumors in mice? To answer this question, groups of 5 mice were inoculated with $5 \times 10^5$ cells per mouse with the following: Mm5mt, Mm5-35 and Mm5-24. The inoculated mice were followed for 100 days. All mice developed tumors. No statistical significant differences in the tumor development was observed when the results were analyzed by the Logrank test comparing either the results observed with Mm5-35 and Mm5mt or Mm5-35 and Mm5-24. Fig. 4 shows the tumorigenicity results obtained with the Mm5-35 and Mm5mt. The tumorigenicity of mice inoculated with Mm5-24 was similar to that of the Mm5mt.

The expression of the MUC1-H23Ag in tumor was also tested. Tumors from the mice inoculated with either Mm5mt, Mm5-24 and Mm5-35 were fixed, embedded in paraffin and then sectioned. Serial sections were assayed by the indirect immunoperoxidase method[4]. MUC1-H23Ag was detected in the tumors derived from Mm5-35 cells but neither the tumors derived from the MM5mt nor the Mm5-24 cells were positive for MUC1-H23Ag. These transfectants (Mm5-35) are therefore suitable to be used in a mouse model system in which anti-human breast cancer immunoprotection was studied.

**Rabbit anti-H23 idiotypic antibodies (RαH23Id)**

Rabbits were immunized with MoAb H23 IgG, and the anti-idiotypic antibodies were purified as described in Methods. The determination of the specificity of the RαH23Id was performed by the indirect ELISA assay. Plates were coated with the

TUMORIGENICITY OF TRANSFECTED CELLS

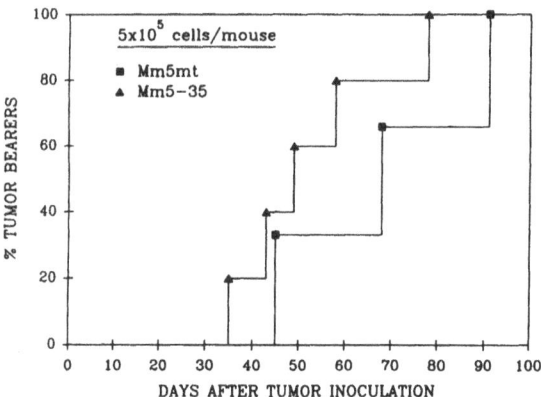

**Figure 4.** Groups of C3Heb mice were each inoculated s.c. either with Mm5mt cells or with Mm5-35. The appearance of palpable tumors was followed up to 100 days.

SPECIFICITY OF ANTI-IDIOTYPIC ANTIBODIES TO THEIR IDIOTYPES

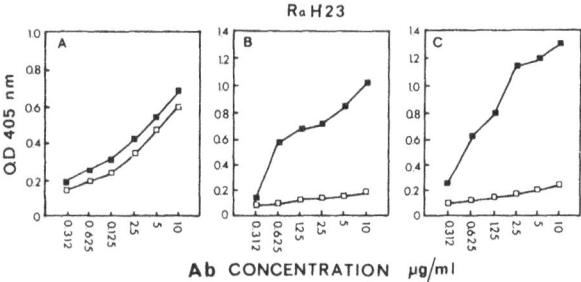

**Figure 5.** Binding of RαH23Id to the H23 idiotype during purification steps. ELISA test was performed using plates coated with either Normal mouse serum or H23 antibodies. The anti-idiotypic antibodies (10μg/ml) were diluted in 0.1% gelatin and incubated at room temperature for 4h.

    A. IgG enriched fraction of RαH23Id from sera of the immunized
       rabbits (40% saturated ammonium sulfate precipitation).
    B. IgG enriched fraction of RαId after intensive adsorption on
       Sepharose-MIgG column.
    C. Affinity purified RαH23Id antibodies (on H23-Sepharose column).

MoAb H23 (IgG1) and P3 IgG as control (IgG1). Serial dilutions of the RαH23Id prior and post purification were added to the coated plates. The binding reaction of the RαH23Id antibodies was measured using goat anti-rabbit IgG coupled to alkaline phosphatase. Fig. 5 shows that RαH23Id after purification recognizes specifically only the H23 idiotype and not the isotype or allotype determinants present on the control mouse IgG.

## Immunization of mice with RαH23Id anti-idiotypic antibodies and irradiated cells

The immunization experiments were performed with purified RαH23Id antibodies or with irradiated Mm5mt and T47D or PBS. Four groups of twenty C3Heb mice each, were immunized as described in Methods.

### Humoral response

Sera of mice immunized with rabbit anti H23-Id antibody or irradiated cells (T47D and Mm5mt) were tested for anti MUC1-H23Ag activity by the ELISA test. Fig. 6 summarizes the results obtained testing individual mice sera at a 1:50 dilution. The results show that sera from the mice immunized with RαH23Id or with the irradiated T47D cells reacted strongly with MUC1-H23Ag. Sera from mice of the control groups immunized with irradiated Mm5tm cells or PBS exhibited no reactivity with the H23Ag.

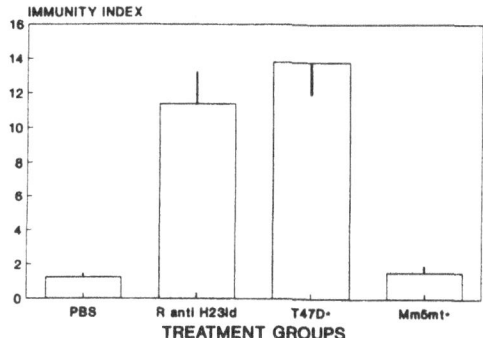

**Figure 6.** Antibody response of vaccinated female mice with anti-Id antibodies to MUC1-H23Ag as measured by ELISA. Four groups of 20 mice each were immunized with (1) PBS (2) rabbit anti-H23Id (3) irradiated T47D cells and (4) irradiated Mm5mt cells. Serum from each mouse was individually tested. the mean binding of each group was calculated. The results are presented as immunity index:

$$\frac{\text{mean binding of experimental group}}{\text{mean binding of the PBS group}}$$

## Cell mediated immune response (T cell proliferation) of mice immunized with rabbit anti H23Id and irradiated T47D cells (MLT)

Ten mice of each group were sacrificed and their spleens removed. The spleen cells were tested for their ability to proliferate upon stimulation with irradiated T47D, Mm-35 or Mm5mt cells. The stimulation was measured by $^3$H-thymidine uptake. Fig. 7 shows that mice immunized either with R$\alpha$H23Id or with T47D cells developed T cell response against the human MUC1-H23Ag (expressed both on T47D and Mm5-35 cells). On the other hand, the mice immunized with the mouse mammary cells developed a better T cell response only to the mouse antigen expressed on both Mm5mt and Mm5-35 cells.

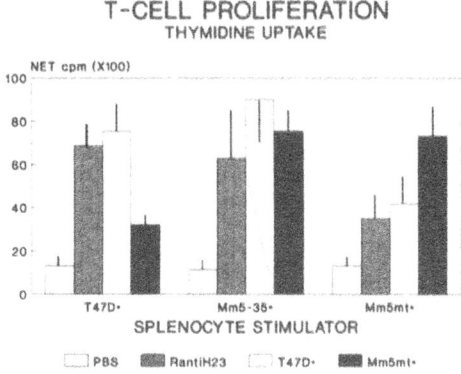

**Figure 7.** Cellular response of immunized mice (as in Fig. 6) was measured as proliferation of sensitized splenocytes with the following cells:
irradiated T47D, irradiated Mm5-35 or irradiated Mm5mt. The proliferation was measured by thymidine uptake.
Spleen cells from individual mice were tested. The mean proliferation of each group was calculated. The results are presented as Net CPM.
Net CPM = [CPM lymphocytes with stimulator cell - (CPM lymphocytes alone + CPM of tumor cells alone)]

## Protection of immunized mice to tumor challenge

Ten of the remaining mice in each group were challenged s.c. with $5 \times 10^6$ Mm5-35 live cells per mouse. At day 35 all the mice in the control group (non-immunized) developed tumors. The tumor incidence in the immunized mice was measured at this time (day 35) (Fig. 8). Sixty percent of the mice immunized with R$\alpha$H23Id were tumor free. In the group immunized with T47D cells 70% of the mice were tumor free, whereas in the group of mice immunized with the syngeneic cells (Mm5mt), 80% were free of tumors.

The results described above demonstrate that immunization with the anti-idiotypic antibodies R$\alpha$H23Id representing the internal image of H23Ag, or with the irradiated T47D cell confers similar protection against tumor challenge in mice.

134

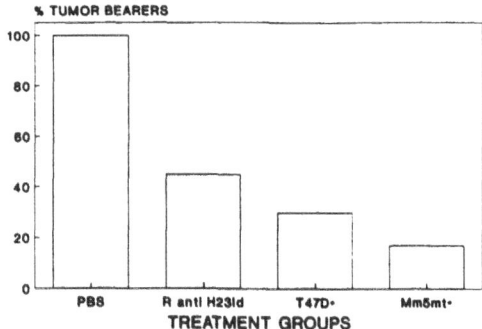

**Figure 8.** Mice were immunized as in Fig. 6 and challenged with $5 \times 10^5$ Mm5-35 live cells per mouse.
Tumor incidence in the immunized groups at day 35 after inoculation,
when 100% of the non-immunized mice developed tumors.

The protection obtained with anti-idiotypic immunization of mice that were never exposed to the tumor antigen or tumor cells, prior to the tumor challenge, was almost as efficient as the immunization with tumor cells.

The results clearly suggest that using anti-Id antibodies as vaccines for cancer immunotherapy is a feasible approach in obtaining immune responses and protection against tumors as compared to the immunization with whole cells.

## DISCUSSION

Tumors often express antigens on the surface of the cells. Studies have been directed to the identification of tumor associated markers that can be used as a target for active or passive immunization[27-32]. As an alternative to the use of tumor antigens, tumor cells or infectious materials, the "internal image" of such antigens has been generated and used to induce anti-tumor immunity[16-19]. According to the immune network hypothesis produced by Jerne[33] certain anti-Id antibodies express structures which resemble the natural antigen[34-36]. It was reported that the anti-Id antibodies bearing the "internal image" of the antigen are able to induce humoral and cellular responses in the immunized animals and furthermore to compete in binding with the antigens[37,38]. It has already been demonstrated that the immune reaction to anti-Id is also expressed as DTH[39]. If an analogy is drawn from viral, bacterial and parasitic infections[13-15,40,41], it seems that anti-Id vaccination could confer a significant and possible beneficial tumor immunity[17,20,42,43].

There are several reports[16,19,42,44] for the production of "internal image" anti-Id which mimic human tumor-associated antigens. Nepon et al.[44] described polyclonal anti-Id antibodies raised in rabbits against murine MoAb 8.2, an antibody specific for human melanoma-associated cell surface marker p97. Mice immunized with the anti-Id demonstrated DTH reaction when challenged with p97+ melanoma cells. Herlyn et al.[16] produced anti-Id antibodies in goat against a mouse MoAb to human gastric carcinoma antigen (GA733). This anti-Id antibody induced a specific immunity to human colon carcinoma[19]. Raychaudhuri et al.[17] have generated anti-Id MoAb against the combining site of an antibody (11c1-Ab1) which recognizes a shared determinant of tumor-associated antigen of lymphoma subline (L1210/GZL) and MMTV gp52. Mice immunized with this anti-Id antibody showed a significant inhibition of L1210/GZL tumor growth. Recently, Bhattacharya-Chatterjee et al.[42] reported that they have generated and characterized syngeneic monoclonal anti-Id mimicking a human T cell leukemia antigen, gp37, which induces anti-human tumor antibody responses in mice. Whether the-Id immunization led to any cell-mediated immune responses in the mice was not reported. Losman et al.[45] suggested that baboon anti-Id antibodies that mimic CEA epitopes may be used as a therapeutic agent in human carcinomas producing CEA.

As previously reported[23], we were able to show that in immunizing mice with the "internal image" of MMTV-gp52 and HuMTV (R$\alpha$4.6/6 and R$\alpha$B11 Id), humoral and cellular immunity against the human breast tumor and the mouse mammary tumor cells was demonstrated.

In previous studies we have reported that MUC1-H23Ag is an excellent marker for human breast carcinomas[4,5]. In this manuscript we have described that R$\alpha$H23Id representing the "internal image" of this antigen is able to immunize mice, produce humoral and T cell immunoresponses and to partially protect mice from tumor challenge. The anti-Id immunotherapy provides a safe way as immunogens since no infectious or genetic materials are involved in the immunization process. Therefore, we suggest that anti-idiotypic vaccines can provide a new framework for therapeutic modalities.

## REFERENCES

1. I.C. Henderson, J.C. Harris, D.W. Kinne and S. Hellman. in: "Cancer Principles and Practice of Oncology," V.I. De Vita, S. Hellman and S.A. Rozenberg, eds., Lippincott Co., Philadelphia (1989).
2. K.E. Hellstrom and I. Hellstrom. in: "Monoclonal Antibodies for Tumor Detection and Drug Targeting," R.W. Baldwin and U.S. Byers, eds., Academic Press, London (1985).
3. K.D. Bageshow. Br. J. Cancer 48:167 (1983).
4. I. Keydar, C.S. Chou, M. Hareuveni, I. Tsarfaty, E. Sahar, G. Selzer, S. Chaitchik and A. Hizi. Proc. Natl. Acad. Sci. USA, 86:1362 (1989).
5. I. Tsarfaty, S. Chaitchik, M. Hareuveni, J. Horev, A. Hizi, D.H. Wreschner and I. Keydar. in: "Breast Cancer Immunodiagnosis and Immunotherapy," R.L. Ceriani, ed., Plenum, New York (1989).
6. M. Hareuveni, D.H. Wreschner, M.P. Kieny, K. Dott, C. Gautier, C. Tomasetto, I. Keydar, P. Chambon and R. Lathe. Vaccine 9:618 (1991).
7. D.M. Swallow, S. Gendler, B. Griffiths, G. Cornay, J. Taylor-Papadmitriou and M. Bramwell. Nature 328:82 (1987).
8. J. Siddiqui, M. Abe, D. Hayes, E. Shani, E. Yunis and D. Kufe. Proc. Natl. Acad. Sci. USA 85:2320 (1988).
9. M. Hareuveni, I. Tsarfaty, J. Zaretsky, P. Kotkes, J. Horev, S. Zrihan et al. Eur. J. Biochem. 189:475 (1990).
10. D.H. Wreschner, M. Hareuveni, I. Tsarfaty, I. Smorodinsky, J. Horev, J. Zaretsky et al. Eur. J. Biochem. 18:463 (1990).
11. D.L. Barnd, M. Lan, R. Metzgar and O.I. Finn. Proc. Natl. Acad. Sci.USA 86:7159 (1989).
12. K.J. Jerome, D.L. Barnd, C.M. Boyer, J. Taylor-Papadimitriou, I.F.C. McKenzie, R.C. Bast Jr. and O.J. Finn. in: "Cellular Immunity and the Immunotherapy of Cancer," UCLA Symposia on Molecular and Cellular Biology, New Series, M.T. Lotze and O.J. Finn, eds., Wiley-Liss (1990).

13. D.L. Sacks, K.M. Esser and A. Sher. J. Exp. Med. 155:1108 (1982).
14. K.E. Stein and T. Soderstrom. J. Exp. Med. 160:1001 (1984).
15. R.C. Kennedy and G.R. Dreesman. J. Exp. Med. 159:655 (1984).
16. D. Herlyn, A.H. Ross and H. Koprowski. Science 232:100 (1986).
17. S. Raychaudhuri, Y. Saeki, H. Fuji and H. Kohler. J. Immunology 137:1743 (1986).
18. V.K. Lee, T.G. Harriott, V.J. Kuchroo, W.J. Halliday, I. Hellstrom and K.E. Hellstrom. Proc. Natl. Acad. Sci. USA 82:6286 (1985).
19. D. Herlyn, A.H. Ross, D. Hiopoulos and H. Koprowski. Eur. J. Immunol. 17:1649 (1987).
20. E. DeFreitas, H. Suzuki, D. Herlyn, M. Lubeck, H. Sears, M. Herlyn and H. Koprowski. Curr. Top. Microb. Immunol. 119:75 (1985).
21. D. Herlyn, M. Lubeck, H.F. Sears and H. Koprowski. J. Immunol. Meth. 85:27 (1985).
22. R.A. Robins, G.W.L. Denton, J.D. Hardcastle, E.B. Austin, R.W. Baldwin and L.G. Durrant. Cancer Res. 51:5425 (1991).
23. N.I. Smorodinsky, Y. Gendler, R. Bakimer, S. Chaitchik, I. Keydar and Y. Shoenfeld. Eur. J. Immunol. 18:1713 (1988).
24. M. Hareuveni, C. Gautier, M.P. Kieny, D.H. Wreschner, P. Chambon and R. Lathe. Proc. Natl. Acad. Sci. USA 87:9498 (1990).
25. C. Gautier, M. Mehtali and R. Lathe. Nucleic Acids Res. 17:8389 (1989).
26. M. Wigler, A. Pellicer, S. Silverstein and R. Axel. Cell 14:725 (1978).
27. R. Sharon and D. Naor. Cancer Immunol. Immunother. 18:203 (1984).
28. H.C. Hoover, M.G. Surdyke, R.B. Dangel, L.C. Peters and M.G. Hanna. Cancer 15:1236 (1985).
29. M.K. Wallack, K. McNally, M. Michaelides, J. Basch, A. Bartolucci, H. Siegler, C. Balch and H. Wanebo. Am. Surg. 52:148 (1986).
30. T. Dalianis. Adv. Cancer Res. 55:57 (1990).
31. D. Talarico, M.. Ittmann, A. Balsari, P. Delli-Bovi, R.S. Basch and C. Basilico. Proc. Natl. Acad. Sci. USA 87:4222 (1990).
32. M.C. Wallack, K.R. McNally, E. Leftheriotis, H. Siegler, C. Balch, H. Wanebo, A.A. Bartolucci and J.Λ. Basch. Cancer 57:649 (1986).
33. N.K. Jerne, Ann. Immunol. 125C:373 (1974).
34. A. Nisonoff and E. Lamoyi. Clin. Immunol. Immunopathol. 21:397 (1981).
35. H. Kohler, S. Muller and C. Bona. Proc. Soc. Exp. Biol. Med. 178:189 (1985).
36. H. Kohler. in: "Idiotype in Biology and Medicine," H. Kohler, J. Urbin and P.A. Cazenave, eds., Academic Press, New York (1985).
37. C. Bona, E. Herber-Katz and W.E. Paul. J. Exp. Med. 153:951 (1981).
38. P.A. Cazenave. Proc. Natl. Acad. Sci. USA 74:5122 (1977).
39. W.R. Thomas, G. Morahan, J.D. Walker and J.F. Miller. J. Exp. Med. 153:743 (1981).
40. M.A. Dichter, H.L. Weiner, B.N. Fields, G. Mitchell, J. Noseworthy, G. Gaulton and M. Greene. Ann. Neurol. 19:555 (1986).
41. R.C. Kennedy, J.W. Eichberg and G.R. Dreesman. Virology 148:369 (1986).
42. M. Bhattacharya-Chatterjee, M.W. Pride, B.K. Seon and H. Kohler. J. Immunol. 139:1354 (1987).
43. S. Raychaudhuri, Y. Saeki, J.J. Chem, H. Iribe and and H. Kohler. J. Immunol. 139:271 (1987).
44. G.T. Nepom, K.A. Nelson, S.L. Holbeck, I. Hellstrom and K.E. Hellstrom. Proc. Natl. Acad. Sci. USA 81:2864 (1984).
45. M.J. Losman, M. Monestier, H.J. Hansen and D.M. Goldenberg. Int. J. Cancer 46:310 (1990).

# ANTI-IDIOTYPE ANTIBODIES AS POTENTIAL THERAPEUTIC AGENTS FOR HUMAN BREAST CANCER

Malaya Bhattacharya-Chatterjee[1], Ewe Mrozek[2], Sonjoy Mukerjee[2], Roberto L. Ceriani[3], Heinz Kohler[1] and Kenneth A. Foon[1]

From the Departments of [1]Lucille Markey Cancer Center, University of Kentucky College of Medicine, Lexington, KY 40536; [2]Molecular Immunology, Roswell Park Cancer Institute, Buffalo, New York and [3]Cancer Research Fund of Contra Costa, Walnut Creek, CA

## INTRODUCTION

Breast cancer is the most common cause of cancer deaths in women. Recurrent breast cancer is not curable by standard therapies and new therapeutic approaches are needed. The goal of this study is to employ an alternative and safe approach to immunotherapy of breast cancer patients using monoclonal anti-idiotype (Id) antibodies in two conceptually different ways. In the first approach, monoclonal anti-Id antibodies which mimic breast cancer tumor-associated antigens (TAA) will be used to actively immunize patients for the production of anti-tumor immunity. In the second approach, monoclonal anti-Id antibodies will be used to remove unwanted excess radioactivity from the circulation of patients previously treated with radiolabeled monoclonal anti-breast TAA antibodies.

Monoclonal antibodies (mAbs) to breast TAA have been studied in diagnosis, prognosis and passive immunotherapy (1-5). Breast TAA shed into the circulation of patients (6) are targets for diagnosis with radiolabeled mAbs which are useful and unique bioprobes (7). Ceriani and colleagues (8,9) have generated a series of murine mAbs that recognize components of human milk fat globule (HMFG) found on the surface membrane of breast cancer cells. Among these mAbs we have selected BrE-1 and BrE-3 for production of anti-Id antibodies.

## HUMAN BREAST TAA IDIOTYPIC CASCADE

According to the immune network hypothesis proposed by Jerne (10), certain anti-Id antibodies (Ab2) express three dimensional shapes which resemble the structures of external antigens. These particular anti-Ids called Ab2$\beta$ (11-14) can induce specific immune responses similar to responses induced by nominal antigen and also can compete with nominal antigens in binding assays. The concept of anti-idiotype immunization

*Antigen and Antibody Molecular Engineering in Breast Cancer Diagnosis and Treatment*, Edited by R.L. Ceriani, Plenum Press, New York, 1994

139

against TAA for patients with BrE-1 positive breast tumors is the subject of this investigation.

mAb BrE-1 was chosen as the Ab1 for production of anti-Id (Ab2) because it defines a unique and specific epitope on high molecular weight HMFG, primarily expressed by human breast tumor cells at high density but not found on normal adult tissues (by immunoperoxidase staining) or peripheral blood lymphocytes (by FACS analysis). BrE-1 reacts with a 400,000 M.W. mucin-like protein present in minute amounts only in human mammary epithelial cells and increased by at least 10-fold on breast carcinoma cells. The restricted specificity of this mAb together with its high binding capacity to representative breast cancer cell lines MCF-7 and SKBR3 makes it an excellent target for generating Ab2 hybridomas.

## Generation of Monoclonal Anti-Idiotype Hybridomas

Syngeneic BALB/c mice were immunized four times with BrE-1 (Ab1) and their spleen cells were fused with the non-secretory mouse myeloma P3-653 cells. Several Ab2 hybridomas were obtained that were specific for the immunizing Id of BrE-1 and did not react with any isotypic or allotypic determinants. To determine whether these Ab2 were directed against the paratope of BrE-1, the binding of radiolabeled BrE-1 to the breast tumor cell line MCF-7 and SKBR3 was studied in the presence of varying amounts of Ab2 hybridoma culture supernatants. Several mAb2s were obtained which were binding site specific. These Ab2s were purified from ascites fluid for further studies. One of these Ab2, 11D10 (IgG1,$\kappa$) appeared to functionally mimic HMFG and had the potential to be used as a network antigen (15) to induce anti-tumor immunity in breast cancer patients.

## Characterization of Ab2 11D10

$^{125}$I-Labeled 11D10 was tested against a panel of mAb of various specificities belonging to major Ig subclasses by a direct binding radioimmunoassay (RIA). Results are shown in Fig. 1. 11D10 bound almost exclusively to BrE-1; there was no crossreactivity with any of the other antibodies tested. Another anti-breast TAA mAb BrE-3, which recognizes a different epitope on HMFG did not bind to 11D10 (Table 1).

To determine conclusively that 11D10 is specific for the BrE-1 idiotype and not against isotype and allotype determinants, we set up an inhibition assay in which the binding of

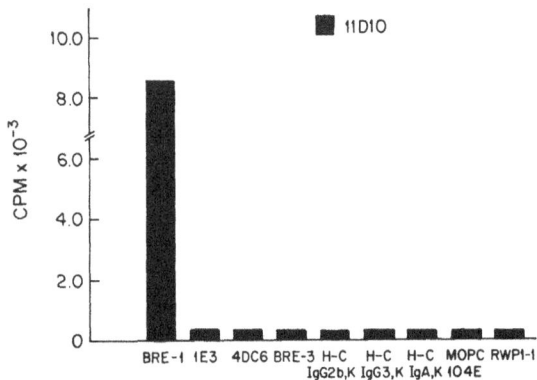

**Figure 1.** Anti-Id specificities of 11D10 (IgG1,$\kappa$). Binding of $^{125}$I-labeled 11D10 ($\sim$25,000 cpm) to various mouse monoclonal proteins and anti-HMFG (breast TAA) antibodies was determined using a direct RIA. The isotypes of the monoclonal proteins are BrE-1 (IgG2b,$\kappa$), 1E3 (IgG1,$\kappa$), 4DC6 (IgG1, $\lambda$), BrE-3 (IgG1,$\kappa$) Hy-Clone IgG2b,$\kappa$; Hy-Clone IgG3,$\kappa$; Hy-Clone IgA,$\kappa$; and MOPC 104E (IgM, $\lambda$), RWP1-1 (IgG2b,$\kappa$). The results are presented as mean cpm (n = 3). The S.D. of the data was less than 10% for each assay.

labeled Ab2 to Ab1 was measured in the presence of different unrelated Ab1, Ab2 or control myeloma proteins. Greater than 90% inhibition was obtained by using the homologous 11D10 (250 ng) and BrE-1 (250 ng), whereas no inhibition was obtained even up to a concentration of 10 $\mu$g with control inhibitors (Table 2).

**Table 1.** Binding of mAb1 BrE-1 and BrE-3 to anti-idiotype (11D10)

| Ab2 | Concentration cpm | BrE-1 (IgG2b) cpm | BrE-3 (IgG1) |
|---|---|---|---|
| | 100 ng | 6,149 ± 301 | 263.0 ± 43.4 |
| 11D10 | 300 ng | 16,731 ± 483 | 260.0 ± 12.3 |
| | 1000 ng | 44,177 ± 1,392 | 374.3 ± 23.8 |

Plates were coated with 100 ng, 300 ng and 1,000 ng of purified Ab2 and reacted with $^{125}$I-BrE-1 IgG2b and $^{125}$I-BrE-3 IgG1 as described in the text.

**Table 2.** Inhibition of idiotype-antiidiotype binding

| Inhibitor | cpm Bound | % Inhibition |
|---|---|---|
| None | 37,071 | 0 |
| 11D10 (Ab2), 0.250 $\mu$g | 1,853 | 95 |
| BrE-1 (Ab1), 0.250 $\mu$g | 2,594 | 93 |
| SN2, 10 $\mu$g | 37,085 | 0 |
| CLL-2, 10 $\mu$g | 37,482 | 0 |
| 4EA2, 10 $\mu$g | 38,904 | 0 |
| RWP 1.1, 10 $\mu$g | 37,082 | 0 |
| 3F3, 10 $\mu$g | 38,132 | 0 |
| MOPC, 10 $\mu$g | 37,161 | 0 |
| 1E3, 10 $\mu$g | 38,523 | 0 |
| 3A4, 10 $\mu$g | 38,064 | 0 |
| F6/32, 10 $\mu$g | 37,904 | 0 |

Purified BrE-1 (Ab1) was used to coat plates (250 ng/well) and the binding of radiolabeled 11D10 ($\sim$50,000 cpm) to BrE-1 was tested for inhibition in the presence of different Ab1, Ab2 or mouse myeloma proteins. The results are presented as mean cpm (n = 3). The SD of the data was <10%. The cpm obtained with excess Ab1 (BrE-1) was considered as background.

To demonstrate that the anti-Id 11D10 is directed against the paratope of BrE-1, the binding of radiolabeled BrE-1 to human breast carcinoma cell lines MCF-7 and SKBR3 was measured in the presence of varying amounts of purified 11D10 (IgG1,$\kappa$). Ab2 11D10 inhibited the binding more than 80% at a concentration of 250 ng while the control Ab2 3H1 (BALB/c IgG1-$\kappa$) did not produce inhibition (Fig. 2). The binding of Ab1 (BrE-1) to Ab2 (11D10) was also inhibited by HMFG antigen (data not shown).

### Induction and Characterization of Monoclonal and Polyclonal Anti-anti-idiotype Antibodies (Ab3)

If the Ab2 11D10 behaves as a network antigen (15), then it should induce the production of Ag-specific Ab3 in the absence of exposure to Ag in a genetically unrestricted way and across species barriers. To confirm this, we immunized mice and rabbits with KLH coupled 11D10 to determine whether we could produce Ab3 that might share idiotopes with Ab1 and exhibit similar binding specificity. The immune sera from both mice and rabbits significantly inhibited the binding of radiolabeled Ab1 to Ab2 suggesting the presence of Ab3 antibodies that share idiotopes with Ab1. Furthermore, we generated monoclonal Ab3 that bound to HMFG in an identical fashion as the Ab1.

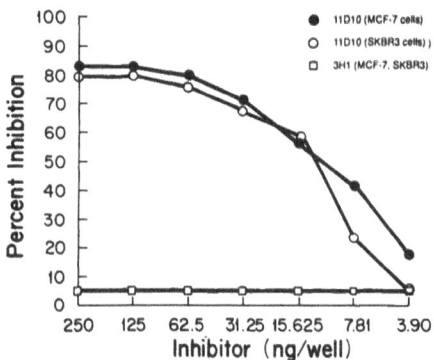

**Figure 2.** Inhibition of BrE-1 binding to MCF-7 and SKBR3 cells by purified Ab2. Confluent monolayer cultures of MCF-7 and SKBR3 cells in 96-well microtiter plates were incubated with different concentrations of purified 11D10 (Ab2) or 3H1 and fixed amount of BrE-1-$I^{125}$ for 2 hrs at room temperature with shaking.

Direct binding with the breast carcinoma cell line SKBR3 of polyclonal mouse and rabbit Ab3 sera and mAb3 at several dilutions is shown in Fig. 3. Anti-isotypic and anti-allotypic antibodies present in the sera were absorbed prior to performing the assay. Monoclonal as well polyclonal Ab3 demonstrated appreciable binding by ELISA while the negative control showed no binding.

## Competition of Ab1 and Ab3 for Binding to SKBR3 Cells

If Ab3 has a similar binding site as Ab1, it should compete with Ab1 for binding to the

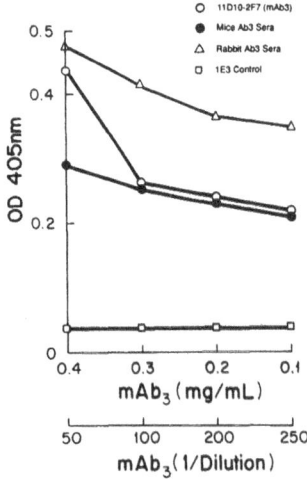

**Figure 3.** Binding of absorbed polyclonal mice and rabbit Ab3 sera as well as mAb3 to breast carcinoma cell line SKBR3 by ELISA.

HMFG Ag present on SKBR3 cells. A fixed amount of radiolabeled BrE-1 was co-incubated with several dilutions of rabbit or mouse Ab3 sera or mAb3 preparations and SKBR3 cells (Fig. 4). Twenty $\mu$g of mAb3 inhibited binding by 25%, whereas the polyclonal Ab3 sera at 1/50 dilution produced 38% and 30% inhibition for rabbit and mouse sera, respectively. This indicated that the polyclonal Ab3 sera bind to the same Ag as Ab1 and therefore contain some antibody molecules with Ab1's properties. The low binding inhibition obtained with these various Ab3 preparations is likely due to lower affinity and avidity as compared to mAb1 for the Ag.

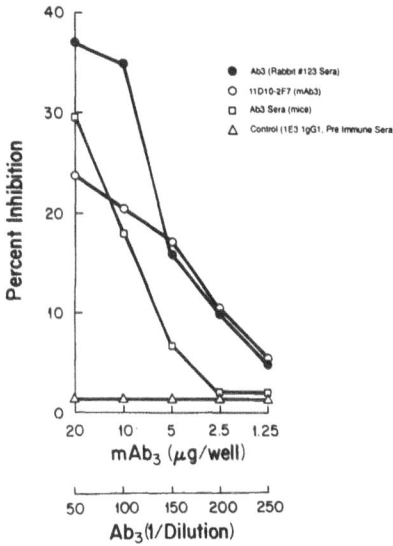

**Figure 4.** Inhibition of BrE-1 (Ab1) binding to SKBR3 cells by mAb3 and polyclonal mouse and rabbit Ab3 sera. Confluent monolayer cultures of SKBR3 cells in microtiter wells were reacted with different concentrations of mAb3 preparations, and different dilutions of rabbit and mouse Ab3 sera and a fixed amount of $^{125}$I-BrE-1 (50,000 cpm). 1E3 mAb and pre-immune sera were used as control.

### Dot Blot Analysis of mAb1 and mAb3

HMFG antigen at different dilutions were transblotted to nitrocellulose filters and reacted with BrE-1 (Ab1) and mAb3 (Fig. 5). The staining was identical but more intense with Ab1 while the control antibody was negative.

### Idiotype Matching Experiment with Ab2 11D10

We studied sera from 50 randomly selected breast cancer patients to determine if any of them had pre-existing matching idiotype which would be recognized by Ab2 11D10. Microtiter plates were coated with F(ab')$_2$ fragment of 11D10 and patient's sera were added at 1:100 dilutions and developed with goat anti-human IgG enzyme labeled antibodies.

As shown in Fig. 6, a small number (8/50) of these breast cancer patients' sera had elevated levels of antibodies reactive with 11D10. The selective criteria in anti-Id therapy is based on the assumption that the disease itself induces a state of priming B cells and T cells in the host. It is hypothesized that in patients who express a corresponding matching Id, Ab2 stimulation would then be able to effectively stimulate such already primed B and

143

T cells. The finding of Id matching sera from breast cancer patients suggest that they may be specially suitable as potential candidates for active anti-Id immunotherapy with Ab2 11D10. We plan on testing this hypothesis.

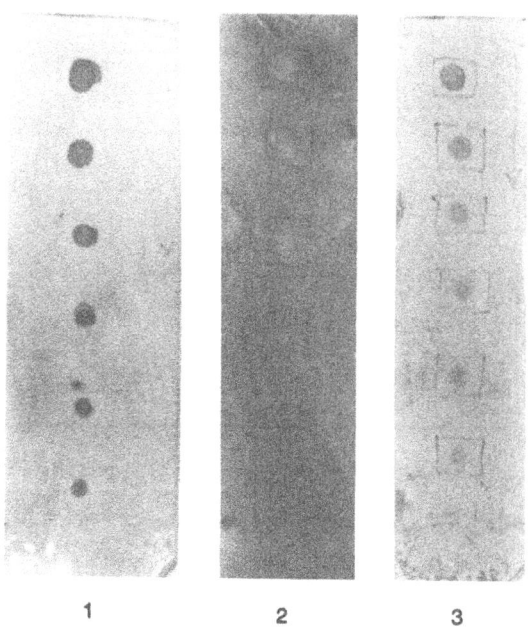

1        2        3

**Figure 5.** Transblot analysis of HMFG on nitrocellulose paper with mAb1 and mAb3. Lanes 1-3 were transblotted with HMFG and incubated with BrE-1, 10 $\mu$g/ml, control 1E3 IgG1, 50 $\mu$g/ml and mAb3 IgG1, 50 $\mu$g/ml, respectively. The reaction was developed by ELISA assay using goat anti-mouse IgG alkaline phosphatase reagents and substrate.

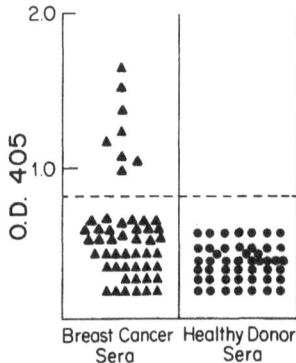

**Figure 6.** Level of expresion of 11D10 anti-Id reactive antibodies in the sera of breast cancer patients. Microtiter plates were coated with 250 ng/well of purified F(ab')$_2$ fragment of 11D10 (Ab2) and incubated with 1:100 dilution of patients' sera and healthy donor's sera. The binding of the sera to Ab2 was detected using alkaline phosphatase conjugated anti-human IgG ($\gamma$ chain specific) antibody and substrate.

## Passive Administration of Anti-Id as a Second Reagent During Radioimmunotherapy

There have been a number of reports indicating a clinical response to antibody targeted radionuclides. Order and his colleagues (16,17) have been using radiolabeled polyclonal antibodies for treatment for carcinoma of the liver. Larson and coworkers performed a Phase I study of [131]I-labeled Fab fragment directed to the P97 glycoprotein in patients with malignant melanoma (18). DeNardo and coworkers (19) observed two complete and 8 partial responses in a Phase I study of 10 B cell lymphoma and chronic lymphocytic leukemia patients treated with radiolabeled Lym-1 antibody. Rosen and coworkers (20) have treated six patients with cutaneous T cell lymphoma with radiolabeled T101 antibody and dramatic response was obtained in two patients with skin and lymph node regression; myelosuppression, however, was the dose limiting toxicity. One problem common to all of these studies has been the presence of excess radioactivity in the system which limits the dosage of radiolabeled antibody for treatment. The aim of this study was to generate monoclonal anti-Ids which will be suitable as second reagents to bind to excess radiolabeled antibody.

## Clearance Study of [111]In-BrE-1 in MX-1 Tumor Bearing BALB/c Nude Mice

Each mouse was injected with 20 $\mu$Ci of 2.9 $\mu$g of [111]In-BrE-1. After 24 hrs 20 $\mu$g of anti-Id 11D10 was injected to one group of six mice to be sacrificed at 30 min and another group at 40 hrs. The control groups of mice at 30 min and 40 hrs were not injected with anti-Id 11D10. After sacrificing the mice, blood and organs were removed for measuring radioactivity levels. The results are shown in Table 3 and expressed as percent dose per gm of [111]In-BrE-1 $\pm$ SEM. At both 30 min and 40 hrs there was significant clearance of radioactivity in almost all organs (specially in blood, kidney, muscle and lung) except liver in experimental groups as compared to controls. The tumor retention was not affected at 30 min, however after 40 hrs there was some clearance in the treated group. Anti-Id 11D10 is an internal image Ab2 which may compete with tumor Ag and may not be ideal for this kind of experiment. These data are very preliminary and need to be verified and standardized with respect to dose and timing. We are planning to use the classical $\alpha$-type anti-Id for this purpose as it does not interfere with antigen binding of Ab1.

## GENERATION OF MONOCLONAL ANTI-IDIOTYPE ANTIBODIES AGAINST mAb BrE-3

Ceriani and colleagues have shown radioimmunolocalization of tumors in breast cancer patients with the BrE-3 mAb. There was negligible localization of radiolabeled BrE-3 in normal tissues or organs (unpublished data). We have used BrE-3 which is an IgG1k for the production of monoclonal anti-idiotype antibodies. Several Ab2 hybridomas have been obtained which are specific for the immunizing Id of BrE-3 and do not react with isotype or allotype matched immunoglobulins. To determine whether these Ab2 are directed against the antigen binding site (paratope) of BrE-3, the binding of radiolabeled BrE-3 to the breast cancer cell line MCF-7 and SKBR3 was studied in the presence of varying amounts of Ab2 hybridoma culture supernatants. Interestingly, three distinct types of anti-idiotype antibodies have been obtained. For example, mAb 2E1 strongly binds to the Id of BrE-3 (Ab1), but does not inhibit the binding of BrE-3 (Ab1) to the target MCF-7 or SKBR3 cells; whereas anti-Id mAb 7C11 inhibits the reaction partially and mAb 5A12 inhibits the reaction completely. All three Ab2s are being purified from ascites fluid for further characterization. The anti-Id 2E1, which is presumably an $\alpha$-type, should be useful as a second antibody to remove unwanted radioactivity from the circulation during high dose radioimmunotherapy of patients with radiolabeled BrE-3. Clearance studies of $^{111}$In-BrE-3 in MX-1 tumor bearing BALB/c nude mice are currently underway. mAb 5A12 will be injected into two different species (mice and rabbits) to see if it can produce an antigen-specific Ab3 response to determine whether it is an Ab2$\beta$. This mAb2 is a possible candidate for direct Ab2 immunization therapy.

**Table 3.** Percent dose per gram of $^{111}$In BrE-1 in BALB/c Nude Mice with MX-1 Tumor*

| | BrE-1 Control 30 min | BrE-1 + anti-Idiotype 30 min | BrE-1 Control 40 HR | BrE-1 + anti-Idiotype 40 HR |
|---|---|---|---|---|
| Blood | 11.38 ± 1.57 | 6.92 ± 1.74 | 6.01 ± 1.13 | 1.34 ± 0.83 |
| Skin | 2.90 ± 0.36 | 3.11 ± 0.54 | 2.49 ± 0.14 | 2.28 ± 0.39 |
| Muscle | 1.23 ± 0.26 | 1.16 ± 0.16 | 1.00 ± 0.07 | 0.59 ± 0.14 |
| Lung | 7.08 ± 1.33 | 3.43 ± 0.80 | 5.48 ± 0.11 | 0.94 ± 0.35 |
| Kidney | 3.59 ± 0.62 | 2.10 ± 0.31 | 3.27 ± 0.29 | 0.97 ± 0.26 |
| Spleen | 2.66 ± 0.49 | 2.13 ± 0.31 | 2.65 ± 0.03 | 1.35 ± 0.47 |
| Liver | 3.73 ± 0.78 | 8.74 ± 3.33 | 3.63 ± 0.11 | 9.12 ± 1.24 |
| Stomach | 0.87 ± 0.21 | 1.23 ± 0.36 | 0.28 ± 0.10 | 0.57 ± 0.06 |
| Intestine | 1.01 ± 0.16 | 0.81 ± 0.02 | 0.80 ± 0.03 | 0.46 ± 0.07 |
| Bone | 1.02 ± 0.12 | 0.84 ± 0.07 | 0.75 ± 0.02 | 0.26 ± 0.04 |
| Marrow | 3.05 ± 0.50 | 1.51 ± 0.17 | 1.83 ± 0.66 | 1.16 ± 0.09 |
| Tumor | 3.28 ± 0.22 | 4.13 ± 0.66 | 4.35 ± 0.27 | 2.51 ± 0.36 |

Each mouse was injected with 20 $\mu$Ci of 2.9 $\mu$g of $^{111}$In-BrE-1. After 24 hrs, 20 $\mu$g of anti-Id 11D10 was injected to one group of mice to be sacrificed at 30 min and another group at 40 hrs. Control mice at 30 min and 40 hrs were uninjected with 11D10.
*Values are expressed as mean % SEM.

## CONCLUSION

In summary, it is our aim to evaluate rationally designed idiotype-based anti-tumor therapies. We are developing monoclonal anti-idiotype antibodies (Ab2) against several different human TAA antibodies (Ab1) and screening them to identify the potential Ab2 candidates which can be used as antigen substitutes for the induction of therapeutic immunity in cancer patients. We have already generated monoclonal idiotypic cascades for three different human tumor-associated antigens. The first cascade originated from a T cell leukemia/lymphoma (21,22), the other from carcinoembryonic antigen (CEA) (23,24) and the third for breast TAA. Recently we have started a Phase I clinical trial with human cutaneous T cell lymphoma and obtained some encouraging results (25). Promising results have also been obtained in clinical trials of melanoma (26,27) and colorectal carcinoma patients (28). Human therapeutic trials with anti-idiotype antibodies are still in the very early stages and its clinical applicability in man remains to be determined.

## Acknowledgements

We thank Susan Morey and Farida Vargas for excellent technical assistance and Cheryl Zuber for typing of the manuscript.
This work was supported in part by NIH Grants RO1 CA 47860, CA 56701, PO1 CA 59306 and CRF Grant PO1 CA42767.

# REFERENCES

1. E. Debus, R. Moll, W.W. Frank, K. Weber, and M. Osborn. Immunohistochemical distinction of human carcinomas by cytokeratin typing with monoclonal antibodies. Am. J. Pathol. 114:121 (1984).

2. A.M. Gown and A.M. Vogel. Monoclonal antibodies to human intermediate filament proteins. III. Analysis of tumors. Am. J. Clin. Pathol. 84:413-424 (1985).

3. G. Pancino, C. Charpin, F. Calvo, M.C. Guillemin, and A. Roseto. A novel monoclonal antibody (7B10) with differential reactivity between human mammary carcinoma and normal breast. Cancer Res. 47:4444-4452 (1987).

4. D.P. Edwards, K.T. Grzyb, L.G. Dressler, R.E. Mansel, D.T. Zava, G.W. Sledge, Jr., and M.L. McGuire. Monoclonal antibody identification and characterization of a MW 43,000 membrane glycoprotein associated with human breast cancer. Cancer Res. 46:1306-1317 (1986).

5. C.A. White, R. Dulbecc, R. Allen, M. Bowman, and B. Armstrong. Two monoclonal antibodies selective for human mammary carcinoma. Cancer Res. 45:1337-1343 (1985).

6. R.L. Ceriani and E.H. Rosenbaum. Breast epithelial antigens in the circulations of breast cancer patients. Immunol. Ser. 53:223-241 (1990).

7. A.D. Thor and S.M. Edgerton. Monoclonal antibodies reactive with human breast or ovarian carcinoma: *in vivo* applications. Semin. Nucl. Med. 19:295-308 (1989).

8. R.L. Ceriani, J.A. Peterson, J.Y. Lee, R. Moncada and E.W. Blank. Characterization of cell surface antigens of human mammary epithelial cells with monoclonal antibodies prepared against human milk fat globule. Somatic Cell Genetics 9:415-427 (1983).

9. J. Taylor-Papadimitriou, J.A. Peterson, J. Arklie, J. Burchell, R.L. Ceriani, and W.F. Bodmer. Monoclonal antibodies to epithelium specific components of the human milk fat globule membrane: production and reaction with cells in culture. Int. J. Cancer 28: 17-21 (1981).

10. N.K. Jerne. Towards a network theory of the immune system. Ann. Immunol. 125C:373-389 (1974).

11. A. Nisonoff and E. Lamoyi. Implications of the presence of an internal image of the antigen in anti-idiotypic antibodies: possible application to vaccine production. Clin. Immunol. Immunopathol. 21:397-406 (1981).

12. H. Kohler, S. Muller, and C. Bona. Internal antigen and the immune network. Proc. Soc. Exp. Biol. Med. 178:189-193 (1985).

13. N.K. Jerne, J. Roland, and A. Cazenave. Recurrent idiotypes and internal images. EMBO J. 1:243-248 (1982).

14. C.A. Bona, and H. Kohler. Anti-idiotpic antibodies and internal images. In: Probes for Receptor Structure and Function, Vol. 4, edited by J.C. Venter, C.M. Fraser and J. Lindstrom, New York: Alan R. Liss, 141-150 (1984).

15. H. Kohler, T. Kieber-Emmons, S. Srinivasan, S. Kaveri, W.J.W. Morrow, S. Muller, C. Kang, and S. Raychaudhuri. Revised immune network concepts. Clin. Immunol. Immunopath. 52:104-116 (1989).

16. S.E. Order, G.B. Stillwagon, J.L. Klein, *et al*. Iodine-131-antiferritin, a new treatment modality in hepatomas: a radiation therapy oncology group study. J. Clin. Oncol. 3:1573-1582 (1984).

17. R.E. Lenard, S.E. Order, J.J. Spunberg, S.O. Asbell, and D.A. Leibel. Isotopic immunoglobulin: a new systemic therapy for advanced Hodgkin's disease. J. Clin. Oncol. 3:1296-1300 (1985).

18. S.M. Larson, J.A. Carrasquillo, K.A. Krohn, *et al*. Localization of I-131-labeled p97 specific Fab fragments in human melanomas as a basis for radiotherapy. J. Clin. Invest. 72:2101-2114 (1983).

19. S.J. DeNardo, L.F. O'Grady, G.L. DeNardo, S.L. Mills, and D.J. Macey. Radioimmunotherapy of lymphoproliferative disease. Blood 72:241 (1988) (abstract).

20. S. Rosen, A.M. Zimmer, R. Goldman-Neiken, *et al*. Radioimmunodetection and radioimmunotherapy of cutaneous T cell lymphomas using an I-131-labeled monoclonal antibody: An Illinois Cancer Council Study. J. Clin. Oncol. 5:562-573 (1987).

21. M. Bhattacharya-Chatterjee, M.W. Pride, B.K. Seon, and H. Kohler. Idiotype vaccines against human T cell acute lymphoblastic leukemia (T-ALL). I. Generation and characterizations of biologically active monoclonal anti-idiotopes. J. Immunol. 139:1354-1360 (1987).

22. M. Bhattacharya-Chatterjee, S.K. Chatterjee, S. Vasile, B.K. Seon, and H. Kohler. Idiotype vaccines against human T cell leukemia. II. Generation and characterization of a monoclonal idiotype cascade (Ab1, Ab2 and Ab3). J. Immunol. 141:1398-1403 (1988).

23. M. Bhattacharya-Chatterjee, S. Mukerjee, W. Biddle, K.A. Foon, and H. Kohler. Murine monoclonal anti-idiotype antibody as a potential network antigen for human carcinoembryonic antigen. J. Immunol. 145:2758-2765 (1990).

24. M. Bhattacharya-Chatterjee, K.A. Foon, and H. Kohler. Anti-idiotype monoclonal antibodies as vaccines for human cancer. Intern. Rev. Immunol. 7: 289-302 (1991).

25. K.A. Foon, L. Vaickus, A. Oseroff, H. Stoll, E. Mrozek, D. Russel, H. Kohler, and M. Chatterjee. Clinical response to anti-idiotype monoclonal antibody vaccine therapy for patients with cutaneous T cell lymphoma. 34th Annual Meeting, Am. Soc. Hematol. 1992 [Abstract].

26. A. Mittelman, Z.J. Chen, T. Kageshita, H. Yang, M. Yamada, P. Baskind, N. Goldberg, C. Puccio, T. Ahmed, Z. Arlin, and S. Ferrone. Active specific immunotherapy in patients with melanoma: A clinical trial with murine anti-idiotypic monoclonal antibodies elicited with syngeneic anti-high-molecular weight melanoma-associated antigen monoclonal antibodies. J. Clin. Invest. 86:2136-2144 (1990).

27. A. Mittelman, Z.J. Chen, H. Yang, G. Wong, and S. Ferrone. Human high molecular weight melanoma-associated antigen (HMW-MAA) mimicry by mouse anti-idiotypic monoclonal antibody MK2-23: Induction of humoral anti-HMW-MAA immunity and prolongation of survival in patients with stage IV melanoma. Proc. Natl. Acad. Sci. USA 89:466-470 (1992).

28. D. Herlyn, M. Wettendorf, E. Schmoll, D. Hopoulos, I. Schedel, U. Dreikhausen, R. Raab, A.H. Ross, H. Jaksche, M. Scriba, and H. Koprowski. Anti-idiotype immunization of cancer patients: Modulation of immune response. Proc. Natl. Acad. Sci. USA 84:8055-8059 (1987).

# THE SIMULTANEOUS EXPRESSION OF c-erbB-2 ONCOPROTEIN AND LAMININ RECEPTOR ON PRIMARY BREAST TUMORS HAS A PREDICTING POTENTIAL ANALOGOUS TO THAT OF THE LYMPH NODE STATUS

Maria I. Colnaghi

Experimental Oncology E
Istituto Nazionale Tumori
20133 Milan, Italy

## INTRODUCTION

Over the past 2 decades the surgical approach to primary breast carcinoma has changed remarkably, passing from radical mastectomy to quadrantectomy and when possible, to a simple tumorectomy. Nevertheless, the dissection of the axillary nodes has not changed due to the unanimous agreement that the status of axillary lymph nodes is the key criterion for assessing prognosis of breast cancer patients. Clinically uninvolved axillary nodes are always dissected despite the fact that several studies[1-5] have shown the irrelevant therapeutic role of axillary node dissection as a "prophylactic" procedure and that surgery on these nodes is responsible for the vast majority of post surgical complications. However, lymph node dissection is still unavoidable today in order to obtain the prognostic information required to plan the future therapeutical treatment of the patient.

The purpose of this work was to investigate whether the biological characterization of primary tumors, such as the evaluation of the expression of molecules involved in the growth and metastatic potential of the tumor cells, can provide us with prognostic information similar to that obtained from the pathological lymph node status.

To this aim two biological markers have been evaluated and their predicting potential compared to that of lymph node status: the c-erbB-2 (neu) oncogene product and the monomeric laminin receptor (LR)[6].

Neu oncogene is a homologue of the EGF-R[7] and has recently been found to be a receptor for a new growth factor[8]. Several reports indicate that neu overexpression, evaluated as DNA, RNA, or protein content, identifies breast cancer patients with a poor prognosis not only among pathologically lymph node positive patients (N+) but also in N- ones[9-11].

The suggested role in the metastatic processes[12] and the recent finding of its impact on breast cancer survival[13] lead us to evaluate the possible predicting potential of the 67 KD LR.

*Antigen and Antibody Molecular Engineering in Breast Cancer Diagnosis and Treatment,* Edited by R.L. Ceriani, Plenum Press, New York, 1994

Neither neu or LR alone are reported to reach the prognostic power of the lymph node status. Nevertheless, no reports are available in which the expression of both of these markers has been evaluated together in order to verify a possible improvement of their prognostic potential in comparison to the evaluation of either of the two.

## PATIENTS, METHODS AND RESULTS

A series of 1117 primary tumors from breast cancer patients, surgically treated in our Institute from January 1968 to December 1971, with 20 years follow up and without any systemic adjuvant therapy, have been evaluated. Among them 679 patients showed no clinical lymph node involvement. Histologic slides of each patient were reviewed for diagnostic reassessment. Pathologically, 494 of these patients were found to be N-.

The evaluation of the expression of neu and LR was carried out by immunohistochemistry in paraffin sections by avidin-biotin indirect immunoperoxidase assay. A polyclonal antiserum directed against a neu synthetic peptide, kindly provided by Dr. D.J. Slamon (UCLA school of Medicine, CA) was used for the analysis of the oncoprotein overexpression. For LR evaluation we produced a monoclonal antibody designated MLuC5, able to identify the relevant epitope on archivial material[14].

Statistical analysis of differences on survival curves was carried out by resorting to the Cox regression model.

The percentage of neu+ and LR+ cases in this series was 23% and 44% respectively. In relation to the lymph node status, the percentage of neu+ and LR+ tumors was respectively 21% and 41% for node-negative patients, versus 24% and 47% for node-positive ones.

**Table 1.** Multivariate analysis of 1117 breast cancer patients

| Criterion | X2 | P. | d.f. | ß | S.E. | R.R. |
|---|---|---|---|---|---|---|
| Axillary lymph.inv. | 82.9 | $10^{-8}$ | 1 | | | |
| N- | | | | -.422 | .048 | 1 |
| N+ | | | | +.422 | - | 2.32 |
| Neu | 15.6 | $8 \times 10^{-5}$ | 1 | | | |
| Negative | | | | -.205 | .050 | 1 |
| Positive | | | | +.205 | - | 1.51 |
| LR | 3.89 | 0.048 | 1 | | | |
| Negative | | | | -.087 | .044 | 1 |
| Positive | | | | +.087 | - | 1.19 |

The univariate analysis showed that lymph node status, neu overexpression and LR expression all significantly affected the patients' survival (P= $10^{-8}$, $2 \times 10^{-5}$ and $6 \times 10^{-3}$ respectively). The multivariate analysis (Table 1) showed that the 3 paramenters were independent prognostic factors.

Among the 1117 primary tumors 101 (9%) expressed both neu and LR, 468 (42%) were double negative, 395 (35%) were LR+ and neu- and 153 (14%) LR- and neu+. As reported in Fig. 1, patients with double positive tumors had a significantly poorer survival in comparison to patients with double negative tumors.

Patients with tumors positive for either LR or neu had an intermediate survival with a poorer prognosis for neu+ LR- patients versus neu- LR+ patients.

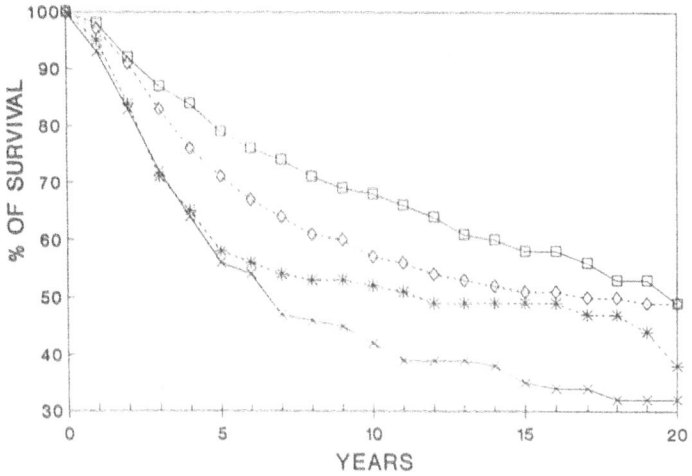

**Figure 1.** Survival of 1117 breast cancer patients according to neu and LR expression on the primary tumor: —☐— LR- NEU- (468); —✗—LR+ NEU+ (101);- ◇- -LR+ NEU- (395);- ✻- -LR- NEU+ (153).

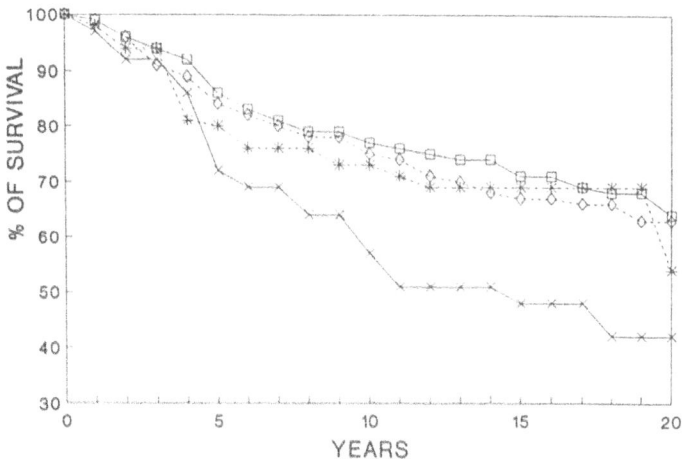

**Figure 2.** Survival of 494 N- breast cancer patients according to neu and LR expression on the primary tumor: —☐— LR- NEU- (226); —✗—LR+ NEU+ (38);- ◇- -LR+ NEU- (163);- ✻- -LR- NEU+ (67).

The survival of patients according to neu and LR was evaluated in 494 N- patients. In these patients, in absence of LR expression, the survivals of neu+ and neu- patients were superimposable, whereas when the tumors were LR+ the overexpression of neu was associated with a poorer prognosis (Fig. 2).

Therefore, the tumor positivity for both markers allows the identification of a subgroup of N- patients with a bad prognosis.

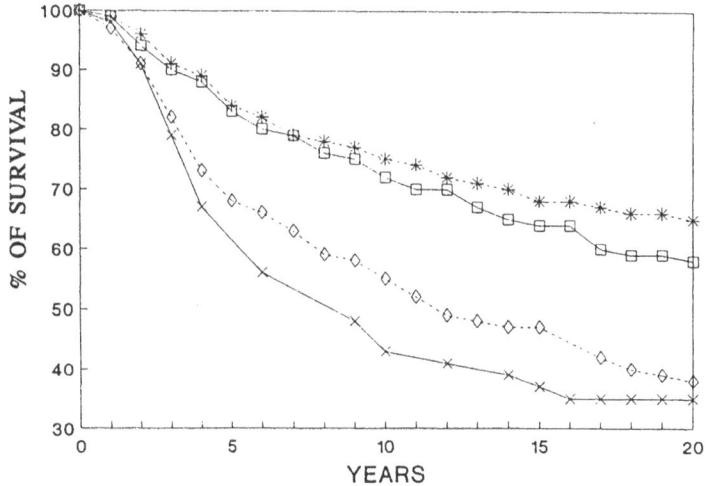

**Figure 3.** Survival of 679 No breast cancer patients according to neu and LR expression on the primary tumor or nodal status:—☐—LR-NEU- (308);—✕—LR+ NEU+ (54);- ✳ -N- (376);- ◇ -N+ (303).

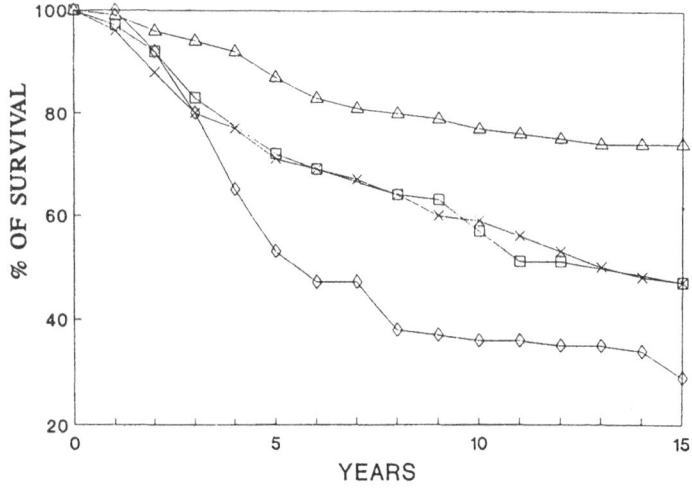

**Figure 4.** Survival of 569 breast cancer patients according to neu and LR expression on the primary tumor and nodal status: —△—LR- NEU- N- (226); —◇—LR+ NEU+ N+ (63); —✕—LR- NEU- N+ (242); —☐— LR+ NEU+ N- (38).

The predicting potential of the pathological assessment of the lymph node status versus the evaluation of the two markers on primary tumors was compared in the group of 679 patients with clinically uninvolved lymph nodes.

As depicted in Fig. 3, the survival of patients with double negative tumors was analogous to the survival of N- patients, whereas the survival of patients with double positive tumors was even worse than that of N+ patients.

Furthermore, the evaluation of the survival according to marker expression and lymph node status allowed the identification of subsets of N+ and N- patients with identical prognosis depending on neu and LR expression. In fact, the survival curves of N- double positive patients and N+ double negative ones are superimposable (Fig. 4).

## DISCUSSION

Our results demonstrated that the biological characterization of the primary tumors was not only superior to the clinical prognostic power and reached a predicting potential analogous to that obtained after microscopic node examination, but also gave additional prognostic information to that obtained by pathologic lymph node evaluation.

In fact, by evaluation of the two markers in the series of 1117 breast cancer examined, subgroups with a different disease aggressiveness among each of the two conventional N- and N+ groups were identified. It was indeed possible to identify N-patients (those positive for both neu and LR) with a prognosis analogous to that of N+ patients (those negative for both markers) as well as N+ patients (those positive for both markers) with a very severe prognosis.

These findings gave a preliminary indication of a future possibility of avoiding node dissection in given subsets of patients according to the marker evaluation of the primary tumor.

## REFERENCES

1. Cancer research campaign (King's/Cambridge) trial for early breast cancer. A detailed update at the tenth year. Cancer Research Campaign Working Party, *Lancet* 1:55 (1980).
2. B. Fisher, N. Wolmark, C. Redmond, M. Deutsch, and E.R. Fisher, Findings from NSABP B-04: Comparison of radical mastectomy with alternative treatments. II. The clinical and biologic significance of medical-central breast cancer, *Cancer* 48:1863 (1981).
3. B. Fisher. A critical commentary on the evaluation of breast cancer surgery. in: *Clinical Trials in Cancer Medicine*, eds. U. Veronesi and G. Bonadonna. Ac.Press Inc., (1985).
4. B. Fisher, C. Redmond, E.R. Fisher, M. Bauer, N. Wolmark, L. Wicherham, M. Deutsch, E. Montague, R. Margolese, and R. Foster, Ten-year resulys of a randomized clinical trial comparing radical mastectomy and total mastectomy with or without radiation, *N. Engl. J. Med.* 312:674 (1985).
5. J.P. Lythgoe, I. Leck, and R. Swindell, Manchester regional breast study. Preliminary results, *Lancet* 1:744 (1978).
6. N. Cascinelli, M.I. Colnaghi, F. Rilke, S. Ménard, R. Bufalino, S. Andreola, M. Greco, L. Mascheroni, and A. Testori, Comparison of the prognostic information of breast cancer patients given by histologic examination of axillary nodes and evaluation of two biological indicators on primary tumor, *Submitted* (1992).

7. W.J. Gullick, 4. The role of the epidermal growth factor receptor and the c-erbB-2 protein in breast cancer, *Int. J. Cancer* 46 Suppl. 5:55 (1990).

8. E. Peles, S.S. Bacus, R.A. Koski, H.S. Lu, D. Wen, S.G. Ogden, R. Ben Levy, and Y. Yarden, Isolation of the neu/HER-2 stimulatory ligand: A 44 kd glycoprotein that induces differentiation of mammary tumor cells, *Cell* 69:205 (1992).

9. T.J. Perren, c-*erb*B-2 oncogene as a prognostic marker in breast cancer, *Br. J. Cancer* 63:328 (1991).

10. W.J. Gullick, S.B. Love, C. Wright, D.M. Barnes, B. Gusterson, A.L. Harris, and D.G. Altman, c-*erb*B-2 protein overexpression in breast cancer is a risk factor in patients with involved and uninvolved lymph nodes, *Br. J. Cancer* 63:434 (1991).

11. F. Rilke, M.I. Colnaghi, N. Cascinelli, S. Andreola, M.T. Baldini, R. Bufalino, G. Della Porta, S. Ménard, M.A. Pierotti, and A. Testori, Prognostic significance of HER-2/*neu* expression in breast cancer and its relationship to other prognostic factors, *Int. J. Cancer* 49:44 (1991).

12. V. Castronovo, C. Colin, A.P. Claysmith, P.H.S. Chen, E. Lifrange, R. Lambotte, H. Krutzsch, L.A. Liotta, and M.E. Sobel, Immunodetection of the metastasis-associated laminin receptor in human breast cancer cells obtained by fine-needle aspiration biopsy, *Am. J. Pathol.* 137:(1990).

13. S. Martignone, S. Ménard, R. Bufalino, N. Cascinelli, R. Pellegrini, E. Tagliabue, S. Andreola, F. Rilke, and M.I. Colnaghi, Prognostic significance of the 67 KDa laminin receptor expression in breast carcinomas, *Submitted* (1992).

14. S. Martignone, R. Pellegrini, E. Villa, N.N. Tandon, A. Mastroianni, E. Tagliabue, S. Ménard, and M.I. Colnaghi, Characterization of two monoclonal antibodies directed against the 67KDa high affinity laminin receptor and application for the study of breast carcinoma progression, *Clin. Exp. Metast.* In press (1992).

# MULTIVARIATE PROGNOSTIC MODEL FOR INFILTRATING DUCTAL CARCINOMA OF THE BREAST IN THE AXILLARY NODE-FREE PATIENT

Roberto L. Ceriani[1], Frank Baratta[1], Ramon J. Gaslonde[1], Carolyn M. De Rosa[2], and Luciano Ozzello[2]

[1]Cancer Research Fund of Contra Costa
2055 N. Broadway
Walnut Creek, CA 94596

[2]College of Physicians and Surgeons, Columbia University
New York, NY 10032

## INTRODUCTION

Antigens present on the human milk fat globule (HMFG) were originally detected with a polyclonal antibody[1], that identified several specific breast glycoproteins[2], some of them later detected in the sera of breast cancer patients[3]. Later, monoclonal antibodies (MoAbs) we created against HMFG first identified a heavy molecular weight glycoprotein[4], later called the breast epithelial mucin. This molecule, recently sequenced[5] possesses heterogeneous amino and carboxyterminal moieties linked by a central moiety constituted by a dodecamer tandem repeat. This tandem repeat sequence is the area of the molecule to which all anti-breast mucin MoAbs are directed to[6] (also see article by Peterson et al, in this publication). The reason for the differential specificity of these anti-mucin MoAbs could be ascribed to diverse glycosylation at the core of these tandem repeat sequences[6].

In previous work[7] a series of anti-mucin MoAbs were created by us. As it was later recognized[6,8] some of these MoAbs bound mucin epitopes with considerable carbohydrate participation to its structure and others (like MoAb BrE-3) bound to an epitope constituted by an unglycosylated peptide sequence. Further, MoAb BrE-3 was shown to be expressed weakly if at all on the normal breast epithelium, but strongly in most breast carcinomas[7,9]. These particular characteristics of this MoAb seemed to indicate that this MoAb binds less glycosylated and hence less mature

*Antigen and Antibody Molecular Engineering in Breast Cancer Diagnosis and Treatment*, Edited by R.L. Ceriani, Plenum Press, New York, 1994

155

forms of the mucin. For this reason, MoAb BrE-3 was chosen to be used in breast cancer prognostic studies.

In a recent paper[10], we established that the epitope of MoAb BrE-3 constitutes a valuable prognostic marker for breast cancer prognosis in patients with infiltrating ductal carcinomas (IDCs) of the breast. (The latter comprise between 80-90% of the carcinomas found at the initial histopathological diagnosis). In this work[10] paraffin-embedded sections of primary lesions of 227 IDCs were immunostained by the immunoperoxidase technique using MoAb BrE-3 as the primary MoAb, and a precise scoring system was developed[10] and tested. This scoring system[10] consisted in measuring the extent of membrane and cytoplasmic binding of BrE-3 to the sections both at the level of intensity and prevalence. Thus, 4 scores were obtained for the expression of the BrE-3 epitope: Membrane intensity (MI), membrane prevalence (MP), cytoplasmic intensity (CI), and cytoplasmic prevalence (CP).

The histopathological scores for the IDCs were then subjected to statistical analysis[10]. It was found both by univariate and multivariate analysis that all of these 4 scores are significantly associated in IDCs with risk for survival time (ST) and relapse time (RT). In addition, the use of this 4-score analysis was enlarged with the addition of traditional variables such as age at diagnosis, histological grade of differentiation of the IDC, axillary lymph node invasion, estrogen receptor status and tumor size. The multivariate analysis performed incorporating the 4-score and traditional variables, demonstrated that the 4-score variables are clearly associated with risk in IDC even in the presence of the traditional variables. The 4-score variables provided non-redundant information to tumor size and axillary node-status (two traditional variables were significantly associated with risk in this study), and all together these constituted a composite prognostic score. These chosen significant variables were used in a Kaplan-Meyer survival analysis that helped to indentify 4 distinct subgroups in terms of survival for IDCs.[10] The prognostic score was employed at the individual level and hence called Individual Linear Composite Prognostic Score (ILCPS).[10] This ILCPS can provide (adapting a formulation proposed by Chevallier[11]), an individualized score or risk for each patient. In this fashion it was possible, with the Kaplan-Meyer curves generated in the multivariable analysis of the ILCPS, to assign to each patient a risk for relapse and survival for her breast cancer.

In view of the success in the assessment of risk for survival for IDCs employing the ILCPS, our attention was drawn to the burning issue of risk in the axillary node-free patient. It is in this type of patient where clear-cut prognosis can lead to the justifiable administration of chemotherapy or chemo-prevention or the avoidance of any adjuvant therapy. Traditionally, evaluation of the axillary lymph status by axillary dissection provided a very definite prognostic indication. The subsequent morbidity associated with axillary dissection (recurrent pains and paresthesia, edema of the arm) and noticeable scaring have presented a problem that newer and stronger prognostic indicators could resolve. For this study we chose to study levels of expression of the BrE-3 epitope on membranes and cytoplasm of 130 primary IDCs of axillary-node negative patients with a maximum follow up of 384 months for individual patients and evaluate the relationship of these variables to patient survivability. Initial tumor size in these patients participated with the 4-score for BrE-3 epitope levels in an ILCPS and provided an individual risk function for survival for each patient.

## MATERIALS AND METHODS

### Patient Population

Paraffin-embedded sections containing tissues of 130 patients with infiltrating ductal carcinoma of the breast who had been treated at the John Muir Medical Center in Walnut Creek, CA, from 1976-81, and at Columbia Presbyterian Medical Center, New York, NY, from 1960-78, and that were found to be axillary-node free by surgical dissection at the time of initial surgery for their primary breast carcinoma were included in the study. Breast carcinomas of special histopathological types (such as lobular, or mucinous, or medullary), were excluded from this study. Clinical patient data were stored in dBASE IV files[12].

### Laboratory Procedures

This retrospective study was conducted on blocks of IDCs of the breast without axillary metastases at the time of their initial surgery. They were fixed in formaldehyde fixative, paraffin embedded and kept in the files of the Pathology department at John Muir Medical Center and Columbia Presbyterian Medical Center. An appropriate number of five micron thick sections were obtained from each block and stored until processing. From each patient, one section was stained by H & E stain, and other sections were separated for staining by immunoperoxidase procedures. These included specimens stained with MoAb BrE-3, and others acting as primary antibody-free controls. Murine MoAb BrE-3 is produced by Coulter Immunology, Hialeah, FL. The ABC method was employed for the immunohistopathological staining of sections with MoAb BrE-3.[10]

The grade of differentiation was expressed as one of three levels: "well", "moderate", and "poorly" differentiated. These grade levels were scored by Dr. Luciano Ozzello on hematoxylin and eosin stained slides of the primary IDCs. The grading was done without knowledge of the clinical follow-up or of the immunohistochemical findings using a modification of Bloom and Richardson's criteria.[13] Briefly, "well" differentiated carcinomas exhibited prominent tubular differentiation and were composed of cells with small, uniform nuclei and only occasional mitotic figures. "Moderately" differentiated carcinomas had inconspicuous or no glandular differentiation, nuclei that were larger and more irregular than those of well differentiated tumors, and infrequent mitotic figures. "Poorly" differentiated carcinomas were characterized by no tubular differentiation, large and pleomorphic nuclei, and frequent mitoses.

### Grading and Rating Procedures

The 4-Score Method[10] is used for defining the prevalence and intensity of staining patterns of cytoplasmic and membrane NPGP expression found in the cytoplasm and on the membranes of breast cancer cells in sections of the infiltrating ductal carcinomas. When scoring for prevalence, a "1" is given if 1-33% of the cells exhibit the attribute (MP or CP), a "2" is given if 34-66% of the cells exhibit the attribute, and a "3" is given if 67-100% of the cells exhibit the attribute. For MI or CI, the most intensely stained specimens at the cell membrane or cytoplasmic site are scored "3" and the least intense "1", while "2" corresponded to intermediate intensity. A "0" is given if the sample does not exhibit any discernible level of expression of antigen. Thus, each specimen receives four scores: two for the degree of "prevalence" (CP and MP) of staining and two for the degree of "intensity" of staining (CI and MI), with each score ranging from a lowest score of "0" to a highest score of "3".

To control for and determine the extent of extraneous sources of undue influence in the scoring of the sections, several measures were instituted as reported.[10]

### Research and Statistical Method

A univariate analysis was conducted to determine the prognostic value of seven parameters. Three of these parameters were suggested by research and clinical data: age (AGE), tumor size (TMSZ), grade of differentiation (GRADE); the 4-Score parameters were suggested by preliminary immunohistopathological studies with MoAb BrE-3.[10] These immunohistopathological variables pertain to the intensity and prevalence of staining pattern attributes: cytoplasmic intensity (CI), cytoplasmic prevalence (CP), membrane intensity (MI), and membrane prevalence (MP). Each of these dimensions is measured by a scale where values of "1", "2" and "3" reflect "low", "medium" and "high" levels respectively.

The **SAS Lifetest** procedure[14], a statistical software program, was used to conduct a univariate analysis. The Lifetest employs the **Kaplan-Meier** (product-limit) method for estimating the survival distribution functions[15], and it uses **Greenwood's formula** for the corresponding estimate of the standard error.[16] Also it provides two rank tests, the **Wilcoxon** and **log-rank** tests, for evaluating the homogeneity of survival functions across patient groups which differ with respect to their standing on prognostic variables.[17] The Wilcoxon test gives greater weight to short survival times, whereas the log-rank test places more weight on longer survival times. The Lifetest is ideally suited for analyzing data that may be right-censored and where minimal statistical assumptions need to be made about the survival distribution function.

The variables evaluated in the univariate analysis were then encoded by the criteria already used[10] and **Table 1**, and submitted to a multivariate analysis. The rationale for the encoding procedure was that those factor levels which were associated with the best prognosis in the univariate analysis were given a value of "0". A "1" was given to the group determined to have the next best prognosis and this was continued until all groups were exhausted.[10] Only 90 cases with complete information on the studied variables were included in this analysis, all with all 4-Score values different from 0. Specifically, **Egret,**[18] an epidemiological statistical software program, was used to conduct a **Cox proportional hazards regression model** analysis with a stepwise procedure[19] on these encoded variables. This model provides a semi-parametric way of modelling failure-time data when there are censored observations. It defines an individual's hazard as his or her risk of dying at a given point of time, given that he or she has survived up to this point in time. The probability of recurrence or death is a function of time from diagnosis and the influence of prognostic variables. Additionally, the model assumes that the baseline hazard function is unknown and that the hazard functions for all other covariate patterns are proportional to this baseline. One implication of this assumption is that the effect of a prognostic variable does not change over time. The survival curve of a group associated with a particular level of a prognostic variable, therefore, is assumed to be above (or below) the survival curve of another such group. In its general form, the Cox model links a failure time and a failure/censoring indicator with a set of fixed covariate values.[19]  Egret was used to check the proportionality function of the Cox model.

Once the multivariate evaluations had been completed, a procedure proposed by Chevallier[11] was adapted to arrive at an **Individual Linear Composite of Prognostic Scores (ILCPS)**.[10]  The ILCPS[10] combines the prognostic value or hazard index of the various factors found to be significant in the multivariate analysis. An ILCPS was computed for the set of factors found to be predictive of RT and for those found to be predictive of ST. The equation used was in the form: ILCPS = ß1*A + ß2*B + ß3*C + ..., where ß1, ß2, and ß3 are the regression coefficients generated by the Cox model for the A, B, and C factors which were found to be significant in the multivariate ST and RT analyses. A patient's standing on each of these factors is thus differentially weighted depending on the association each factor has with RT or ST.  Given the manner in which these factors were coded and weighted, a high ILCPS could only mean a poor prognosis.

**Table 1.** Encoding of the 4-Score and traditional variables used for the Cox proportional hazard analysis of node negative patient survival time.

| | | |
|---|---|---|
| Age: | AGE >0 and ≤50, | then 1 |
| | AGE >50 and ≤75, | then 0 |
| | AGE >75, | then 1 |
| Tumor Size: | TMSZ ≥0 and ≤2.5, | then 0 |
| | TMSZ >2.5, | then 1 |
| Grade: | GRADE=P, | then 2 |
| | GRADE=M, | then 1 |
| | GRADE=W, | then 0 |
| CP: | CP=1 or CP=2, | then 0 |
| | CP=3, | then 1 |
| CI: | CI=1 or CI=2, | then 0 |
| | CI=3, | then 1 |
| MP: | MP=1, | then 1 |
| | MP=2 or MP=3, | then 0 |
| MI: | MI=1 or MI=2, | then 1 |
| | MI=3, | then 0 |

Once an ILCPS was calculated for all patients, a distribution histogram was obtained. The points on this distribution which sorted the scores into the most distinct groups were used to form patient groups which were then analyzed using the Lifetest procedure.[14]

This **a posteriori** analysis sought to compare the prognostic value of the 4-Score Method variables with the prognostic value of traditionally used variables in relation to RT and ST. To make this comparison, ILCPS values were determined for three sets of variables: (a) **ILCPS(Trad)**, developed with the traditional variables alone; (b) **ILCPS(4-Score)**[10], developed using the 4-Score variables alone; and (c)

**ILCPS(Comb)**[10] developed using a combination of traditional and 4-Score variables. Kaplan Meier analysis was used to evaluate the association of each of the different sets of ILCPS values with respect to ST and RT. Following this analysis, each set was then reanalyzed using the Cox model with a stepwise procedure to determine which set of variables yielded the ILCPS which was most significantly associated with either RT or ST.

All data processing and statistical analyses were performed on an IBM PS/2 Model 50, IBM PS/2 Model 80, and on a Compaq 386 PC. Each work station thus served to control for potential computer or software artifacts and to cross-validate findings.

## RESULTS

### Patient Population

The average age at diagnosis of the breast cancer patients in this study was 56 years. The average tumor size was 2.7 centimeters in diameter with 60% of all tumors being 2.50 centimeters in diameter or less at time of surgery. All patients did not have axillary dissemination at the start of this study. The grade of differentiation had a distribution where 59% of the tumors were graded "moderate", 18% were graded "poor", and 23% were graded "well".

**Table 2** summarizes the clinical data obtained from the Tumor Board at John Muir Medical Center and Columbia Presbyterian Medical Center. Survival time (ST) was defined to be the period of time in months from the date of diagnosis to the date of death due to breast cancer. Patients who died from causes other than those relating to breast cancer were included for study and data from these records were treated as right-censored cases for evaluation purposes. Relapse time (RT) was defined as the period of time in months from the date of diagnosis to the date at which relapse was clinically identified. Data from patients who were dropped out of the study for reasons other than a breast cancer relapse were considered right censored for these analyses.

Seven parameters (AGE, TMSZ, GRADE and the 4-Score parameters) were used to separate patients into groups to determine the prognostic value of the sorting variable on patient RT and ST. The groups formed for this purpose are listed in **Table 2**. Preliminary analyses on a sample of patients determined the particular levels of each variable which were used to sort patients into different groups. These levels were selected because they maximized the number of observations which could be used for analysis and appeared to be the most discriminating.

### Univariate Analysis

The univariate Kaplan-Meier analysis for ST for each of the variables under study is summarized in **Table 3**. Tumor size of less than 2.5 cm in diameter, a low cytoplasmic prevalence, a low cytoplasmic intensity, a high membrane prevalence and a high membrane intensity are each significantly associated with a good prognosis for ST, **Table 3**. Age at diagnosis and grade of differentiation were not found to be associated with ST. In contrast, none of the variables under study were significantly associated with relapse time in this population.

**Table 2.** Distribution variables in the axillary node-negative patient population.

| | |
|---|---|
| Number of patients | 130 |

**Traditional Variables**

| | |
|---|---|
| Age at diagnosis (AGE) | |
|     1-50 | 45 |
|     51-75 | 75 |
|     >75 | 10 |
| Tumor Size (TMSZ) in cm diameter | |
|     ≤2.5 cm | 75 |
|     >2.5 cm | 50 |
| Grade of differentiation (GRADE) | |
|     Poor | 20 |
|     Moderate | 65 |
|     Well | 26 |

**4-Score Variables**

Cytoplasmic prevalence (CP) of breast epithelial mucin antigen by immunoperoxidase staining with MoAb BrE-3

| | |
|---|---|
| 0 | 5 |
| 1 | 10 |
| 2 | 35 |
| 3 | 78 |

Cytoplasmic intensity (CI) of breast epithelial mucin antigen by immunoperoxidase staining with MoAb BrE-3

| | |
|---|---|
| 0 | 5 |
| 1 | 46 |
| 2 | 60 |
| 3 | 17 |

Membrane prevalence (MP) of breast epithelial mucin antigen by immunoperoxidase staining with MoAb BrE-3

| | |
|---|---|
| 0 | 22 |
| 1 | 45 |
| 2 | 40 |
| 3 | 21 |

Membrane intensity (MI) of breast epithelial mucin antigen by immunoperoxidase staining with MoAb BrE-3

| | |
|---|---|
| 0 | 22 |
| 1 | 4 |
| 2 | 35 |
| 3 | 67 |

Data points from some of the variables are missing due to insufficient record keeping (TMSZ) or were not determinable (GRADE, CP, CI, MP, MI).

## Multivariate Analysis

The variables TMSZ, GRADE, AGE, CP, CI, MP, MI were recorded using the coding scheme shown in **Table 1**. Cox multivariate analysis of these recorded variables determined that TMSZ, CP, CI, MP and MI have a high association with the prediction of ST. AGE and GRADE did not contribute any significant information to the prediction of ST when the other variables were placed in the model first. The results of the Multivariate Cox Analysis of the individual variables are shown in **Table 4**.

## ILCPS Development

β-coefficients determined in the multivariate analysis were used to develop ILCPS values for three sets of variables (**Table 4**): (a) ILCPS(Trad), (b) ILCPS(4-Score), and (c) ILCPS(Comb). Those variables having significant association with ST were included in the development of ILCPS values. The ILCPS(Trad) comprised TMSZ, the ILCPS(4-Score) comprised CP, CI, MP and MI and the ILCPS(comb) comprised TMSZ, CP, CI, MP and MI.

**Table 3.** Summary of Kaplan-Meier univariate analyses of sub-groups of studied variables for survival time (ST) of axillary-node-negative patients. The long-rank test is sensitive to deviations earlier in the study. The Wilcoxon test is sensitive to deviations later in the study.

| Studied Variable | p-value | |
|---|---|---|
| | log-rank | Wilcoxon |
| **Traditional Variables** | | |
| Age at Diagnosis (AGE) (1-50, 51-75, >75) | n.s. | n.s. |
| Tumor Size in cm diameter (TMSZ) (≤2.5 cm, **>2.5 cm**) | <0.01 | <0.01 |
| Grade of Differentiation (GRADE) (Poor, Moderate, Well) | n.s. | n.s. |
| **BrE-3 4-Score Method Variables** | | |
| Cytoplasmic Prevalence of breast mucin by MoAb BrE-3 (CP) (1 or 2, **3**) | 0.06 | 0.05 |
| Cytoplasmic Intensity of breast mucin by MoAb BrE-3 (CI) (1 or 2, **3**) | <0.01 | <0.01 |
| Membrane Prevalence of breast mucin by MoAb BrE-3 (MP) (**1**, 2 or 3) | 0.13 | 0.04 |
| Membrane Intensity of breast mucin by MoAb BrE-3 (MI) (1 or **2**, 3) | 0.13 | 0.05 |

n.s. - survival curves for the studied strata within the variable group do not significantly differ at the p<0.05 level.
Boldface strata were determined to be the worst prognostic group.

For encoding for the Cox multivariate analysis, those strata within a variable which was considered to have the best prognosis were given a 0. The strata with the next best prognosis was given a 1, and this was continued until all strata were exhausted.

The ILCPS(Trad) which was significantly associated with the prediction of ST (**Table 4**) used the following linear combination of variables: ILCPS(Trad) = (1.4*TMSZ), with observed values ranged from zero (best prognosis) to 1.4 (worst prognosis).

The ILCPS(4-Score) which was significantly associated with the prediction of ST

(**Table 4**) took the following linear form: ILCPS(4-Score) = (2.1*CP) + (1.2*CI) + (1.4*MP) + (0.9*MI). Values for the ILCPS(4-Score) associated with ST range from 0 to 5.6.

When a combination of variables (Traditional and 4-Score) was analyzed (**Table 4**), the linear form ILCPS(Comb) = (1.6*TMSZ) + (1.8*CP) + (1.1*CI) + (1.5*MP) + (1.4*MI) was found to be significantly associated with the prediction of ST. The observed values of the ILCPS(Comb) associated with ST ranges from 0 to 7.4.

**Table 4.** Summary of multivariate Cox Proportional Hazards model analysis using a stepwise procedure evaluating survival time for study variables of axillary-node-negative patients.

| Studied Variable | p-value | Survival Time $\beta$-coefficient | Risk |
|---|---|---|---|
| | | **Traditional Variables Only** | |
| TMSZ | <0.01 | 1.4 | 4.0 |
| GRADE | n.s. | - | - |
| AGE | n.s. | - | - |
| | | **4-Score Method Variables Only** | |
| CP | <0.01 | 2.1 | 8.3 |
| CI | 0.01 | 1.2 | 3.3 |
| MP | <0.01 | 1.4 | 3.9 |
| MI | 0.04 | 0.9 | 2.6 |
| | | **Traditional and 4-Score Variables** | |
| TMSZ | <0.01 | 1.6 | 5.2 |
| GRADE | n.s. | - | - |
| AGE | n.s. | - | - |
| CP | 0.03 | 1.8 | 6.0 |
| CI | 0.03 | 1.1 | 2.9 |
| MP | <0.01 | 1.5 | 4.5 |
| MI | <0.01 | 1.4 | 6.0 |

Kaplan-Meier univariate analysis utilizing the various ILCPS models determined that the ILCPS model has a strong association to ST (**Table 5**). Cutoff points for the different ILCPS models were determined by analysis of distribution histograms for the ILCPS models.

The Kaplan-Meier ST curve based upon risk groups assigned by the combined ß-coefficients of the 4-Score values, or ILCPS(4-Score) was obtained. Three different groups, also with statistically significant different survival distribution functions were identified (not shown).

A traditional variable (TMSZ) participates in the ILCPS(Trad). A Kaplan-Meier analysis (not shown) of the ILCPS(Trad) shows that it can identify 2 risk groups with statistical significance (p < 0.0001) and that visually are clearly separated.

The parameter involved in the ILCPS(Trad) is then merged with those in the ILCPS(4-Score) to create the ILCPS(Comb). With it, a very high statistical significance (p < 0.001) is obtained for ST and the Kaplan-Meier curve (**Figure 1**) based on it shows 4 distinct groups with clear cut different outcomes.

## Comparison of ILCPS Values by Cox Analysis

Cox multivariate analysis of the three ILCPS models were analyzed with respect to ST. This analysis determined that each of the individual models was significantly associated with ST when tested alone. However, the ILCPS(Comb) was the model most significantly associated with ST, and no other model was able to contribute any significant information to the ILCPS(Comb) value when the 3 ILCPS models were tested together (**Table 5**).

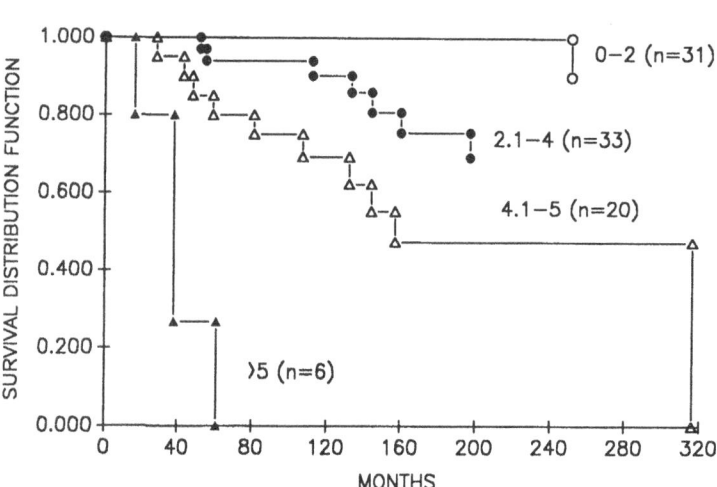

**Figure 1.** Kaplan-Meier survival curve based upon risk groups assigned by the ILCPS(Comb). Lower ILCPS(Comb) values are associated with a better prognosis.

## DISCUSSION

The present work supports our previous findings indicating the ability of the 4-Score method of immunohistopathological prognosis to separate those patients at higher risk among surgically treated axillary node-free breast cancer patients. In addition, it provides a stronger experimental basis to be added to our previous report[10] for the use of the ILCPS(Comb) not only with those parameters studied here, but with many others that can be incorporated in the future. The statistical treatment developed by us for this purpose[10] clearly separates those prognostic markers with significant association with risk for the patient studied and, even as important, eliminates those markers providing redundant information to the other stronger markers participating in the ILCPS(Comb). This latter ability to eliminate redundant input reduces significantly the level of diagnostic indecision provided by the expected variability of markers that can be obtained for each individual patient.

164

**Table 5.** Summary of stepwise analysis of multivariate Cox Proportional Hazards model on the Individual Linear Composite of Prognostic Scores (ILCPS) for patient survival time of axillary-node-negative patients.

| Studied Variable | p-value | Survival Time $\beta$-coefficient | Risk |
|---|---|---|---|
| | | **ILCPS SCORES TESTED INDIVIDUALLY** | |
| ILCPS(TRAD) | <0.01 | 1.4 | 4.0 |
| ILCPS(4-SCORE) | <0.01 | 1.3 | 3.8 |
| ILCPS(COMB) | <0.01 | 1.5 | 4.4 |
| | | **ILCPS SCORES COMPARISON** | |
| ILCPS(COMB) | <0.01 | 1.5 | 4.4 |
| ILCPS(TRAD) | n.s. | - | - |
| ILCPS(4-SCORE) | n.s. | - | - |

ILCPS(TRAD)-->TMSZ
ILCPS(4-SCORE)-->CP, CI, MP, MI
ILCPS(COMB)-->TMSZ, CP, CI, MP, MI

In the present case, both the univariate and multivariate analyses identify immunohistopathological parameters participating in the 4-Score method that have very strong association to ST in the axillary node free-patient. The level of association is comparable to that of TMSZ, which was clearly demonstrated before to be of high prognostic association with survival in the axillary node-free breast cancer patient.[20]

It is significant that in a recent review[21], the integration of available prognostic markers into a panel for the establishment of prognosis in axillary node-free patient is shown to be very desirable. However, a demonstrable useful approach had not yet been employed until then. Our introduction of the ILCPS(Comb) approach[10] bridges this gap and provides a versatile statistical instrument with which to profit from available and forthcoming prognostic factors.

In this study, ILCPS(Comb) could separate 4 groups in the axillary node-free patient population in terms of their association with ST risk. It will be left then to the oncologist to decide as to what level of risk can be sustained without therapeutic intervention. At a practical level, the ILCPS(Comb) score will help the oncologist make this choice as follows: If the 10-year ST is desired for a patient having the following variable standings: TMSZ, >2.5 cm, CP=2, CI=1, MP=2 and MI=2, is calculated by the following formula: ILCPS(Comb) = (1.6 x 1) + (1.8 x 0) + (1.1 x 0) + (1.5 x 0) + (1.4 x 1) = 3.0. This ILCPS(Comb) value places the hypothetical patient in the group corresponding to the ILCPS(Comb) ranging from 2.1 to 4.0. Examination of the Kaplan-Meier plot (Fig. 1) corresponding to the ILCPS(Comb) with respect to ST indicates that the probability of survival at 10 years is 90%. This can be compared to the probability of survival at 10 years for the other groups, which is 100%, 69% and 0% respectively. The reliability of this prognostic procedure will be greatest when the analysis referenced in Figure 1 is based on a larger sample than the one for this pilot study.

A better understanding of the use of comparative statistical analysis will open the door to more accurate prognosis on an individualized patient basis. The small number of axillary node-free patients to which this model has been applied with success suggests that as larger patient numbers could be studied, it will be possible to establish these findings and approaches as valuable and providing a sound basis for the individual analysis of risk for the axillary node-free patient.

The demonstrated validity of the 4-Score method for assessment of risk in the axillary node-free breast cancer patient, and its higher association with risk when added to TMSZ to compose the ILCPS(Comb)[10], provides the surgical pathologist an economical and easy to perform procedure. Results of the 4-Score method in the present analytical set up can be integrated with other prognostic markers available with relative ease. Therefore, these results indicate the need for the extension of these studies into a larger retrospective study and eventually into a prospective one.

## REFERENCES

1. R.L. Ceriani, K.E. Thompson, J.A. Peterson, and S. Abraham, Surface differentiation antigens of human mammary epithelial cells carried on the human milk fat globule. Proc. Nat. Acad. Sci. USA, 74:582-586 (1977).

2. M. Sasaki, J.A. Peterson, and R.L. Ceriani, Quantitation of human mammary epithelial antigens in cells cultured from normal and cancerous breast tissues. In Vitro, 17:150-158 (1981).

3. R.L. Ceriani, M. Sasaki, H. Sussman, W.M. Wara, and E.W. Blank, Circulating human mammary epithelial antigens in breast cancer. Proc. Natl. Acad. Sci. USA, 79:5420-5424 (1982).

4. R.L. Ceriani, J.A. Peterson, J.Y. Lee, R. Moncada, and E.W. Blank, Characterization of cell surface antigens of human mammary epithelial cells with monoclonal antibodies prepared against human milk fat globule. Somat. Cell Genet., 9:415-427, 1983.

5. M.J.L. Ligtenberg, H.L. Voss, A.M.C. Gennisen, and J. Hilkens, A carcinoma associated mucin is generated by a polymorphic gene encoding splice variants with alternative amino termini. J. Biol. Chem. 265:5573-5578 (1990).

6. J.A. Peterson, D. Larocca, G. Walkup, R. Amiya, and R.L. Ceriani, Molecular analysis of epitopic heterogeneity of the breast mucin NPGP, in: Breast Epithelial Antigens: Molecular Biology to Clinical Applications. R.L. Ceriani ed., Plenum Publishing, New York, (1991).

7. J.A. Peterson, D.T. Zava, A.K. Duwe, E.W. Blank, H. Battifora, and R.L. Ceriani, Biochemical and histological characterization of antigens preferentially expressed on the surface and cytoplasm of breast carcinoma cells identified by monoclonal antibodies against human milk fat globule. Hybridoma, 9:221-235 (1990).

8. R.L. Ceriani, J.A. Peterson, E.W. Blank, and D. Lamport, Epitope expression on the breast epithelial mucin. Breast Cancer Res. Treat., 24:103-113 (1992).

9. E.W. Blank, K.D. Pant, C.M. Chan, J.A. Peterson, and R.L. Ceriani, A novel anti-breast epithelial mucin MoAb (BrE-3). Characterization and experimental biodistribution and immunotherapy. Cancer J., 5:38-44 (1992).

10. R.L. Ceriani, C.M. Chan, F.S. Baratta, L. Ozzello, C.M. DeRosa, and D.V. Habif, Levels of Expression of breast epithelial mucin detected by monoclonal antibody BrE-3 in breast cancer prognosis. Intl. J. Cancer, 51:343-354 (1992).

11. B. Chevallier, V. Mosseri, J.P. Dauce, P. Bastit, J.P. Julien, and B. Asselain, A prognostic score in histological node-negative breast cancer. Br. J. Cancer 61:436-440 (1990).

12. Ashton Tate Corp. Dbase IV, Ashton Tate Corp, Torrance CA (1988).

13. H.J.G. Bloom and W.W. Richardson, Histological grading and prognosis in breast cancer. Brit. J. Cancer 11:359-366 (1957).

14. SAS Institute Inc. The Lifetest Procedure. SAS Technical Report: P-179, Additional SAS/STAT Procedures, Release 6.03. SAS Institute Inc., Cary NC, (1988).

15. E.L. Kaplan, P. Meier, Nonparametric estimation form incomplete observations. J. Am. Statist. Assn. 53:457-481 (1958).

16. M. Greenwood. The natural duration of cancer, *in:* "Reports on Public Health of Medical Subjects," Her Majesty's Station Office, London (1926).

17. J.D. Kalbfleish and R.L. Prentice, The statistical analysis of failure time data, John Wiley and Sons, New York (1980).

18. Statistics and Epidemiology Research Corporation Egret. Statistics and Epidemiology Research Corporation, Seattle WA (1990).

19. D.R. Cox and D. Oakes, Analysis of survival data, *in:* Monographs on Statistics and Applied Probability. Chapman and Hall, New York (1988).

20. B. Fisher, N.H. Slack, I.D.J. Bross, et al, Cancer of the breast: size of neoplasm and prognosis. Surg. Gynecol. Obstet. 163:1311-1316 (1986).

21. W.L. McGuire, A.K. Tandon, D.C. Allred, G.C. Chamness, and G.M. Clark, How to use prognostic factors in axillary node negative breast cancer patients. J. Nat. Cancer Inst. 82:1006-1015 (1990).

# THE USE OF MONOCLONAL ANTIBODY IMMUNOCONJUGATES IN CANCER THERAPY

Geoffrey A. Pietersz, Kenia Krauer, and Ian F.C. McKenzie

The Austin Research Institute
The Austin Hospital
Studley Road
Heidelberg VIC 3084
Australia

## INTRODUCTION

The conventional therapeutic approaches to breast cancer, including surgery, radiotherapy and cytotoxic drugs, has led to a certain degree of responsiveness which has not significantly changed in the last 20 years. Because of the high incidence of breast cancer, there is a real need to use additional forms of therapy which could potentially lead to a cure of this disease. In this light, new therapeutic approaches using antibodies (either alone or as immunoconjugates as discussed herein), or antigen (as in vaccination procedures) are receiving close attention. The current status of vaccines for breast cancer is considered elsewhere in this volume, and here we review the use of antibody based therapy. It should be noted that while antibodies are discussed in this chapter as a means of conveying toxic moieties to tumors, other carriers such as serum proteins (eg transferrin), cytokines (eg. IL-2) and other moieties have been used; these have been reviewed elsewhere[1]. At this time, there is some pessimism regarding the value of antibody immunoconjugates for the therapy of cancer, and at the outset we would like to dispel this pessimism for the following reasons: a) few, if any trials have progressed beyond Phase I/II and a formal comparison with other modes of therapy has not been done; b) as these are early studies, most of the patients used for therapeutic purposes had very large lesions and it would be most unlikely that complete responses could be obtained (as will be discussed below, it is our belief that immunoconjugates will find a place, and control the treatment of small metastic deposits arising from the treatment of large volume disease); c) the treatment of solid tumors usually has to be curtailed because of the occurrence of human anti-mouse antibody (HAMA) responses, and the maximum tolerated dose of immunoconjugate has rarely been achieved.

*Antigen and Antibody Molecular Engineering in Breast Cancer Diagnosis and Treatment*, Edited by R.L. Ceriani, Plenum Press, New York, 1994

169

It is our belief that immunoconjugates do and will work. In a simple experiment we used ricin conjugated to whole antibody, the conjugation being performed under circumstances which led to the B chain being blocked and at least *in vitro*, the conjugate was entirely specific for the cancer cells[2]. This highly toxic compound was injected directly into subcutaneous tumors in mice and within a few days these had disappeared; by contrast, the same immunoconjugate injected into tumors which were non-reactive grew progressively[3]. The point of this experiment was that *if a specific antibody containing a highly toxic moiety is delivered to the appropriate site, then large tumors can be eradicated.* The key features of this simple experiment were: a) specificity of the antibody; b) using a highly toxic immunoconjugate containing ricin; and c) having sufficient amount of material in the right place; if these three moieties could be put into clinical practice, there is no reason why immunoconjugates should not be a powerful new immunotherapeutic tool. This review will describe the use of monoclonal antibodies alone for therapy, and the use of immunoconjugates containing isotopes, drugs, toxins and enzymes with a focus particularly on drug-antibody conjugates, as we have had the most experience with these. The use of toxin and enzyme-antibody conjugates is reviewed elsewhere[4,5], and isotope-antibodies in breast cancer are discussed elsewhere in this volume. We note that in breast cancer few preclinical studies have been performed, and virtually no formal clinical trials with drug, enzyme or toxin-antibody immunoconjugates. The review will therefore refer to data accrued from other cancers.

## THE USE OF ANTIBODIES ALONE FOR THERAPY

For an antibody to be an effective therapeutic agent, it should have some persistence in the circulation, reach the target and at that site, invoke the usual secondary mechanisms which lead to either cell lysis or phagocytosis including complement fixation and ADCC. The most effective antibodies are those that react with a high density of antigen on the target, leading to the binding of greater amounts of complement and evoking greater phagocytosis or possibly cell lysis. With the exception of the OKT3 antibody[6] (used successfully in transplantation) and of the Campath 1 rat antibody[7], murine monoclonal antibodies used alone have failed to have any therapeutic effect as they satisfied few of the criteria listed above. In general, murine antibodies in humans have a short half life, little reaches the tumor, they have poor biological activity, they may have poor specificity and for solid tumors (but not usually lymphoma), the human anti-mouse or HAMA response occurs within a few days leading either to serum sickness, but also preventing the immunoconjugate reaching its target. At this time, we can state fairly categorically that murine antibodies used alone for the treatment of cancers, such as breast cancer, have been a failure and should not be used.

**Table 1.** Problems with murine monoclonal antibodies as therapeutic agents for cancer.

| Problem | Solution |
|---|---|
| • Short 1/2 life | - human Mab[1] |
| • <1-2% in tumors | - human Mab<br>- improve access |
| • Poor biological activity<br>(complement; ADCC) | - human Mab<br>- immunconjugates[2] |
| • HAMA | - human Mab |
| • Poor specificity | - improved selection [1] |

[1]see elsewhere in the volume
[2]discussed herein

The solutions to these problems (Table 1) are to use human antibodies and/or immunoconjugates. The human antibodies will have an improved half-life, more should reach the tumor, they should activate the appropriate inflammatory response and the HAMA response should be greatly reduced. The use of murine antibody based immunoconjugates will suffer from a number of these problems, but will have appropriate activity. At this time, most of the murine antibody based studies are either winding down or being completed while awaiting the production of chimaeric, CDR-grafted or totally human antibodies, and in essence, the clinical use of immunoconjugates is "marking time" while the appropriate tests are done with these new antibodies prior to using them either alone or as immunoconjugates. Indeed, in our laboratory, we are now performing comparative studies with murine and chimaeric anti-MUC1 antibodies. The production and use of chimaeric small totally human antibodies is described elsewhere in this volume and includes variations such as bispecific antibodies.

## MUC1 AS A TARGET FOR ANTIBODY AND ANTIBODY-DRUG IMMUNOCONJUGATES

We have recently performed preclinical studies using Idarubicin-BC2 (anti-MUC1) antibodies for the therapy of MUC1+ 3T3 cells (obtained from Dr D Wreschner). In contrast to other antibodies and other systems (eg. CEA, Ly-2, Ly-3, transferrin receptor), the Idarubicin-antibody conjugate had little activity *in vivo*. Further studies revealed that: a) the BC2 antibody bound satisfactorily, *in vitro*, at 4°C and indeed, *in vitro* the Idarubicin-antibody conjugate was active; b) at 37°C *in vitro* ~70-80% of the antibody dissociated from the cell surface and only 20% of cell bound BC2 was internalised. By contrast, using the transferrin receptor as a target ~80% of the antibody was internalised; c) the binding affinity of the antibody decreased dramatically at 37°C.

At present, we have reservations regarding MUC1 as a suitable target for antibody based therapy. Perhaps with very high affinity antibodies there will be better internalisation of the drug or toxin. However, the nature of the MUC1 molecule is such that it tends to cycle through the endoplasmic reticulum rather than to lysosomes - and cleavage of immunoconjugates may not occur. Possibly MUC1 will be a suitable target for agents that do not require internalisation such as enzymes and isotopes.

In a different study, using MUC1+ 3T3 cells, we tested the effects of antibody together with complement on the growth and survival of tumors in BALB/c mice. The murine BC2 antibody was entirely without effect - a not surprising finding given usually lack of effect of murine antibodies in mice. The addition of complement did nothing to this even though the antibody was able to fix complement. When a chimaeric cBC2γ1 antibody was used there was still no effect on the tumors (early results). These studies indicate that MUC1 may not be a suitable target for antibodies. Thus, in most cases, antibodies will need to be "armed" with either isotopes, drugs or toxins to produce a local, focussed, anti-tumor effect. With enzymes the concept is a little different as a 2-stage procedure is involved: i) the enzyme is localised to the tumor; ii) a prodrug is given which is cleaved by the enzyme at the site of release, to produce a toxic drug.

## PRODUCTION OF IMMUNOCONJUGATES

There have been many preclinical studies described using isotopes, drugs, toxins or enzymes conjugated to antibody (Tables 2-4). Clearly with so many agents being used no single agent stands out as being substantially better than others. A comparison of the advantages and disadvantages of each type of conjugate is listed (Table 5) and a few general comments will be made on these.

**Table 2.** Isotopes coupled to MoAb

| Gamma | Beta | Alpha |
| --- | --- | --- |
| Iodine - 125, 131 | Yttrium - 90 | Bismuth - 212 |
| Technetium - 99m | Phosphorus - 32 | Astatine - 211 |
| Gallium - 67 | Rhenium - 186, 188 | |
| Indium - 111 | Palladium - 109 | |

a) At present more trials have been done with isotope-antibody conjugates than with the other moieties; this is probably a reflection of the ease of conjugation and extensive use has been made of [131]I-mAb and [90]Y-mAb.

b) There have been few studies conducted with drug-antibody conjugates as it is difficult to conjugate hydrophobic drugs to hydrophilic antibodies and there is a limit on the amount of drug that can be conjugated.

**Table 3.** Drugs conjugated to Mab

| Antimetabolites | - | methotrexate | Antimitotic agents | - | vinca alkaloids |
| | - | aminopterin | | - | podophyllotoxin |
| | - | cytosine arabinoside | | - | colchicine |
| | - | 5'-fluorodeoxyuridine | | | |
| Alkylating agents | - | melphalan | Miscellaneous | - | bleomycin |
| | - | chlorambucil | | - | macromomycin |
| | - | phenylenediamine mustard | | - | neocarzinstatin |
| | - | mitomycin C | | - | calicheamycin |
| Anthracyclines | - | doxorubicin | | | |
| | - | daunorubicin | | | |
| | - | Idarubicin | | | |
| | - | morpholino doxorubicin | | | |

c) The antigen target is crucial - for isotope-antibody conjugates the behaviour of the antigen is not so critical, ie.whether it internalizes, but for drugs and toxins, the antigen and therefore the complex, must be internalised;  enzymes work at the cell surface and internalisation is not required.

d) Isotope or drug containing antibody conjugates do not usually lead to an immune response to the toxic moiety - the rare exception is the description of antibodies to the linkage used when vincristine was attached to antibody[8];  by contrast, enzymes (if of a different origin than that of the species being treated) and toxins can lead to significant antibody responses which are likely to curtail therapy.

**Table 4.** Toxins or enzymes linked to MoAb

| Toxins | Enzymes |
| --- | --- |
| Plant | |
| ricin | carboxypeptidase G2 |
| abrin | glucouronidase |
| gelonin | cytoidine deaminase |
| saporin | |
| modecin | |
| Bacterial | |
| diphtheria | |
| pseudomonas exotoxin | |
| Fungal | |
| amanitin | |
| Animal | |
| cobra venom factor | |

The use of isotope antibodies is discussed elsewhere in this volume, but we also draw attention to the use of [90]Y-MUC1 antibodies for the treatment of ovarian cancer[9]. In an extensive trial, Epenetos and colleagues treated minimal residual disease of ovarian cancer with this therapeutic regime and of the patients able to be adequately assessed 14/15 are in remission some 5 years after debulking treatment. These results are extraordinary, and if this trend can be continued, this would certainly be a favoured mode of therapy.

**Table 5.** A comparison of immunoconjugates used for cancer therapy

| Parameter | Isotope | Drug | Toxin/Enzyme |
|---|---|---|---|
| chemistry of conjugation | easy | difficult | easy |
| yields | high | medium | low |
| stability/half life | low (depends on isotope | good | good |
| handling | difficult | easy | easy |
| tumor heterogeneity | good | not good | not good |
| antigen internalization required | no | yes no (enzyme) | yes (toxin); |
| cocktail of Mab | good | good | good |
| damage to surrounding tissues & tumors | yes | no | no |
| damage elsewhere | yes | no | yes |
| antibody to moiety | no | no | yes |
| access to tumors | good | good | not as good |

Antibody-enzyme and antibody-toxin conjugates have been extensively reviewed[4,5] and will not be discussed further here, but we will concentrate on the use of drug-antibody conjugates and make some comments regarding toxin antibody conjugates.

## USE OF DRUG-ANTIBODY CONJUGATES FOR THE TREATMENT OF CANCER

With the use of many drugs (Table 3) in different labs a number of general principles have been derived which apply to the use of drug-antibody conjugates. These are: a) loss of drug activity on conjugation; b) conjugation leads to a specific form of therapy; c) large amounts of drug-antibody conjugate can be given without toxicity; d) there is increased accumulation of drug in the tumor compared with free drug when given as an immunoconjugate; e) the serum half life of the drug is longer when conjugated to antibody.

**Loss of Drug Activity on Conjugation.** The chemistry of conjugating drugs to antibodies is difficult - basically as a hydrophobic substance (the drug) is conjugated to hydrophilic antibody. Various methods have been used and described in detail elsewhere[10]. However, there is almost always a 10 fold loss of drug activity on conjugation. There are several exceptions, for instance, idarubicin (an anthracycline derivative) varies between two and ten fold loss of activity[11], but the major exception is with the use of alkylating agents where there can be an increase in drug activity on conjugation to antibody.

**Conjugates are Specific**. In many different test systems both *in vitro* and *in vivo* the immunoconjugates retain the specificity of the antibody. ie. *in vitro* will kill cells to which the antibodies bind, but not cells to which the antibody does not bind - the "specificity ratio" obtained from such experiments varies from 5-50 so that highly specific agents can be produced by immunoconjugation. However, with some drugs, particularly *in vitro*, specificity is difficult to demonstrate. For example, aminopterin[12], 5FUDR[13] and podophyllotoxin[14], have low specificity *in vitro*, however *in vivo,* tumor non-reactive conjugates are inactive compared with the activity of the specific immunoconjugates.

**Large amounts of drug antibody can be given without toxicity**. With most drug antibody conjugates large amounts of the immunoconjugate can be given without drug toxicity. Indeed, we have found it difficult with drugs such as N-acetyl melphalan to determine the toxicity of the immunoconjugate, as sufficient antibody cannot be given. A nice example of this is the comparison of the toxicity of free idarubicin with the same amount of idarubicin given in the conjugate ~ our studies demonstrated that all the mice given the free drug died of drug toxicity, whereas those given the drug antibody immunoconjugate survived[15]. In analysing these results one must bear in mind that there is a significant loss of drug activity on conjugation, however, when this is taken into consideration, it is still clear that the immunoconjugates are, in general, non-toxic.

**Increased accumulation of drug occurs in tumors**. These experiments are difficult to do as it requires large amounts of radiolabelled free drug to determine their uptake by tumors. However, with doxorubicin, methotrexate, idarubicin and melphalan, approximately 3-5 times as much drug is found in the tumor when given as an immunoconjugate as when given as free drug. These findings substantiate the use of drugs in the form of immunoconjugates. However, in all of these studies it should be noted that only a small amount of the administered immunoconjugate reaches the tumor - perhaps only 1-2% in humans, although 10-20% has been achieved in mice.

**The serum half life of drugs is prolonged when conjugated to antibody.** There is a substantial increase in half-life of a drug when conjugated to antibody and this should lead to a more prolonged therapeutic effect.

In the light of these principles it is clear that immunoconjugates should provide preferential treatment of tumors over the use of free drugs.

# EXAMPLES OF SOME DRUG-ANTIBODY IMMUNOCONJUGATES

As indicated earlier, a large number of drugs have been conjugated to antibody - we will describe two of our most potent immunoconjugates as examples of the principles described above. In the first, 5FUDR was conjugated to antibody using an active ester of the succinyl derivative and a large number of residues bound - however, beyond 20 residues there was a substantial loss of antibody activity. The immunoconjugates were highly specific both *in vitro* and *in vivo*, and *in vivo* cause a delay in tumor growth or shrinkage of mouse tumor allografts and or human grafts in nude mice[16]. These examples have not been tested in breast cancer models. In the second example, the use of idarubicin - a potent anthracycline gave similar results - anti-tumor effects led to disappearance of 60% of the tumors growing in nude mice[17].

As the cytotoxic drugs have not been toxic to mice when conjugated to antibodies, and greater potency would be desirable, there is now a tendency to use more toxic drugs - even those which are too toxic to use in the clinic. For example, aminopterin (not used because of its toxicity) is substantially better than methotrexate for anti-tumor activity *in vivo*[18]. Highly potent derivatives of anthracycline such as the morpholino compounds and other compounds such as calcheamycin - which are far too potent and toxic to use alone are now also being used in preclinical studies with significant effects.

## CLINICAL TRIALS

A number of clinical trials have been done with drug-antibody conjugates, but at this time fewer trials have been done than with isotopes and toxins. The clinical trials include the use of doxorubicin, N-acetylmelphalan, mitomycin C, neocarzinostatin, methotrexate, VLB - in ~ 150 patient's. However, these studies were Phase I and we expect more results on Phase I/II studies to appear within the next few years. In our own Phase I/II study using melphalan-anti-CEA in colon cancer we noted: a) the absence of side effects; b) amounts of drug in excess of the MTD (maximum tolerated dose) could be given; c) large amounts of antibody (in excess of 2gm) could be given without side effects; d) some subjective improvement was noted and some tumor shrinkage - none of which could be accorded a partial or complete response; e) anecdotal evidence that one patient with minimal residual disease was cured by the therapy; f) the occurrence of HAMA curtailed treatment[19]. At this time, it is clear these trials should be repeated using potent drugs, chimaeric or human antibodies and after appropriate Phase I/II studies, then we would recommend trials in patients with minimal residual disease, ie. an adjuvant setting. We are pessimistic that with large tumors, greater than 1cm in diameter, that sufficient antibody can be given to eradicate larger tumors.

## TUMOR ACCESS

One way of increasing the potency of immunoconjugates is to increase the amount which reaches the tumor. As indicated above, the maximum levels obtained are only 1-2% of the injected dose in the tumor. We have tried to increase this amount using several approaches which really attack the tumor vasculature. In the first, vasoactive agents were used - in the belief that these act primarily on the peripheral vasculature and spare vessels in tumors. Thus, propranolol was able to potentiate the value of immunoconjugates[20]. In a second study, tumor necrosis factor (TNF) was able to substantially increase the effect of immunoconjugates provided it was given at the same time as the immunoconjugate[21]. Indeed, up to 4 times as much immunoconjugate could be found in the tumor when TNF was given at the same time as the immunoconjugate; if there was a delay in the use of immunoconjugate after giving TNF, less amounts were found in the tumor. We attribute these effects as being due to TNF acting directly on the endothelium - if given too early, then intravascular thrombosis occurs preventing the influx of immunoconjugate into the tumor. In humans, TNF is toxic, but could possibly be used as TNF-antibody immunoconjugates.

## THE FUTURE

There is clearly much more to be done with clinical trials with immunoconjugates. At this time most laboratories will be preparing drug-antibody conjugates with a new round of antibodies - be they chimaeric or fully human antibodies. These will be more potent, have a longer half life and many of the antibodies alone may be effective. More toxic drugs should be sought and improvements in the linker technology to enable the conjugation of more drug or isotope. By genetic engineering techniques it may be possible to engineer better or more linkage sites on antibodies for hydrophobic drugs. Once these agents are proven to be non-toxic, we predict that they will form part of the treatment of cancer in patients. Our prediction would be that these agents will be most potent when used at the time of surgery for minimal residual disease, for example, in patients with breast cancer undergoing surgery (and therefore with little evidence of extensive spread) would receive (say) a gram of antibody conjugate over several days and a repeat some months later to "mop up" microscopic deposits of cancer spread throughout the body. However, such predictions are of no value without the appropriate clinical trials and these will take several years to complete.

# REFERENCES

1.  G.A. Pietersz, A. Rowland, M.J. Smyth and I.F.C. McKenzie, Conjugated antibodies: chemoimmunoconjugates, *in*: "Therapeutic Applications Of Monoclonal Antibodies In Cancer", Ed. R.O. Dillman, Marcel-Dekker Inc, California In press (1992).

2.  G.A. Pietersz, J. Kanellos and I.F.C. McKenzie, Novel synthesis and *in vitro* characterization of a disulfide linked ricin-monoclonal antibody conjugates devoid of galactose binding activity, *Cancer Res.* 48:4469 (1988).

3.  J. Kanellos, I.F.C. McKenzie and G.A. Pietersz, Intratumor therapy of solid tumors with the use of ricin-antibody conjugates, *Immunol. and Cell Biol.* 67: 89 (1989).

4.  P.D. Senter, P.M. Wallace, H.P. Svensson, D.E. Kerr, I. Hellstrom, and K.E. Hellstrom, Activation of prodrugs by antibody-enzyme conjugates, *Adv. Exp. Med. Biol.* 303:97 (1991).

5.  J.W. Uhr, R.J. Fulton, M.A. Till and E.S. Vitetta, Monoclonal antibodies as carriers of toxins, *Prog. Clin. Biol. Res.* 288:403 (1989).

6.  P. Vigeral, N. Chkoff, L. Chatenoud et al, Prophylactic use of OKT3 monoclonal antibody in cadaver kidney recipients: utilization of OKT3 as the sole immunosuppressive agent, *Transplantation.* 41: 730 (1986).

7.  R. Willemze, D.J. Richel, J.H. Falkenburg, G. Hale, H. Waldmann, F.E. Zaan et al, In vivo use of Campath-1G to prevent graft-vs-host disease and graft rejection after bone marrow transplantation, *Bone Marrow Transpl.* 9:255 (1992).

8.  B.H. Peterson, S.V. Deherdt, D.W. Scheck and T.F. Bumol, The human immune response to KS1/4-desacetylvinblastine (Ly256787) and KS1/4-dacetylvinblastine hydrazide (Ly203728) in single and multiple dose clinical trials, *Cancer Res.* 51:2286 (1991).

9.  A.A. Epenetos (personal communication).

10. G.A. Pietersz, The linkage of cytotoxic drugs to monoclonal antibodies for the treatment of cancer, *Bioconj. Chem.* 1:89 (1990).

11. G.A. Pietersz, M.J. Smyth and I.F.C. McKenzie, Immunochemotherapy of a murine thymoma with idarubicin - monoclonal antibody conjugates, *Cancer Res.* 48:926 (1988).

12. K.G. Krauer, R. Bell and G.A. Pietersz, Aminopterin-monoclonal antibody conjugates. Antitumor activity and toxicity, *Drug Targeting and Delivery.* In press (1992).

13. A. Goerlach, K.G. Krauer, I.F.C. McKenzie and G.A. Pietersz, *In vitro* antitumor activity of 5-fluoro-2-deoxyuridine-monoclonal antibody conjugates, *Bioconj. Chem.* 2:96 (1991).

14. G.A. Pietersz, K.G. Krauer, H. Holessis and I.F.C. McKenzie, Conjugation *in vitro* and *in vivo* efficacy of highly cytotoxic anti cancer drugs-aminopterin (AMN), 5-fluoro-2-deoxyuridine (5-FUDR) and podophyllotoxin, Abstract P-85 *in* "Proc. of 5th international conference on monoclonal antibody immunoconjugates for cancer", *Antib. Immunoconj. Radiopharm.* 4:226 (1991).

15. G.A. Pietersz, M.J. Smyth and I.F.C. McKenzie, The use of anthracycline antibody complexes for specific antitumor therapy *in*: "Targeted Diagnosis And Therapy", Ed J.D. Rodwell, Marcell Dekker Inc, California, 1:25 (1988).

16. K.G. Krauer, I.F.C. McKenzie and G.A. Pietersz, The anti-tumor effect of 2'-deoxy-5'-fluorouridine conjugates against a murine thymoma and colon carcinoma xenografts, *Cancer Res.* 52:132 (1992).

17. A.J. Rowland, I.F.C. McKenzie and G.A. Pietersz, Preclinical investigation of the antitumor effects of anti-CD19-idarubicin immunoconjugates, *Cancer Immunol. Immunother.* Submitted (1992).

18. J. Kanellos, G.A. Pietersz, Z. Cunningham and I.F.C. McKenzie, Antitumor activity of aminopterin-monoclonal antibody conjugates; *in vitro* and *in vivo* comparison with methotrexate-monoclonal antibody conjugates, *Immunol. Cell Biol.* 65:483 (1987).

19. J.J. Tjandra, L. Ramadi and I.F.C. McKenzie, Development of human anti-murine antibody (HAMA) response in patients, *Immunol. Cell Biol.* 68:367 (1990).

20. M.J. Smyth, G.A. Pietersz and I.F.C. McKenzie, Use of vasoactive agents to increase tumor perfusion and the antitumor efficacy of drug-monoclonal antibody conjugates, *J. Natl. Cancer Inst.* 79:1367 (1987).

21. S.M. Russell, K.G. Krauer, I.F.C. McKenzie and G.A. Pietersz, Effect of tumor necrosis factor on the antitumor efficacy and toxicity of aminopterin-monoclonal antibody conjugates. Parameters in optimization of therapy, *Cancer Res.* 50:6028 (1990).

# RADIOIMMUNOLOCALIZATION OF BREAST CANCER USING BrE-3 MONOCLONAL ANTIBODY

Elissa L. Kramer[1], Sally J. DeNardo[2], Leonard Liebes[1], Marilyn E. Noz[1], Linda Kroger[2], Stephan D. Glenn[3], Philip Furmanski[4], and Roberto Ceriani[5]

[1]New York University Medical Center/Bellevue Hospital Center 560 First Avenue, New York, NY 10016

[2]Section of Radiodiagnosis and Therapy, Univ. of California at Davis, Sacramento, CA

[3] Coulter Immunology, Hialeah, FL 33010

[4] Department of Biology, New York University, New York, NY 10003

[5]Cancer Research Fund of Contra Costa, Walnut Creek, CA 94596

## INTRODUCTION

Radioimmunolocalization for detection or therapy of breast cancer has undergone only limited investigation. Successful targeting of breast tumors with radiolabeled antibodies has awaited the identification of the optimal antigen targets, the appropriate antibodies, as well as the linking chemistry necessary to produce stable radioimmunoconjugates. Radioimmunodetection trials in breast cancer have employed both the intravenous and interstitial administration routes. Sensitivity of intravenously administered immunoconjugates for metastatic disease has ranged from 50-78% in small series of patients [1-3]. The antibodies used in these trials were directed against various breast cancer associated antigens including human milk fat globule membrane (HMFG) or breast epithelial mucin and CEA. Excellent sensitivity for primary breast tumors using an antibody directed against TAG-72 has been reported[3], but in the same patients,

*Antigen and Antibody Molecular Engineering in Breast Cancer Diagnosis and Treatment*, Edited by R.L. Ceriani, Plenum Press, New York, 1994

181

axillary lymph node involvement was not detected accurately. Radioimmunotherapy using [131]Iodine L6 antibody has met with some successful results, but the antigen is not always present in breast tumors[4]. Although radioimmunotherapy with [131]I-L6 holds great promise, other radioimmunoconjugates will be needed.

The highly prevalent tumor-associated breast epithelial mucin antigens in breast cancer are logical targets for radioimmunoconjugates. Recently, a series of antibodies directed against the 400kD epitope of HMFG, also known as breast epithelial mucin, has been developed[5, 6]. These antibodies react with over 90% of breast cancer cell lines against which they have been tested[7] and on immunohistochemistry react with most breast carcinoma specimens[6]. On the basis of preclinical studies in nude mice which have shown excellent localization and effective radioimmunotherapy in breast tumor xenografts[8-10] preliminary clinical trials with one of these antibodies, Mc5, were initiated[11]. Despite immunohistochemical demonstration of the antigen in tumor, little localization of [131]Iodine- Mc5 was observed after intravenous administration. The high levels of antigen-antibody complexes were noted in the serum of these patients suggesting that the circulating epitope may have blocked radioiodinated antibody delivery to tumor.

On the basis of these results, another antibody in this series, BrE-3, which recognizes an epitope less frequently and less abundantly present in serum of patients with breast cancer, was selected as a more promising antibody for targeting tumor in vivo[12]. A Phase I clinical study using [111]In MX-DTPA BrE-3 was performed to study the localization, pharmacokinetics and toxicity of this radioimmunoconjugate as a preliminary step toward developing this immunoconjugate for both radioimmunodetection and radioimmunotherapy. On the basis of the results of this trial, a second Phase I radioimmunotherapy trial was begun. The data fromthe initial Phase I trial as well as the imaging data from the ongoing therapy trial are reported.

## METHODS

### Subjects

We studied 15 women with metastatic or recurrent breast carcinoma under the first Phase I clinical protocol. An additional patient was studied at the first dose level of a radioimmunotherapy trial which involved co-infusion of both [111]Indium-MX-DTPA BrE-3(5 mCi) and [90]Yttrium-MX-DTPA BrE-3 (6.25 mCi/m$^2$). The average age of these patients was 59 years. All had undergone conventional therapy including hormonal therapy, chemotherapy and/or radiotherapy for their recurrent or metastatic disease. None of the patients had previously received murine monoclonal antibodies. All subjects had an adequate performance status and normal renal, hepatic, hematologic and cardiac function as assessed by standard blood tests and electrocardiograms. The extent of their disease was established by physical examination or conventional radiographic and scintigraphic examinations. In all patients, the expression of the epitope recognized by BrE-3 antibody was established by immunohistochemical staining of previously obtained tumor specimens. Written informed consent was obtained from each subject according to the guidelines established by the institutional review boards at the two respective clinical sites.

**Serum levels of breast epithelial mucin reactive with BrE-3 antibody**

Before administration of the antibody, serum was obtained to measure the level of circulating antigen reactive with BrE-3 antibody. Circulating BrE-3 epitope was determined by a competitive serum assay with the BrE-3 epitope on the solid phase.

**BrE-3 antibody**

BrE-3, developed at the Cancer Research Fund of Contra Costa is a murine IgG$_1$ monoclonal antibody reacting with the polyepitopic moiety of breast epithelial mucin[6]. The antibody was provided by Coulter Immunology (Division of Coulter Corporation, Hialeah, FL) in a sterile and pyrogen free form as the nonconjugated antibody as well as conjugated to the (1,4) methyl-benzyl isothiocyanate DTPA (MX-DTPA) for labeling with [111]Indium ([111]In) chloride or [90]Yttrium ([90]Y) chloride. The study was performed under a U.S. IND sponsored by Coulter Immunology.

For each administration in the localization study, approximately 5 mCi of pharmaceutical grade [111]Indium chloride (Amersham Corporation) was buffered in acetate. For labeling, 2 mg MX-DTPA BrE-3 was incubated with the [111]In Chloride for 20 minutes. The mixture was then challenged with 5 mM EDTA. Radiolabeling efficiency for the [111]In-MX-DTPA BrE-3 was assessed by instant thin layer chromatography and averaged 97$\pm$ 6%. [90]Yttrium chloride was incubated with 2 mg MX- DTPA BrE-3 and separated by column chromatography. The radiolabeled MX-DTPA BrE-3 was then mixed with 8 mg of unconjugated BrE-3, filtered through a 0.22 $\mu$ filter, and diluted to 200 ml in 5% human serum albumin in normal saline. Pyrogen and sterility testing were performed for all radiolabeled preparations. Sterility testing of each preparation was negative. Pyrogen levels were always within acceptable limits, i.e., < 5 endotoxin units/ kg/ hour of infusion. Immunoreactivity evaluated using BrE- antigen coated beads averaged 71%.

Three different dose levels of antibody were tested in the localization protocol.

Cohorts of 5 patients received total doses of 10 mg, 50 mg, or 100 mg. At the lowest dose level the radiolabeled antibody mixture was administered over 1 hour. For the two subsequent dose levels the additional unlabeled, nonconjugated BrE-3 antibody (40 mg or 90 mg) was diluted in 5% human serum albumin and administered intravenously at the rate of 1-2 mg/min. Once the unlabeled antibody infusion was complete, 30 minutes were allowed to elapse and the radiolabeled mixture was infused as described. For the radioimmunotherapy protocol, the patient received a total of 50 mg of antibody. The $^{111}$In-MX-DTPA BrE-3 and the $^{90}$Y-MX-DTPA BrE-3 were infused simultaneously.

Vital signs were monitored during the infusion for a minimum of 3 hours. Also, routine blood chemistries, complete blood count, prothrombin time, partial thromboplastin time, and urinalysis were obtained 72 hours after antibody administration to evaluate for subacute toxicity.

**Imaging**

Quantitative planar imaging was performed to obtain pharmacokinetics in normal organs and to assess tumor localization. $^{111}$Indium transmission scans were performed prior to antibody administration. Conjugate regional anterior and posterior gamma camera views of the head, chest, abdomen and pelvis were obtained at 4, 24, 72 hours and approximately 8 days after antibody administration using a large field of view gamma camera fitted with a medium energy collimator. Dual 20% energy windows centered on 173 and 247 keV, the two photopeaks of $^{111}$Indium, were employed for the acquisitions. In addition, anterior and posterior whole body images were acquired at these time points. At 72 hours and 8 days after antibody administration SPECT imaging was performed whenever possible.

Images were interpreted by the Nuclear Medicine physician with full knowledge of the extent and sites of disease.

Region of interest analysis with background subtraction and correction for attenuation and gamma camera sensitivity and efficiency was used to determine percent injected activity in normal organs and measurable tumors. The geometric mean of the anterior and posterior regions was used for liver, spleen and lung calculations. For the kidneys and tumors the counts from a single planar view were used[13,14]. Monoexponential modeling was used to determine the biological half life of the radiolabeled antibody in each organ, whole body, and measurable tumors. The cumulative activity was calculated using the effective half life and the fraction injected activity.

**Pharmacokinetics**

Serial blood sampling was performed at 5, 30, 60, 120 minutes, 4, 6, 24 hours and daily to 8 days after antibody administration. Timed urine collections were also obtained throughout this period. Total radioactivity in serum and urine samples was measured using a 1282 LKB gamma counter. Serum samples were further subjected to gel permeation high pressure liquid chromatography. Collected fractions were subjected to UV detection at 280 nm and gamma radioactivity counting to determine the association of radioactivity with antigen-antibody complexes, intact antibody, and breakdown products in serum.

Pharmacokinetic parameters for radiolabeled antibody in blood were determined. The half-time of clearance was described using nonlinear biexponential modeling. Alpha and beta half-lives, area under the curve (AUC), clearance, and percentages AUC cleared with the beta half-life were obtained. Also, the total radioactivity excreted in the urine was calculated.

**Radiation dosimetry**

Radiation dosimetry was estimated for $^{111}$In-MX-DTPA BrE-3. Extrapolation of the biodistribution data from $^{111}$In-MX-DTPA BrE-3 was made to obtain radiation dose estimates for $^{90}$Y-MX-DTPA BrE-3. Using the cumulative activity from the region of interest analysis, the MIRD formalism was applied to estimate radiation dose for whole body, lung, liver, kidneys, and spleen. For bone marrow, it was assumed that one fourth of the marrow volume was blood. The activity in this volume of blood was taken as the activity in the marrow and the "S" factor for marrow to marrow dose (non-penetrating) was applied. For $^{111}$Indium the dose to marrow from marrow was added to the penetrating dose to marrow from other organs. For $^{90}$Yttrium estimates the radiation dose from the whole body and other organs was not included since the penetrating radiation from these sites would contribute < 1% of the total marrow dose. For measurable tumors, the radiation dose was calculated using the appropriate "S" factors based on the size and geometry of the lesions.

**Human anti-mouse antibody (HAMA)**

HAMA responses in these patients were assessed prior to administration of radiolabeled antibody, at one week, at 1 month, and up to 3 months post antibody administration. Serum samples were assayed by capturing serum IgG on Staph A particles, saturating with normal human immunoglobulin and incubating with $^{125}$I BrE-3 antibody to assess anti-idiotype and anti-isotype HAMA. IgE HAMA was measured by capturing serum IgE on beads coated with specific goat anti-human IgE, and then incubating with either $^{125}$I labeled specific goat anti-human IgE immunoglobulin or with $^{125}$I BrE-3 antibody[15].

## RESULTS

### Serum levels of breast epithelial mucin reactive with BrE-3 antibody

In 14 of 16 patients the serum level of the epitope recognized by BrE-3 was less than 10 µg/ml. In two patients the baseline levels were quite elevated (>40 µg/ml) (Figure 1).

### Imaging

Seventy-two separate sites of disease were identified by conventional diagnostic modalities. Of these, 43 were in the skeleton; 7 were chest wall lesions; 8 in lymph nodes; 6 in the liver; and 8 in other organs including lung. Overall, 62 (86%) of the known lesions were detected. This included 2 of 6 liver metastases, 3/4 lung metastases, and 7/8 lymph nodes. Thirty-nine (91%) of the known skeletal metastases were detected. In addition, 11 previously unsuspected lesions were identified in the skeleton and 2 unsuspected soft tissue tumors were seen. Five of the skeletal metastases could be confirmed by conventional imaging modalities (plain film, MRI or scintigraphy). The two soft tissue tumors were confirmed subsequently at a follow-up physical examination (Figure 2).

### Pharmacokinetics

A biexponential pharmacokinetic model was used to describe the levels of radiolabeled antibody in blood over time. The half life of distribution ($T_{1/2\alpha}$) was found to average $9.5 \pm 2.7$ hours and the half-life of elimination ($T_{1/2\beta}$) averaged $56 \pm 25.4$ hours across all patients. The average clearance of radiolabeled antibody from serum was $0.52\pm0.09$ ml/min/m$^2$. No significant difference in these parameters was found among the three dose levels ($p>0.2$). The area under the curve (AUC) did increase with antibody dose level administered showing a significant correlation ($R^2= 0.99$) (Figure 3). The percentage of the AUC that was cleared from the serum with the $T_{1/2\beta}$ averaged 83.7%.

### Radiation dosimetry

The percent injected dose (%ID) accumulated in the liver averaged $11.9 \pm 5.2\%$ at 72 hours after injection. Lesser amounts were measured in the spleen and kidneys. The %ID in the lungs averaged of $5.0\pm 3.4\%$. By region of interest analysis of images, the %ID seen in tumors at 24 hours after antibody administration ranged from 0.02-2.56%.

Radiation dose estimates for [111]In-MX-DTPA BrE-3 were made for normal organs. The liver and spleen received the highest doses, $1.30 \pm 0.46$ rads/mCi (mean ± S.D.) and $1.48\pm 0.85$ rads/mCi, respectively. The average whole body dose was $0.45\pm 0.11$ rads/mCi.

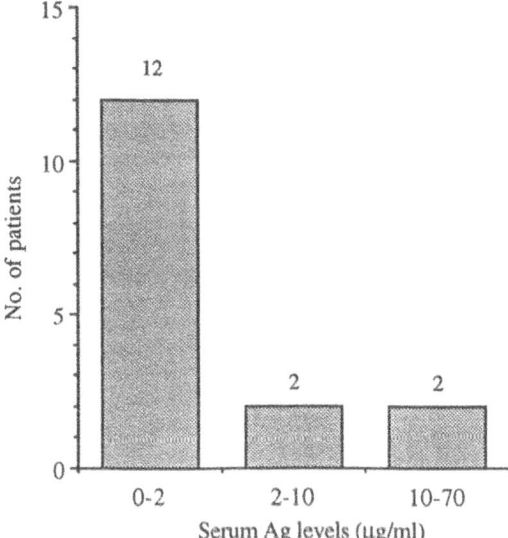

**Figure 1.** Baseline serum levels of antigen reactive with BrE-3 monoclonal antibody

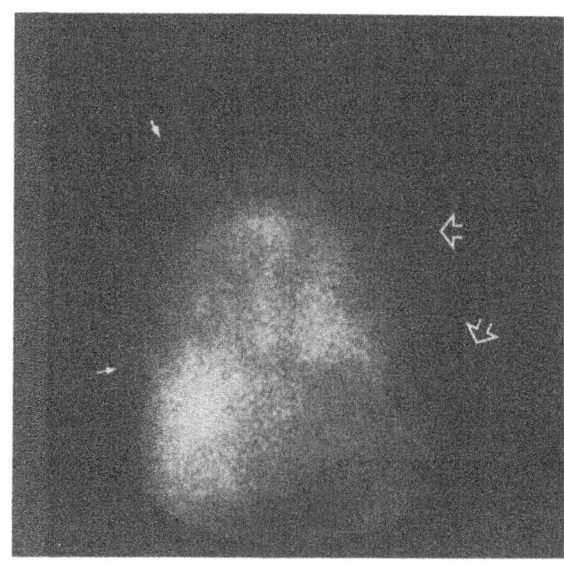

**Figure 2.** Anterior view of the chest obtained 72 hours after administration of 5 mCi $^{111}$In-MX-DTPA BrE-3 in a patient who is status post right mastectomy with recurrent right chest wall disease(small arrows). Concentration of radioactivity is also present in the left axilla and in the left breast (open arrows). Although physical examination in these areas was unremarkable at the time of antibody administration, palpable tumor was detected three weeks later.

The biodistribution data for [111]In-MX-DTPA BrE-3 was extrapolated to make radiation dose estimates for [90]Y-MX-DTPA BrE-3. Again, the liver and spleen doses were the highest with the liver estimated to receive 9.22± 3.67 rads/mCi and the spleen estimated to receiv 15.36 ± 10.96 rads/mCi. Whole body dose estimates averaged 2.03 ± 1.6 rads/mCi and the marrow dose using the contribution from blood was estimated to be 2.10 ± 0.97 rads/mCi.

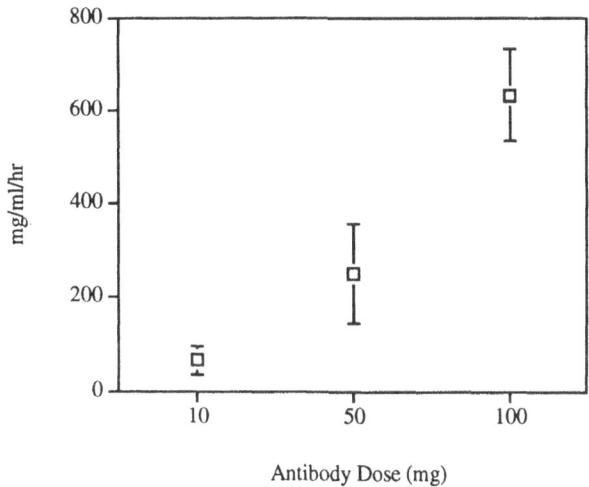

**Figure 3.** Mean (± S.E.) area under the curve for radiolabeled antibody over time.

## DISCUSSION

These preliminary results suggest that [111]In-MX-DTPA BrE-3 has significant potential in radioimmunolocalization of breast cancer for diagnosis as well as therapy. The high detection rates in this series of patients are comparable to or exceed the detection rates for breast cancer reported in the literature[1, 3, 16-23]. The high detection rate found here may be partly explained by the abundance and frequency with which the epitope recognized by BrE-3 antibody is expressed on breast tumors. All tumors screened by immunohistochemistry in these trials have expressed the antigen. This agrees with the experience reported in earlier studies with these antibodies[6].

Detection rates were highest in chest wall, lymph node, and skeletal metastases. In fact, for skeletal metastases immunoscintigraphy was slightly more sensitive than bone scintigraphy. In addition, immunoscintigraphy detected an axillary lymph node metastasis and a breast tumor before they became evident on physical examination. Although only one third of the liver lesions were detected, the relatively low %ID (approximately 12%) accumulated in the normal liver in these patients compares favorably with other [111]Indium immunoconjugates. This relatively low %ID in the liver suggests that there is potential for detection of liver metastases with this radioimmunoconjugate. This was a relatively small series of patients with nonuniform activity of disease in the liver; more extensive trials are warranted to better evaluate detection rates in the liver.

Radioimmunodetection in breast cancer has the potential to play a useful contributory role in the management of both primary and metastatic disease. In primary breast cancer, no adequate noninvasive technique exists to accurately stage lymph nodes. Although radiation therapy may adequately treat the axillary nodes reducing the incidence of local recurrence to about 3% [24], surgical sampling of these nodes is still required to adequately stage the axilla and obtain the necessary prognostic information. Accurate staging of axillary lymph nodes by radioimmunodetection might modify the need to do extensive axillary dissections in all patients. Although initial attempts at immunolymphoscintigraphy suffered from lack of specificity[20,21], more recently techniques have been refined to improve both sensitivity and specificity[25]. To date intravenously administered TAG-72 specific radiolabeled antibodies (B72.3) used in primary breast cancer have not been accurate in staging the axilla[3]. [111]In-labeled B72.3 was very sensitive for the detection of primary tumors[3]. In our therapy patient, [111]In-MX-DTPA BrE-3 localized a breast tumor as well as axillary node disease before they became apparent on physical examination.

Conceivably, immunoscintigraphy might play a role in defining multicentric disease or in clarifying or augmenting the information from mammography. If the sensitivity of radioimmunodetection with [111]In-MX-DTPA BrE-3 proves to be more sensitive than currently available modalities for detection of distant metastases, radioimmunodetection may be helpful in better staging patients with more advanced primary tumors. Given the ubiquity of the antigen recognized by BrE-3 antibody, intravenously administered [111]In MX-DTPA BrE-3 might have greater sensitivity than previously evaluated antibodies, but this, too, requires evaluation.

As more effective therapies for recurrent and metastatic breast cancer are developed the role for sensitive radioimmunodetection will grow. Early detection of disease when tumor burden is small theoretically will offer an advantage in achieving effective therapeutic responses whether it be through dose-intensified chemotherapy or by other novel therapeutic modalities.

Finally, a radioimmunoconjugate that localizes frequently and with high concentration may have potential for delivering therapeutic levels of radiation. Radioimmunoimaging in this situation will play a crucial role in therapy planning: providing evidence that the immunoconjugate will target as expected and quantitative information concerning radiation dose to tumor and normal organs. The therapeutic trial that will help determine the utility of using radioimmunoimaging to predict radiation dosimetry from a similar immunoconjugate labeled with [90]Yttrium is now underway.

# ACKNOWLEDGEMENTS

This work was funded by the National Cancer Institute primarily through 3PO1-CA42767 awarded to the Cancer Research Fund of Contra Costa.

# REFERENCES

1. R. Rainsbury, The localization of human breast carcinomas by radiolabelled monoclonal antibodies, Br JSurg 71:805 (1984).

2. P. Riva, G. Moscatelli, G. Paganelli and e. al, Antibody-guided diagnosis: An Italian experience on CEA-expressing tumours, Int J Cancer 2(Suppl):114 (1988).

3. L. Lamki, A. Buzdar, S. Singletary, M. Rosenblum, V. Bhadkamkar, L. Esparza, D. Podoloff, A. Zukiwski, G. Hortobagyi and J. Murray, Indium-111-labeled B72.3 monoclonal antibody in the detection and staging of breast cancer: A Phase I Study, J Nucl Med 32:1326 (1991).

4. S. DeNardo, K. Warhoe, L. O'Grady, I. Hellstrom, K. Hellstrom, S. Mills, D. Macey, J. Goodnight and G. DeNardo, Radioimmunotherapy for breast cancer: treatment of a patient with I-131 L6 chimeric monoclonal antibody, Int J. Biol Markers 6:221 (1991).

5. R. Ceriani, J. Peterson, J. Lee, R. Moncada and E. Blank, Characterization of cell surface antigens of human mammary epithelial cells with monoclonal antibodies prepared against human milk fat globule, Somat Cell Genet 9:415 (1983).

6. J. Peterson, D. Zava, A. Duwe and e. al, Biochemical and histological characterization of antigens preferentially expressed on the surface and cytoplasm of breast carcinoma cells identified by monoclonal antibodies against the human milk fat globule, Hybridoma 9:221 (1990).

7. R. Ceriani, J. Peterson, E. Blank, C. Chan and R. Cailleau, Development and characterization of breast carcinoma cell lines as in vitro and in vivo models for breast cancer diagnosis and therapy, In Vitro (In press).

8. R. Ceriani, E. Blank and J. Peterson, Experimental immunotherapy of human breast carcinomas implanted in nude mice with a mixture of monoclonal antibodies against human milk fat globule components, Cancer Res 47:532 (1987).

9. R. Ceriani, M. Sasaki, D. Orthendahl and L. Kaugman, Localization of human breast tumors grafted in nude mice with a monoclonal antibody directed against a defined cell surface antigen of human mammary epithelial cells, Breast Cancer Res Treat 12:177 (1988).

10. R. Ceriani and E. Blank, Experimental therapy of human breast tumors with 131 I-labeled monoclonal antibodies prepared against the human milk fat globule, Cancer Res 48:4664 (1988).

11. R. Gonzalez, D. Dienhart, R. Kasliwal and e. al, A Phase I study of a radiolabeled monoclonal antibody 131 Mc5 in breast cancer, (Submitted for publication).

12. E. Blank, K. Pant, C. Chan, J. Peterson and R. Ceriani, A novel anti-breast epithelial mucin

MoAb (BrE-3). Characterization and experimental biodistribution and immunotherapy, Cancer J 5:38 (1992).

13. D. Macey, S. DeNardo, G. DeNardo, J. Goodnight and M. Unger, Uptake of Indium-111-labeled monoclonal antibody ZME-018 as a function of tumor size in a patient with melanoma. Uptake of Indium-111-labeled monoclonal antibody ZME-018 as a function of tumor size in a patient with melanoma, Am J Phys Imag 3:1 (1988).

14. D. Macey, G. DeNardo and S. DeNardo, A Treatment Planning Program for Radioimmunotherapy. In: " Frontiers of Radiation Therapy and Oncology," J. Vaeth and J. Meyer, ed., Karger, Basel (1990). pp 123-131.

15. D. Dienhart, D. Bloedow, C. Hartmann and e. al., A phase I trial of KC-4 monoclonal antibody serotherapy of advanced non-small cell lung and breast cancers: Clinical, pharmacokinetic, and immunologic results., Cancer Res ( Accepted for publication).

16. K. Ryan, R. Dillman, S. DeNardo, G. DeNardo, J. Beauregard, P. Hagan, D. Amox, M. Clutter, K. Burnett, C. Rulot, R. Sobol, I. Abramson, R. Bartholomew, J. Frincke, C. Birdwell, D. Carlo, L. O'Grady and S. Halpern, Breast Cancer Imaging with In-111 human IgM monoclonal antibodies: preliminary studies, Radiology 167:71 (1988).

17. R. Rainsbury, J. Westwood, R. Coombes, A. Neville, R. Ott, T. Kalirai, V. McCready and J.-C. Gazet, Location of metastatic breast carcinoma by a monoclonal antibody chelate labelled with indium-111, Lancet ii:934 (1983).

18. R. Mandeville, N. Pateisky, K. Philipp, E. Kubista, F. Dumas and B. Groux, Immunolymphoscintigraphy of axillary lymph node metastases in breast cancer patients using monoclonal antibodies: first clinical findings, Anticancer Res 6:1257 (1986).

19. K. Kairemo, Immunolymphoscintigraphy with 99m Tc--labeled monoclonal antibody (BW431/26) reacting with carcinoembryonic antigen in breast cancer, Cancer Res (Suppl) 50:949 (1990).

20. F. Deland, E. Kim, R. Corgan and e. al, Axillary lymphscintigraphy by radioimmunodetection of carcinoembryonic antigen in breast cancer, J Nucl Med 20:(1979).

21. F. Deland, E. Kim, D. Goldenberg and e. al, Lymphoscintigraphy with radionuclide-labeled antibodies to carcinoembryonic antigen, Cancer Res 40:2997 (1980).

22. A. Athanassiou, D. Pectasides, K. Pateniotis and e. al, Immunoscintigraphy with 131I-labelled HMFG2 and HMFG1 F(ab')2 in the pre-operative detection of clinical and subclinical lymph node metastases in breast cancer patients, Int J Cancer 2(Suppl):89 (1988).

23. A. Epenetos, S. Mather, M. Granowska and e. al, Targeting of iodine-123-labelled tumour-associated monoclonal antibodies to ovarian, breast, and gastrointestinal tumours, Lancet 2:999 (1982).

24. B. Fisher, C. Redmond, E. Fisher, M. Bauer, N. Wolmark and e. al, Ten-year results of a randomized clinical trial comparing radical mastectomy and total mastectomy with or without radiation, N Engl J Med 312:674 (1985).

25. J. Tjandra, I. Russell, J. Collins, J. Andrews, M. Lictenstein, D. Binns and I. MacKenzie, Immunolymphoscintigraphy for the detection of lymph node metastases from breast cancer, Cancer Res 49:1600 (1989).

# SUPPRESSION OF HUMAN ANTI-MOUSE ANTIBODY RESPONSE TO MURINE MONOCLONAL ANTIBODY L6 BY DEOXYSPERGUALIN: A PHASE I STUDY

Kapil Dhingra[1], Herbert Fritsche[2], James L. Murray[3], Albert F. LoBuglio[4], M.B. Khazaeli[4], Susan Kelley[5], Mark Tepper[5], Douglas Greene[5], Daniel Booser[1], Aman Buzdar[1], Martin Raber[1], Lia Gutierrez[1], and Gabriel Hortobagyi[1]

Departments of [1]Medical Oncology, [2]Laboratory Medicine and [3]Clinical Immunology and Biological Therapy, The University of Texas M.D. Anderson Cancer Center, 1515 Holcombe Boulevard, Houston, Texas 77030, [4]Comprehensive Cancer Center, University of Alabama at Birmingham, Birmingham, Alabama 35294 [5]Bristol-Myers Squibb Company, Wallingford, Connecticut 06492

## INTRODUCTION

The concept of using monoclonal antibodies (MAbs) to localize and treat human tumors has become a clinical reality over the last few years. Antibodies have been used to modulate the host immune system to activate tumoricidal effector mechanisms and are being used as targeting vehicles for delivery of exogenous cytotoxic molecules such as radioisotopes, chemicals and biologicals. Their ability to selectively target tumor cells also makes them attractive for radioimmunoimaging and for assessing tumor response to therapy[1].

### Human Anti-mouse Antibody (HAMA) Response

The majority of MAbs undergoing clinical trials have been developed by hybridoma technology in which B-lymphocytes from mice immunized with the relevant tumor antigen are fused with malignant plasma cells[2]. These murine antibodies are recognized as foreign proteins by the human immune system and elicit the production of HAMA. HAMA usually appear in the circulation 2 - 3 weeks after administration of the murine antibody. HAMA are usually of the IgG class and may be directed against the

*Antigen and Antibody Molecular Engineering in Breast Cancer Diagnosis and Treatment*, Edited by R.L. Ceriani, Plenum Press, New York, 1994

193

constant region (anti-isotypic), the variable region (anti-idiotypic), or the antigen binding region (anti-paratopic) of the murine antibody. Once such a sensitization has occurred, subsequent doses of the MAb complex rapidly with the neutralizing antibodies and are cleared from the circulation by the reticuloendothelial cells, impeding localization of the MAb to the target cells. Readministration of MAb to such presensitized individuals can result in an anamnestic response and, more importantly, the immune complexes thus formed may lead to serious allergic reactions including serum sickness[3].

The frequency and intensity of the HAMA response is related to the inherent immunogenicity of the MAb as well as a number of host parameters, some of which remain poorly characterized. HAMA are seldom encountered in patients with B-cell malignancies (e.g. CLL) but are frequent in patients with T-cell malignancies[4-6]. Because of the differences in their peptide structure, some antibodies can be expected to be more immunogenic than others. Mouse whole antibodies are more immunogenic than the Fab fragment alone. The dosage of MAb administered may also be a relevant factor. In addition, the number of injections, the time interval between injections, and the route of administration have also been suggested to be important determinants of HAMA response.

Several approaches have been tried to suppress the HAMA response (reviewed in 7). Concurrent administration of the MAb and chemotherapeutic agents such as cyclophosphamide or azathioprine, and radiotherapy may have a modest inhibitory effect on HAMA response[8,9]. Administration of large, frequent doses of MAb has also been tried with some success[10,11] although this remains controversial[3]. Immunosuppressive agents such as cyclosporin A have shown potential in limited trials for suppressing HAMA although delayed appearance of HAMA was observed[12,13]. Genetic engineering has provided the tools for generation of chimeric antibodies in which the murine variable region of the antibody is coupled to the human constant region. Chimeric antibodies are associated with a somewhat lower incidence of HAMA, although the potential for development of neutralizing anti-idiotypic antibodies remains. Other potential and theoretical approaches to prevent HAMA response include intradermal antigen desensitization, use of radioimmunoconjugates, and immunotoxins. An agent that suppresses HAMA may have widespread application as an adjunct to diagnostic and therapeutic application of MAbs.

We are conducting a phase I clinical trial using a novel immunosuppressive drug, deoxyspergualin (DSG), to suppress HAMA response to the murine MAb L6. The initial experience from this trial is reported here.

## DSG

Deoxyspergualin (DSG) is a derivative of spergualin, a fermentation product isolated from Bacillus laterosporus. Early studies showed activity of this agent against some hematologic tumors, however, presently its most promising properties relate to its immunosuppressive effects. DSG has demonstrated excellent immunosuppressive activity when administered either prophylactically or therapeutically in many animal models of

194

transplant rejection[14-17]. Preliminary studies also suggest similar efficacy in humans[18]. In vivo studies also demonstrate a potent immunosuppressive effect in autoimmune models[19-21].

A large number of in vitro studies of DSG have been performed in an attempt to determine the mode of action. These studies suggest that this agent acts through mechanisms which are quite distinct from those of other immunosuppressive agents including cyclosporin A. It does not inhibit IL-2 synthesis and has only minor effects on expression of IL-2 receptors. It has been shown to inhibit the generation of antigen-specific cytotoxic T-lymphocytes and variable results have been reported for effects on LAK cell activity[22,23].

One of the most striking features of the in vivo activity of DSG is its ability to block humoral antibody responses against both T-cell-dependent and T-cell-independent antigens[24]. It has been reported to inhibit the antibody response to highly immunogenic proteins including Keyhole Lympet Hemocyanin (KLH)[25], sheep red blood cell antigens[26] and pseudomonas exotoxin immunoconjugates[27]. The mechanism of this humoral inhibition is believed to be via effects on the antigen presenting cell and/or the B-cell.

## L6 Antibody

L6 is a murine MAb antibody of the $IgG_{2a}$ class that binds to the cell surface of most human adenocarcinomas and non-small cell lung carcinomas. The nature of its target antigen has not been fully characterized yet. The antibody is capable of mediating antibody-dependent cellular cytotoxicity (ADCC) and complement-dependent cytotoxicity (CDC) in vitro[28].

In two previous phase I studies (one using L6 alone and another employing a combination of L6 and interleukin-2)[29,30], administration of L6 induced a HAMA response in approximately two-thirds of patients (13/18 and 9/14, respectively). In one of these studies, eight of the thirteen patients developing HAMA also developed anti-idiotypic antibodies. HAMA typically appeared around day 14, although antimouse antibodies were first detected as late as 70 days after the initiation of treatment in rare instances. The frequency of HAMA response did not appear to be related to the dosage of MAb administered. The absolute level of HAMA ranged from less than 100 ng/ml to greater than 38,000 ng/ml, as measured by a double antigen ELISA assay using polyclonal mouse immunoglobulin (Immunomedics, Inc., New Jersey) (for details of the assay, see below).

## STUDY DESIGN

Patients with metastatic colon, ovarian, breast, and non-small cell lung cancer who have failed standard therapy for their disease are eligible for this phase I study. The dose levels of the two drugs are as follows.

**Table 1.** Study Design

| Dose level | L6<br>mg/m$^2$ (d.1-5) | DSG<br>mg/m$^2$ (d.1-7) | Schedule |
|:---:|:---:|:---:|:---:|
| I | 200 | 50 | q 6 weeks |
| II | 200 | 150 | q 6 weeks |
| III | 200 | 150 | q 3 weeks |

DSG is administered by intravenous infusion over three hours followed by L6 infusion over one hour. Patients are followed for toxicity, HAMA, alteration in peripheral blood lymphocyte subsets, quantitative immunoglobulins, and clinical response. The study is designed to exclude a reduction of HAMA response to 20% by concomitant administration of DSG at any given dose. Initially, three patients are enrolled at a dose level. If two or more of these patients develop HAMA, that dose level is considered ineffective. If none or one of three develop HAMA, accrual continues to a total of eight patients. If four or more of eight patients at a given dose level develop HAMA, that dose level may be considered ineffective.

## HAMA Assays

HAMA levels are measured by a commercial ELISA kit supplied by Immunomedics, Inc., (New Jersey) and by a radiometric assay technique[31]. Both assays utilize a "double antigen" format but differ in several ways. The ELISA assay uses polyclonal mouse immunoglobulin as the antigen and thus detects human antibodies to murine constant regions. The results of the assay are compared to a standard curve made from an affinity purified primate anti-mouse immunoglobulin and reported as ng/ml antibody "equivalents". The radiometric assay utilizes murine L6 as the antigen and thus detects HAMA to either constant or variable region of L6. The results of this assay are reported as nanograms of L6 bound/ml serum.

The lower limit of sensitivity of the ELISA assay is reported to be 37 ng/ml antibody "equivalents" and a positive assay is defined at $\geq$ 74 ng/ml according to the manufacturer's instructions. By the radiometric method, a positive assay is defined as a value of at least twice the pre-therapy value and greater than 2 S.D. above the mean binding in normal donors. Eighteen normal donors had $9 \pm 5$ ng/ml binding values, therefore, in order to be considered positive, the anti-L6 antibody level in the patient sample must exceed 19 ng/ml.

## Drug Assays

**DSG.** A high pressure liquid chromoatographic (HPLC) method has been developed and validated for the determination of DSG in serum and plasma. The internal standard is added to the serum sample and then the sample is processed using a solid phase extraction technique. The extracted sample is then reconstituted in mobile phase and injected on an HPLC. Measurement of DSG and the internal standard was performed by post-column derivatization with o-phthalaldehyde and fluorescence detection. The assay was validated over the concentration range of 5-1,000 ng/mL with an inter-assay variability below 3%.

**L6.** Murine monoclonal antibody L6 in serum was measured by an enzyme immunoassay (ETA. An L6 specific murine anti-idiotype monoclonal antibody, 1B, was adsorbed onto polystyrene assay plates and used to capture L6 from serum samples. The captured L6 was then detected using a biotinylated murine anti-idiotypic antibody (13B) with specificity for murine L6 and avidin-linked horseradish peroxidase. The assay has been validated over the concentration range of 10-50 ng/ml. Samples above 50 ng/mL are diluted to the linear range and re-assayed. The inter-assay variability is below 15%.

## RESULTS

### Patient Characteristics

A total of 16 patients (15 F, 1 M) have been treated with this combination so far, nine at dose level I and seven at dose level II. Their median age is 49 years (range, 32-72). The primary diagnoses include breast carcinoma (14 patients) and colon carcinoma (2 patients). All patients had failed extensive prior systemic therapy including six who had failed more than three prior chemotherapy regimens.

### HAMA Response

Fifteen of the sixteen patients enrolled on the study are evaluable for HAMA (Table 2) by ELISA assay. One patient received L6 MAb for six days instead of five and is therefore considered inevaluable as a protocol violation even though no anti-mouse antibodies were detected in her serum up to 6 weeks after treatment. At dose level I, two of the eight patients developed detectable HAMA beginning on d. 42 and 125, respectively. The highest HAMA levels in these individuals were 160 ng/ml and 54 ng/ml, on day 99 and 145, respectively. The first individual received two courses of treatment uneventfully and then had to discontinue treatment, despite a lack of any evidence of tumor progression, due to the occurrence of anaphylactoid reaction during the third course. Interestingly, there was no difference in the L6 pharmacokinetics between the first and second course in this patient, despite the presence of circulating HAMA during the administration of second course of treatment. Thus, the degree of HAMA response was not high enough to alter the kinetics of this large dose of L6. The second individual was taken off-study after two courses due to progressive disease. HAMA were first detected in her serum approximately 2.5 months after the last dose of L6. It should be noted that the highest level of HAMA observed in this individual would not be considered positive according to the manufacturer's criteria. At dose level II, one of the seven individuals has developed HAMA so far (level 150 ng/ml).

The same serum samples were also analyzed using a double antigen radiometric assay. Serum samples from the first twelve patients have been analyzed so far. Of these, samples from 9 patients showed qualitatively similar results by both methods (two patients positive, and seven negative). In three patients, samples that were negative for HAMA by ELISA assay, were positive for anti-L6 antibodies at a modest level (40, 73, and 23 ng/ml), positive value being a level of greater than 19 ng/ml.

**Table 2.** Induction of HAMA in patients treated with L6 and DSG

| DSG Dose Level | No. of patients (Evaluable) | HAMA[*] (+) | (-) | Anti-L6 antibody[**] (+) | (-) |
|---|---|---|---|---|---|
| I | 9 (8) | 2 | 6 | 4 | 4 |
| II | 7 (7) | 1[***] | 6 | 0 | 3 |

\* ELISA Assay
\*\* Double Antigen Radiometric Assay
\*\*\* Radiometric assay of corresponding sample pending

## Pharmacokinetics

Preliminary data on the plasma concentrations of DSG and L6-MAb are available in six patients treated at dose level I (DSG 50 mg/m$^2$ as a three hour infusion on days 1-7). Mean (S.D.) values of Area Under the Plasma Concentration Curve (AUC) were 1697 (352) ng.hr/ml and 1225 (346) ng.hr/ml on days 1 and 7, respectively. The mean (S.D.) total body clearance of DSG was 940 (140) ml/min on day 1 and 1226 (346) ml/min on day 7, respectively. The mean (S.D.) elimination half-life for DSG was 1.09 (0.31) hours on Day 1 and 0.91 (0.18) hours on Day 7. There was no observable accumulation of DSG after dosing for 7 days, nor change in the disposition of DSG after 7 days of therapy. In contrast, the disposition of L6 appeared to change after receiving daily doses for 5 days (in combination with DSG). There were increases in L6 mean (S.D.) AUC from 1436

(745) μg. hr/ml on Day 1 to 5212 (1557) μg. hr/ml on Day 5. The mean L6 half-life increased from 11.9 (4.6) hours on Day 1 to 36.7 (6.5) hours on Day 5. In addition, the total body clearance of L6 decreased over ten-fold from 5.08 (2.03) ml/min on day 1 to 0.33 (0.1) ml/min on Day 5. There was no evidence of increased clearance of monoclonal antibody L6 from course 1 to course 2 in patients for whom repeat course data are available.

## Toxicity

The treatment has been generally well tolerated. There has been only one instance of WHO grade III toxicity - hypersensitivity reaction, described earlier, during the third course of treatment in an individual who had circulating HAMA. The symptoms were promptly reversed by diphenhydramine and epinephrine, but recurred on resumption of treatment and the patient was taken off-study. All other toxicities observed so far are $\leq$ WHO Gr II and include fatigue/headache (9 patients), nausea/vomiting (9 patients), fever/chills (6 patients), hypersensitivity reactions (3 patients), and granulocytopenia (3 patients). No significant changes in serum BUN, creatinine, bilirubin, or SGOT have been observed.

## Immunologic Effects

Rapid decrease in serum complement levels has been observed in all patients during each course consistent with complement fixation by L6 MAb. $C_4$ decreased to undetectable limits by day 4 and returned to normal by day 14 - 21. Decreases in $C_3$ and CH50 have also been noted in all patients, although these have tended to normalize before day 14. Mean $C_3$ level was 161.2 mg/dl prior to treatment and 103.5 mg/dl after treatment. Mean pre-and post-treatment CH50 was 154 mg/dl and 7 mg/dl respectively. No significant changes in serum immunoglobulin levels have been observed. Phenotyping of peripheral blood lymphocytes has not revealed any consistent changes. Mean ($\pm$S.D.) T4/T8 ratio prior to and after treatment was 1.22 ($\pm$0.54) and 1.01 ($\pm$0.56), respectively.

## Anti-tumor Activity

Although clinical response determination is not the primary objective of this phase I study, all patients have been closely followed for potential anti-tumor effects of the combination. No patient has achieved a major response (partial or complete remission) so far.

## SUMMARY AND FUTURE DIRECTIONS

The early experience with the combination suggests that DSG can be safely combined with the L6 MAb. The early data also suggest that DSG may suppress HAMA response to murine L6 administration in humans. Accrual on the study continues. The observations made so far also highlight the necessity to standardize HAMA assay methodologies, and to gain a better understanding of clinically significant HAMA and to better delineate the anti-isotypic HAMA response from anti-idiotypic response. Further studies are also needed to assess the effect of DSG on ADCC and CDC as mediators of MAb action. Other obvious questions that need to be answered are: What is the optimum dose of DSG? Can DSG suppress secondary HAMA responses? What is the long-term toxicity of DSG? The answers to all these questions await definitive trials of DSG for HAMA prevention.

## Acknowledgements

We wish to thank Judy Vance for preparation of the manuscript. This study is sponsored by the National Cancer Institute and supported, in part, by Bristol-Myers Squibb Company, Wallingford, Connecticut.

Kapil Dhingra is a recipient of a Clinical Oncology Career Development Award from the American Cancer Society.

## REFERENCES

1. Blakely DC. Drug targeting with monoclonal antibodies--A review. **Acta Oncol** 1992; **31**: 91-97.
2. Kohler S, Milstein G. Continuous cultures of fused cells secreting antibody of predefined specificity. **Nature** 1975; **256**: 495-497.
3. Tjandra JJ, Ramadi L, McKenzie IFC. Development of human anti-murine antibody (HAMA) response in patients. **Immunol Cell Biol** 1990; **68**: 367-376.
4. Shawler DL, Bartholomew RM, Smith LM, Dillman RO. Human immune response to multiple injections of murine monoclonal IgG. **J Immunol** 1985; **135**: 1530-1535.
5. Dykewicz MS, Cranberg JA, Patterson R, Rosen ST, Shaughnessy MA, Zimmer AM. Human IgE, IgG and IgA antibody responses to T101, a murine monoclonal antibody against human lymphocytes: implications for pathogenesis, risk and avoidance of adverse immunologic reactions. **Int Arch Allergy Appl Immunol** 1990; **92**: 131-137.
6. Schroff RW, Foon KA, Beatty SM, Oldham RK, Morgan AC. Human anti-murine immunoglobulin responses in patients receiving monoclonal antibody therapy. **Cancer Res** 1985; **45**: 879-885.
7. Van Kroonenburgh MJPG, Pauwels EKJ. Human immunological response to mouse monoclonal antibodies in the treatment or diagnosis of malignant diseases. **Nucl Med Commun** 1988; **9**: 919-930.
8. Jaffer GJ, Fuller TC, Cosimi AB, Russell PS, Winn HJ, Colvin RB. Monoclonal Antibody Therapy: Anti-idiotypic and non-idiotypic antibodies to OKT3 arising depsite intense immunosuppression. **Transplantation** 1986; **41**: 572-578.
9. Thistlethwaite JR,Jr., Cosimi AB, Delmonico FL, et al. Evolving use of OKT3 monoclonal antibody for treatment of renal allograft rejection. **Transplantation** 1984; **38**: 695-701.
10. Sears Hf, Bagli DJ, Herlyn D. Human immune response to monoclonal antibody administration is dose-dependent. **Arch Surg** 1987; **122**: 1384-1388.

11. Sears Hf, Herlyn D, Steplewski Z, Koprowski H. Effects of monoclonal antibody immunotherapy on patients with gastrointestinal adenocarcinoma. **J Biol Response Modifiers** 1984; **3**: 138-150.

12. Ledermann JA, Begent RHJ, Bagshawe KD. Cyclosporin A prevents the anti-murine antibody response to a monoclonal anti-tumor antibody in rabbits. **Br J Cancer** 1988; **58**: 562-566.

13. Ledermann JA, Begent RHJ, Bagshawe KD, et al. Repeated antitumor antibody therapy in man with suppression of the host response by Cyclosporin A. **Br J Cancer** 1988; **58**: 654-657.

14. Engemann R, Gassel HJ, Lafrenz E, Stoffregen C, Thiede A. Transplantation tolerance after short-term administration of 15-Deoxyspergualin in orthotopic rat liver transplantation. **Transplant Proc** 1987; **XIX**: 4241-4243.

15. Amemiya H, Suzuki S, Manabe H, et al. 15-Deoxyspergualin in an immunosuppressive agent in dogs. **Transplant Proc** 1988; **XX**: 229-232.

16. Kaufman DB, Field MJ, Gruber SA, et al. Extended functional survival of murine islet allografts with 15-deoxyspergualin. **Transplant Proc** 1992; **24**: 1045-1047.

17. Collier DStJ, Caine R, Thiru S, Kohno H, Levickis J. 15-Deoxyspergualin in experimental dog renal allografts. **Transplant Proc** 1988; **XX**: 240-241.

18. Amemiya H, Suzuki S, Ota K, et al. A novel rescue drug, 15-deoxyspergualin: first clinical trials for recurrent graft rejection in renal recipients. **Transplantation** 1990; **49**: 337-343.

19. Schorlemmer HU, Bartlett RR, Schleyerbach R, Dickneite G, Seller FR. Immunosuppressive therapy of experimental autoimmune diseases like rheumatoid arthritis and systemic lupus erythematosus by 15-deoxyspergualin. **Int J Immunotherapy** 1989; **1**: 9-20.

20. Schorlemmer HU, Seller FR. Therapeutic effects of 15-deoxyspergualin in acute and chronic relapsing experimental allergic encephalomyelitis (EAE) as models for multiple sclerosis (MS). **Drugs Exptl Clin Res** 1991; **XVII**: 461-469.

21. Schorlemmer HU, Bartlett RR, Seller FR. 15-Deoxyspergualin (15-DSG) has a curative effect on the development of SLE-like autoimmune disease in MRL/1 mice. **Agents and Actions** 1991; **34**: 151-155.

22. Kerr PG, Atkins C. Deoxyspergualin inhibits cytotoxic T lymphocytes but not NK or LAK cells. **Immunol Cell Biol** 1991; **69**: 177-183.

23. Thomas F, Matthews C, Pittman K, Thomas J. 15-Deoxyspergualin produces inhibition of lymphokine-activated killer cell activity. **Transplant Proc** 1992; **24**: 712-713.

24. Fujii H, Takada T, Nemoto K, et al. Deoxyspergualin directly suppresses antibody formation *in vivo* and *in vitro*. **J Antibiot** 1990; **43**: 213-219.

25. Tepper M, Petty B, Bursuker I, Pasternak R, Schacter BZ. Inhibition of antibody production by immunosuppressive agent, deoxyspergualin. **Transplant Proc** 1991; **23**: 328-331.

26. Nemoto K, Hayashi M, Abe F. Immunosuppressive activities of 15-deoxyspergualin in animals. **J Antibiot** 1987; **40**: 561-562.

27. Pai LH, Fitzgerald DJ, Tepper M, Schacter B, Spitainy G, Pastan I. Inhibition of antibody response to Pseudomonas exotoxin and an immunotoxin containing pseudomonas exotoxin by 15-deoxyspergualin in mice. **Cancer Res** 1990; **50**: 7750-7753.

28. Hellstrom I, Garrigues U, Lavie E, et.al.. Antibody-mediated killing of human tumor cells by attached effector cells. **Cancer Res** 1988; **48**: 624-627.

29. Goodman GE, Hellstrom I, Brodzinsky L, et al. Phase I trial of murine monoclonal antibody L6 in breast, colon, ovarian, and lung cancer. **J Clin Oncol** 1990; **8**: 1083-1092.

30. Ziegler LD, Palazzolo P, Cunningham J, et al. Phase I trial of murine monoclonal antibody L6 in combination with subcutaneous interleukin-2 in patients with advanced carcinoma of the breast, colorectum, and lung. **J Clin Oncol** 1992; **10**: 1470-1478.
31. LoBuglio AF, Wheeler RH, Trang J, et al. Mouse/human chimeric monoclonal antibody in man: kinetics and immune response. **Proc Natl Acad Sci USA** 1989; **86**: 4220-4224.

# OVERVIEW OF RADIOIMMUNOTHERAPY IN ADVANCED BREAST CANCER USING I-131 CHIMERIC L6

S.J. DeNardo, L.F. O'Grady, C.M. Richman, and G.L. DeNardo

Department of Internal Medicine
University of California Davis Medical Center
Sacramento, California

## SUMMARY ABSTRACT

[131]I chimeric L6 (ChL6) monoclonal antibody (MoAb) therapy has been performed in 12 patients with advanced, metastatic breast cancer. The protocol was designed to determine the maximum tolerated dose (MTD) of radioimmunotherapy that could be administered at 4 intervals. Ten patients received 20 - 70 mCi/m$^2$ of [131]I ChL6. Two of the patients received granulocyte colony stimulating factor (GCSF) on days 10-20 post therapy. The MTD for two doses was 60 mCi/m$^2$ and thrombocytopenia was the dose limiting toxicity in the absence of marrow reconstitution with stem cells. Two patients received 150 mCi/m$^2$ with autologous peripheral blood stem cell support 7 and 9 days post treatment. The MTD has not been reached for [131]I-ChL6 with autologous stem cell support. In the 12 patients treated with [131]I ChL6, six patients (50%) had measurable tumor regressions greater than 30% of the sum of the largest two dimensional products for measurable tumors. Four of these 6 patients had a partial response (PR), i.e., ≥ 50% reduction in tumor size.

These therapeutic responses associated with modest clinical toxicity in heavily pretreated patients suggest that clinically relevant radioimmunotherapeutic approaches can be devised for metastatic breast cancer.

## INTRODUCTION

Over the last 50 years, despite improved diagnostic technology, earlier detection, new chemotherapy agents and more aggressive treatment regimens with autologous bone marrow rescue,[1,2,3] there has been no change in survival rate of adult patients who develop metastatic breast cancer.[4] Efforts to treat cancer patients with monoclonal antibodies (MoAb) have met with variable success, and no benefit has been demonstrated in breast cancer thus far.[5-10] We approached the treatment of breast cancer using the chimeric form of the L6 monoclonal antibody (ChL6), radioiodinated with [131]I. Patients were given unconjugated L6 or ChL6 in

*Antigen and Antibody Molecular Engineering in Breast Cancer Diagnosis and Treatment*, Edited by R.L. Ceriani, Plenum Press, New York, 1994

203

amounts sufficient to cover nontumor targets and to activate biologic systems at the tumor site so that subsequently administered [131]I ChL6 would achieve maximum targeting of the breast cancer.[11] The treatment dose of [131]I ChL6 was preceded by an imaging study with the same radiopharmaceutical in order to assure tumor targeting and absence of normal tissue targeting. Using treatment doses of [131]I ChL6 given at 4-6 week intervals, responses were observed in 6 of the 12 patients with advanced breast cancer and were associated with acceptable toxicity. We believe that these promising results were made possible because the pretreatment infusion of unconjugated L6 and ChL6 induced an inflammatory response at the tumor site, enhancing delivery and efficacy of the subsequently administered [131]I ChL6.[12]

## MATERIALS AND METHODS

The MoAb L-6, an $IgG_{2a}$ mouse antibody, targets a membrane bound antigen found on human adenocarcinoma cells of the lung, colon, ovary and breast.[13] It possesses tumoricidal activity manifested by antibody dependent cellular cytotoxicity (ADCC) in the presence of human peripheral blood mononuclear cells and complement dependent cytotoxicity (CDC) in the presence of human complement.[14,15] A chimeric human-mouse antibody was produced in which mouse constant domains C-G2a and C-kappa were replaced by the human C-G1 and C-kappa.[16] Chimeric and murine L-6 antibodies bind adenocarcinoma cells with the same avidity, but ChL6 is 50 to 100 times more effective at mediating ADCC.[15,16]

The radiopharmaceutical was prepared using chloramine-T radioiodination with [131]I (ICN Biomedicals, Inc., Irvine, CA) and the final products were sterile and pyrogen-free.[17,18] HPLC TSK 3000 chromatography and cellulose acetate electrophoresis demonstrated that greater than 95% of the radioactivity was associated with the antibody. Immunoreactivity of each preparation had greater than 70% direct binding to a live human breast tumor cell line in vitro (HBT 3477).[19] The radiopharmaceutical contained 10 mCi of [131]I per mg of antibody, 1 mCi of [131]I per ml, and human serum albumin 4% weight to volume.

Twelve patients with advanced metastatic breast cancer who had failed aggressive standard therapy and had rapidly progressing disease were treated with [131]I ChL6. Their metastatic tumor had tested L-6 positive by immunopathology. These patients were selected to assess the toxicity of this treatment approach and the maximum tolerated [131]I dose that could be given as [131]I ChL6. Previous pharmacokinetic studies of murine L-6 in breast cancer patients revealed the need to give a 200 mg infusion of unconjugated antibody before the [131]I labeled antibody to achieve maximum tumor and minimal lung uptake.[11] All imaging and therapy doses were therefore given after slow infusion of 200 mg L6 or 200 mg ChL6. In 11 of the 12 patients, the imaging study was performed the day prior to the therapeutic dose as final assessment for therapy and to determine the potential for enhanced tumor uptake of the therapeutic dose given after the biologic activation seen from the imaging dose.[12] After each therapeutic dose, quantitative gamma camera imaging was performed for at least one week to obtain pharmacokinetics for dosimetric analysis.[20]

Serum and plasma samples were drawn prior and during MoAb infusions, immediately after the infusion, 2-4 hours post dose and daily for 3-5 days for pharmacokinetics and quantitation of serum mediators. Serum albumin (normal range 3.8 - 5.1 g/100/ml) levels were determined by the colorimetric bromcresyl purple method.[21] Serum C3 (normal range 88 - 186 mg/100 ml) and C4 (normal range 14 - 54 mg/100ml) levels were determined by nephelometry.[22] IL-2 levels were determined by a similar radioimmunoassay from Advanced Magnetics Inc. IL-2 is normally undetectable in serum as IL-2 bound to soluble IL-2 receptor (sIL-2R) is undetectable by this assay. The tracer was incubated overnight with duplicate

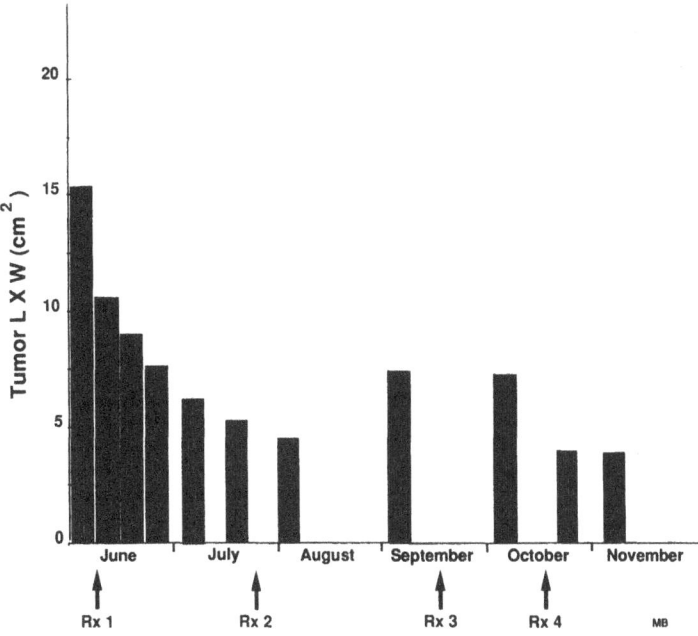

Figure 1. Therapy course of patient three demonstrated regression of her tumor in response to [131]I ChL6 therapy doses (Rx 1 - 4). All measurable tumor areas are graphically shown as the sum of the products of their longest diameter and the greatest perpendicular diameter obtained from caliper measurements taken by two physicians before therapy and at frequent intervals after each of her therapy doses.

samples and rabbit anti-human IL-2 for 4 hours at room temperature. The complexes were precipitated by centrifugation and the pellets were washed one time with supplied wash buffer prior to counting the pellet. The IL-2 levels were calculated by comparison to supplied IL-2 standards and controls.

Soluble IL-2R levels in patient serum or plasma were determined by an enzyme immunoassay kit from T Cell Diagnostics (Cambridge, MA). Our normal values were less than 480 U/ml which agrees with literature referenced levels.[23] Fifty microliters of each duplicate sample along with 100ul of supplied horse radish peroxidase conjugated anti-human sIL-2R were added to duplicate wells already coated with another anti-human sIL-2R monoclonal antibody which recognizes a non-overlapping epitope and incubation for 3 hours at room

TABLE 1. Three Arms of [131]I ChL6 Protocol: Summary of Response

| | NO. OF PATIENTS | PR | SR | HAMA | MTD |
|---|---|---|---|---|---|
| 1. [131]I ChL6 | 8 | 4 | 0 | 4 | $60 \text{ mCi/m}^2$ |
| 2. [131]I ChL6/GCSF | 2 | 0 | 2 | 2 | $60 \text{ mCi/m}^2$ |
| 4. [131]I ChL6 Autologous Peripheral Blood Stem Cells/GCSF | 2 | 0 | 0 | 2 | open $\geq 150$ $\text{mCi/m}^2$ |

temperature. Chromogen was added to each well for 30 minutes and the reaction was stopped with 2N sulfuric acid and the absorbance read at 490nm. The sIL-2R level was determined by comparison to recombinant sIL-2R standards and controls supplied by the manufacturer.

Therapy doses were given as close to 4 week intervals as tolerated by the patient for treatment levels of 20, 60 and 70 mCi/m$^2$ and the second or subsequent therapy doses for any patient were adjusted downward in steps dictated by hematologic toxicity. The patients were treated on three protocol arms. In the first, the escalating doses were given to 8 patients to determine the maximum tolerated dose (MTD) which would not produce grade 3 or 4 marrow toxicity. The second protocol arm was added to determine if the use of GCSF on days 10 to 20 post therapy dose could increase the MTD. Since the use of GCSF alone did not raise the MTD, a third arm was then designed to determine the MTD of [131]I ChL6 with autologous peripheral blood stem cell support of marrow function.[24] Stem cells were obtained by 4 to 6 daily apheresis procedures beginning 4 days after initiating GCSF to mobilize precursors into the circulation.[25] After sufficient cells were obtained to support three treatments and the patient had been off GCSF for one week, [131]I ChL6 was given at an initial dose level of 150 mCi/m$^2$ (more than twice the non stem cell supported MTD). Following the radioimmunotherapy dose, when the whole blood level was less than 1μCi/ml, 5 x 10$^8$ cryopreserved mononuclear cells/kg were transfused, and a 2 week course of GCSF was given to stimulate the progenitors. Hematopoietic colony forming units were determined for each stem cell infusion.[24,25]

## RESULTS

Nine of the 12 patients received at least 2 and as many as 4 treatment doses of [131]I ChL6. The remaining 3 patients received only one treatment dose. Six of the 12 patients had measurable tumor regression calculated to be greater than 30% of the sum of the products of greatest dimensions of all measurable disease and 4 of these patients had partial responses (PR) lasting one to five months (Table 1) (Fig. 1). Calculated tumor radiation dose ranged from 3 to 70 rads per administered mCi of I-131. Eight of the 12 patients developed antibodies (HAMA) to the ChL6, limiting further therapy since doses given when high levels of HAMA was present resulted in rapid clearing of the therapy dose from the patient's blood, not allowing the dose to reach tumor. Ten of the 12 patients developed transient grade 3 or 4 hematologic toxicity during the course of therapy doses but none of these patients had bleeding or infections (Table 2).

Two patients reported here were in the autologous stem cell support arm of the protocol. Two doses of [131]I ChL6 (150 mCi/m$^2$) were given to one patient with a six week interval. Stem cells were infused within 10 days of each dose but not until the blood level of [131]I had become less than 1 μCi/ml. Since the success of the stem cells to quickly engraft would diminish if they received a cytotoxic dose of radiation from radioactivity in the blood, it is relevant that the infused stem cells given at this [131]I blood level successfully expanded the blood cell population and prevented significant hematologic toxicity. However, the first 150mCi/m$^2$ dose of [131]I ChL6 given with stem cell support to a second patient resulted in thrombocytopenia and required a second stem cell infusion. This patient received the same level of mononuclear cells/kg as the initial patient but stem cell cultures revealed that they contained fewer (less than half) colony forming units (CFUs) than the stem cells given the prior patient who experienced only minimal myelo-suppression. After the second stem cell infusion, platelet recovery occurred.

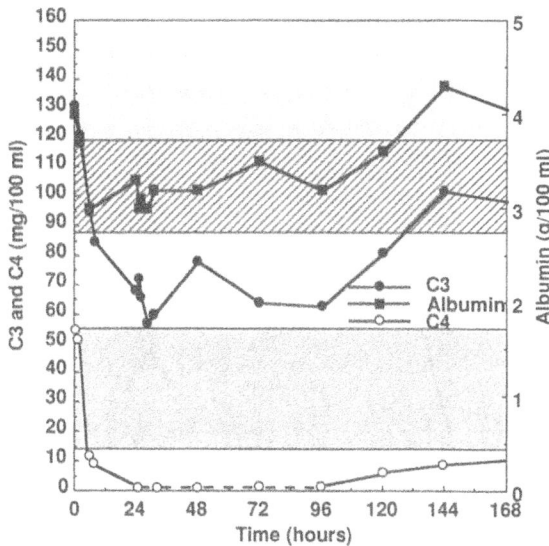

Figure 2. An example of the temporal sequence of changes in serum C3, C4 and albumin which occurred after MoAb infusion in patients. A second infusion of MoAb was started 24 hours after the first infusion. Time 0 is the baseline value obtained immediately prior to the start of the first antibody infusion. All patients have shown a decrease in complement and albumin values during and subsequent to the infusion. Recovery to normal levels varied from patient to patient but most measurements became normal within 7 - 10 days after infusion. Shaded and stippled areas indicate normal ranges (see text) for C3 ($/\!/\!/$), C4 (■) and albumin ( ).

In the 12 therapy patients C3, C4, and albumin levels fell during L6 and ChL6 infusions and remained below normal for hours to days post therapy (Fig. 2). The 11 patients receiving their imaging and therapy infusions on sequential days demonstrated a dose and time dependent pattern of sIL-2R levels in serum when compared to their preinfusion level. IL-2 levels were elevated shortly after initiation of the infusion of L6 or ChL6 in 2 patients (Fig. 3). IL-2 levels, however, could not be measured by this assay once the IL-2 receptor level had risen.

## DISCUSSION

This is the first radiolabeled MoAb therapy which has produced objective responses in patients with metastatic breast cancer. This is also the first radioimmunotherapy in which autologous peripheral blood stem cells have been used as supportive therapy to enable administration of higher doses of radioactivity. Measurable tumor regression was observed in 6 of the 12 patients. The longest duration of response was 5 months and the latter patient could not be further treated because she developed a high HAMA titer. Her response included a reduction in tumor volume and a significant reduction in bone pain allowing her to resume a normal life after having been restricted to a wheelchair because of pain.

The mechanisms by which the tumoricidal effect was achieved may relate both to the activation of the patients immune systems by the biologically potent chimeric antibody as well as to radiation received by the tumor from the targeted [131]I. The preload of unconjugated L6 or ChL6 was given to cover endothelial targets demonstrated by prior studies,[11] as well as to utilize the immunologic effects of this biologically active antibody.[15,16] The decrease in serum complement (C3) levels during and immediately after the unlabeled antibody infusion

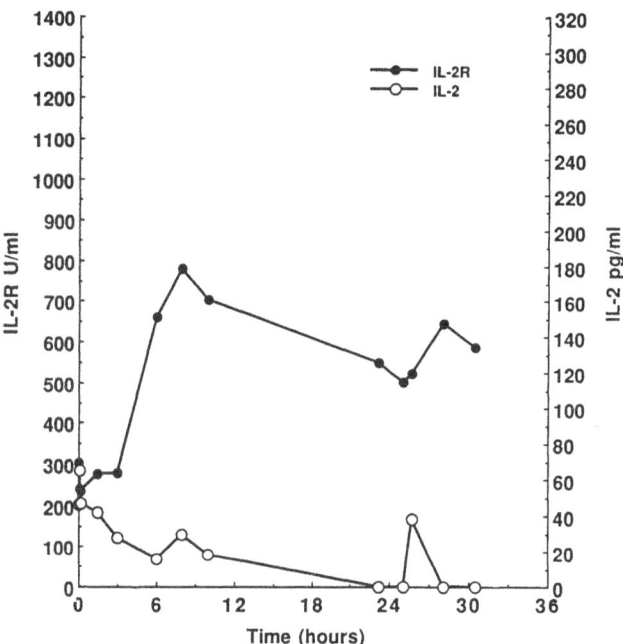

Figure 3. An example of changes seen in IL2 and sIL2R levels which occur with MoAb infusion in patients. This data was obtained from the same patient MoAb infusions shown in Figure 2. An immediate short-lived rise in IL2 was seen after initiation of each 200 mg infusion (0-4 hrs; 24-28 hrs). A marked rise in sIL2R, peaking shortly after the end of each infusion occurred in patients who subsequently demonstrated clinical tumor regression.

indicates that complement was consumed by biologic activities initiated by this antibody (Fig. 2).[12,26] Clinical evidence of inflammation at superficial tumor sites after each dose also suggested antibody activation of immune effector cells, release of cytokines, and increased local vascular permeability which enhanced the uptake of the therapy dose. As we have previously reported, patients demonstrating the best clinical responses have most frequently had significant rise in their serum sIL-2R levels during infusion of the unlabeled MoAb.[12] It is unlikely, however, that the therapeutic response seen in these patients was due to this immunologic activity alone, since therapy studies using large amounts of unlabeled L6 or ChL6 in patients with breast cancer have demonstrated little or no responses.[27,28] The radiation doses to tumor were calculated to be 3 to 70 rads per administered mCi of [131]I and are considered to be the primary mechanism for these responses. We postulate that responses have been secondary to synergy between enhanced delivery of the targeted radiation and tumor sensitization caused by activated immune cell mechanisms.

The hematologic toxicity observed at these doses of radiopharmaceutical were transient (Table 2). The radiation effect on the red blood cell line was minimal but the effect on platelet production was dose-limiting similar to that previously observed in patients receiving radioimmunotherapy for lymphoma.[29] The patient receiving 70 mCi/m$^2$ had a grade 4 hematologic toxicity two weeks after the second therapy dose but one week later had recovered to grade 3 toxicity and at 5 weeks had recovered to normal. In the two patients receiving GCSF on days 10 to 20 post therapy, one patient had no hematologic toxicity, but the second patient had reached a transient grade 4 thrombocytopenia four weeks after the second dose and recovered to grade one at five weeks. It appears that the nadir of platelets and neutrophils may become more severe after repeat doses of [131]I ChL6 therapy and usually occurs between two to four weeks after administration of 60-70 mCi/m$^2$ of this radiopharmaceutical. Recovery time and degree of recovery were variable, probably relating to the patient's marrow reserve after previous radiation and chemotherapy.

We conclude that responses were achieved in 6 of 12 patients with advanced metastatic breast cancer after treatment with radiolabeled ChL6 MoAb. Because these patients were refractory to chemotherapy and primarily selected to determine the toxicity associated with this therapeutic approach, the clinical responses are more remarkable. Manageable levels of toxicity occurred in these patients. Unfortunately, due to initiation of treatment late in the disease course and onset of HAMA titers in most patients that limited further therapy, the responses were transient. Future therapeutic efforts will focus on metastatic breast cancer patients with less extensive disease using drugs such as cyclosporin A [30] to reduce HAMA response and predetermined numbers of stem cell CFUs to support dose intensification of the [131]I ChL6 therapy. These more aggressive approaches will help to determine whether clinically useful radioimmunotherapy can be delivered to breast cancer, and if this therapy can be effectively combined with agents using different and complementary cancer cytotoxic mechanisms.

TABLE 2.  Effects of [131]I ChL6 Therapy Dose Level and Number on Hematologic Toxicity and Tumor Response

| Patient | mCi/m$^2$ | Marrow Support | # of Doses | Hematoxicity Per Dose | Response |
|---------|-----------|----------------|------------|-----------------------|----------|
| 1 | 20 | 0 | 3 | 0,3,4 | PR |
| 2 | 60 | 0 | 1 | 3 | NR |
| 3 | 60 | 0 | 4 | 2,2,0,3 | PR |
| 4 | 60 | 0 | 2 | 2,4 | NR |
| 5 | 60 | 0 | 1 | 0 | NR |
| 6 | 60 | 0 | 2 | 2,4 | P |
| 7 | 60 | 0 | 3 | 1,2,0 | PR |
| 8 | 70 | 0 | 2 | 0,4 | PR |
| 9 | 60 | GCSF | 2 | 0,3 | SR |
| 10 | 60 | GCSF | 2 | 2,4 | SR |
| 11 | 150 | stem cell/ GCSF | 2 | 2,2 | NR |
| 12 | 150 | stem cell/ GCSF | 1 | *4 | NR |

PR = Partial response, ≥ 50% sum of products of tumor L and W
SR = Some response, decrease < 50% and ≥ 30% sum of products of tumor L and W
NR = No response, decrease < 30% and progression of ≤ 25% in any existing lesion
P  = Progression, increased by > 25% in any existing lesion
*  = Stem cell colony forming units too low

## ACKNOWLEDGEMENT

This research was supported by grants from the National Cancer Institute (PHS NIH CA47829) and the Department of Energy (DE FG03-84ER60233). Mouse and Chimeric L6 were provided by ONCOGENE, Seattle, WA.

## REFERENCES

1. I.C. Henderson, J.R. Harris, D.W. Kinne, and S. Hellman. Cancer of the breast, in: V.T. Devita, S. Hellman, S.A. Rosenberg, eds., Cancer Principles and Practice of Oncology. JB Lippincott, Philadelphia 1197-1261 (1989).

2. E. Silverberg, C.C. Boring, and T.S. Squires. Cancer statistics. CA 40:9-26 (1990).

3. K.H. Antman. Dose intensive therapy in breast cancer, in: "High-Dose Cancer Therapy: Pharmacology, Hematopoietins, Stem Cell," J.O. Armitage, K.H. Antman, eds., Williams & Wilkins, Baltimore 701-718 (1992).

4. M.S. Fox. On the diagnosis and treatment of breast cancer. JAMA 241:489-494 (1979).

5. J.J. Tjandra and I.F.C. McKenzie. Murine monoclonal antibodies in breast cancer: an overview. Br J Surg 75:1067-1077 (1988).

6. A. Thor, M.O. Weeks, and J. Schlom. Monoclonal antibodies and breast cancer. Seminars in Oncology 13:393-401 (1986).

7. L.M. Weiner, J. O'Dwyer, J. Kitson, R.L. Comis, A.E. Frankel, R.J. Bauer, M.S. Konrad, and E.S. Groves. Phase I evaluation of an anti-breast carcinoma monoclonal antibody 260F9-recombinant ricin A chain immunoconjugate. Cancer Res 49:4062-4067 (1989).

8. J. Malamitsi, D. Skarlos, S. Fotiou, P. Papakostas, G. Aravantinos, D. Vassilarou, J. Taylor-Papadimitriou, K. Koutoulidis, G. Hooker, and D. Snook. Intracavitary use of two radiolabeled tumor-associated monoclonal antibodies. J Nucl Med 29:1910-1915 (1988).

9. B.J. Gould, M.J. Borowitz, E.S. Groves, P.W. Carter, D. Anthony, L.M. Weiner, and A.E. Frankel. Phase I study of antibreast immunotoxin by continuous infusion. J of the NCI 81:775-781 (1989).

10. B.P. Avner, S.K. Liao, B. Avner, K. DeCall, and R.K. Oldham. Therapeutic murine monoclonal antibodies developed for individual cancer patients. J of Biological Resp Mod 8:25-36 (1989).

11. S.J. DeNardo, L.F. O'Grady, D.J. Macey, L.A. Kroger, G.L. DeNardo, K.R. Lamborn, N.B. Levy, S.L. Mills, I. Hellstrom, and K.E. Hellstrom. Quantitative imaging of mouse L-6 monoclonal antibody in breast cancer patients to develop a therapeutic strategy. Nucl Med Biol 18:621-631 (1991).

12. S.J. DeNardo, G.R. Mirick, L.A. Kroger, L.F. O'Grady, K.L. Erickson, A. Yuan, K.R. Lamborn, I Hellstrom, K.E. Hellstrom and G.L. DeNardo. The biologic window for ChL6 radioimmunotherapy. Cancer (1994).

13. I. Hellstrom, D. Horn, P. Linsley, J. P. Brown, V. Brankovan, and K.E. Hellstrom. Monoclonal antibodies raised against human lung carcinomas. Cancer Res 46:3917-23 (1986).

14. I. Hellstrom, P.L. Beaumier, and K.E. Hellstrom. Antitumor effects of L-6, an IgG2a antibody that reacts with most human carcinomas. Proc Natl Acad Science USA 83:7059-7063 (1986).

15. G.P. Adams, S.J. DeNardo, A. Amin, L.A. Kroger, G.L. DeNardo, I. Hellstrom, and K.E. Hellstrom. Comparison of the pharmacokinetics in mice and the biological activity of murine L-6 and human-mouse chimeric Ch L6 antibody. Antibod Immunoconjug Radiopharm 5:81-95 (1992).

16. A.Y. Liu, R.R. Robinson, K.E. Hellstrom, E.D. Murray, Jr., C.P. Chang, and I. Hellstrom. Chimeric mouse-human IgG1 antibody that can mediate lysis of cancer cells. Proc Natl Acad Science USA 84:3439-3443 (1987).

17. W.M. Hunter and F.C. Greenwood. Preparation of iodine-131 labelled growth hormone of high specific activity. Nature 194:495 (1962).

18. S.L. Mills, S.J. DeNardo, G.L. DeNardo, A.L. Epstein, J-S. Peng, and D. Colcher. I-123 radiolabelling of monoclonal antibodies for in vivo procedures. Hybridoma 5:265-275 (1986).

19. P.L. Beaumier, D. Neuzil, H-M. Yang, E.A. Noll, R. Kishore, J.F. Eary, K.A. Krohn, W.B. Nelp, K.E. Hellstrom, and I. Hellstrom. Immunoreactivity assay for labeled anti-melanoma monoclonal antibodies. J Nucl Med 27:824-828 (1986).

20. D.J. Macey, G.L. DeNardo, and S.J. DeNardo. A treatment planning program for radioimmunotherapy. Front Radiat Ther Oncol 24:123-131 (1990).

21. A. Louderback, E.H. Mealy, and P.H. Wiernik. A new dye-binding technique using bromocresyl purple for determination of albumin in serum. Clin Chem 14:793-794 (1968).

22. P. Yam L.D. Petz, and N.R. Cooper. The relationship between hemolytic and immunodiffusion methods for measurement of C4 in patients with immunologic disorders. Am J Clin Path 64:351-357 (1975).

23. A. Linde, B. Anderson, S.B. Svenson, H. Ahrne, M. Carlsson, P. Forsberg, et al. Serum levels of lymphokines and soluble cellular receptors in primary Epstein-Barr virus infection and in patients with chronic fatigue syndrome. J Infec Dis 165:994-1000 (1992).

24. A. Kessinger, J.O. Armitage, J.D. Landmark, D.M. Smith, and D.D. Weisenberger. Autologous peripheral hematopoietic stem cell transplantation restores hematopoietic function following marrow ablative therapy. Blood 71:723-727 (1988).

25. A. Elias, L. Ayash, K. Anderson, C. Wheeler, G. Schwartz, I. Teppler, C. Lynch, M. Hunt, S. Pap, J. Deary, J Pelaez, L. Schnipps, J Griffin, E. Frei, and K. Antman. Hematologic support during high dose intensification for breast cancer: Recruitment od peripheral blood progenitor cells by GM-CSF and chemotherapy. Blood 76 (suppl):536a (1990).

26. S.J. DeNardo, K.A. Warhoe, L.F. O'Grady, G.L. DeNardo, I. Hellstrom, K.E. Hellstrom, and S.L. Mills. Radioimmunotherapy with I-131 chimeric L-6 in advanced breast cancer. in: "Breast Epithelial Antigens," R.L. Ceriani, eds., Plenum Press, New York, pp. 227-232 (1991).

27. G.E. Goodman, I. Hellstrom, C. Nicaise, L. Brodzinsky, D. Hummel, and K.E. Hellstrom. Phase I trial of murine monoclonal antibody L-6 in breast, colon, ovarian,and lung cancer. J Clin Oncol 50:2449-2454 (1990).

28. G.E. Goodman, I. Hellstrom, D.E. Yelton, J.L. Murray, S. O'Hara, E. Meaker, L. Zeigler, P. Palazollo, C. Nicaise, J. Usakewicz, et al. Phase I trial of chimeric (human-mouse) monoclonal antibody L-6 in patients with non-small-cell lung, colon, and breast cancer. Cancer Immunol Immunother 36(4):267-273 (1993).

29. G.L. DeNardo, S.J. DeNardo, N. Levy. Treatment of B cell malignancies with $^{131}$I-Lym-1 and mechanisms for improvement. in: "Monoclonal Antibodies 2, Applications in Clinical Oncology," A. Epenetos, ed., Chapman & Hall Medical, New York, pp. 355-367 (1993).

30. J.A. Ledermann, R.H.J Begent, K.D. Bagshawe, S.J. Riggs, F. Searle, M.G. Glaser, A.J. Green and R.G. Dale. Repeated antitumor antibody therapy in man with suppression of the host response by cyclosporin A. Brit J Cancer 58:654-657 (1988).

# CONTRIBUTORS

J.R. Adair, Oncology Biology, Celltech Research Division, 216 Bath Road, Slough, Berks., U.K. SL1 4EN

V. Apostolopoulos, The Austin Research Institute, The Austin Hospital, Studley Road, Heidelberg VIC 3084, Australia

M. Baker, Toronto General Hospital, Dept. of Medicine, University of Toronto

T.S. Baker, Oncology Biology, Celltech Research Division, 216 Bath Road, Slough, Berks., U.K. SL1 4EN

F. Baratta, Cancer Research Fund of Contra Costa, 2055 N. Broadway, Walnut Creek, CA 94596

A. Baruch, Dept. of Cell Research and Immunology, Tel Aviv University, Ramat Aviv, Tel Aviv 69978, Israel

M. Bhattacharya-Chatterjee, Lucille Markey Cancer Center, University of Kentucky College of Medicine, Lexington, KY 40536

E.W. Blank, Cancer Research Fund of Contra Costa, 2055 N. Broadway, Walnut Creek, CA 94596

D. Booser, Dept. of Medical Oncology, The University of Texas M.D. Anderson Cancer Center, 1515 Holcombe Blvd., Houston, TX 77030

C.C. Bose, Oncology Chemistry, Celltech Research Division, 216 Bath Road, Slough, Berks., U.K. SL1 4EN

A. Buzdar, Dept. of Medical Oncology, The University of Texas M.D. Anderson Cancer Center, 1515 Holcombe Blvd., Houston, TX 77030

K. Cantell, National Public Health Institute, SF-00280 Helsinki, Finland

L. Carmon, Dept. of Cell Research and Immunology, George S. Wise Faculty of Life Sciences, Tel Aviv University, Tel Aviv 69978, Israel

P. Carter, Dept. of Protein Engineering, Genentech, Inc., 460 Point San Bruno Blvd., So. San Francisco, CA 94080

H.M. Caskey-Finney, Oncology Biology, Celltech Research Division, 216 Bath Road, Slough, Berks., U.K.  SL1 4EN

R.L. Ceriani, Cancer Research Fund of Contra Costa, 2055 N. Broadway, Walnut Creek, CA  94596

M.I. Colnaghi, Experimental Oncology E, Istituto Nazionale Tumori, 20133 Milan, Italy

J.R. Couto, Cancer Research Fund of Contra Costa, 2055 N. Broadway, Walnut Creek, CA  94596

G.L. DeNardo, Dept. of Internal Medicine, University of California Davis Medical Center, Sacramento, CA

S.J. DeNardo, Dept. of Internal Medicine, University of California Davis Medical Center, Sacramento, CA

J.W. Dennis, Samuel Lunenfeld Research Institute, Mount Sinai Hospital, 600 University Ave., Toronto, Ontario, Canada  M5G 1X5

C.M. DeRosa, College of Physicians and Surgeons, Columbia University, New York, NY  10032

K. Dhingra, Dept. of Medical Oncology, The University of Texas M.D. Anderson Cancer Center, 1515 Holcombe Blvd., Houston, TX  77030

B. Fernandez, Samuel Lunenfeld Research Institute, Mount Sinai Hospital, 600 University Ave., Toronto, Ontario, Canada  M5G 1X5

I. Figari, Dept. of Endocrinology, Genentech, Inc., 460 Point San Bruno Blvd., So. San Francisco, CA  94080

K.A. Foon, Lucille Markey Cancer Center, University of Kentucky College of Medicine, Lexington, KY  40536

H. Fritsche, Dept. of Laboratory Medicine, The University of Texas M.D. Anderson Cancer Center, 1515 Holcombe Blvd., Houston, TX  77030

P. Furmanski, Dept. of Biology, New York University, New York, NY  10003

R.J. Gaslonde, Cancer Research Fund of Contra Costa, 2055 N. Broadway, Walnut Creek, CA  94596

S.D. Glenn, Coulter Immunology, Hialeah, FL  33010

P. Goss, Toronto General Hospital, Dept. of Medicine, University of Toronto

D. Greene, Bristol-Myers Squibb Company, Wallingford, Connecticut 06492

L. Gutierrez, Dept. of Medical Oncology, The University of Texas M.D. Anderson Cancer Center, 1515 Holcombe Blvd., Houston, TX  77030

D.V. Habif Sr., College of Physicians and Surgeons, Columbia University, New York, NY 10032

M. Hareuveni, Sourasky Medical Center, Tel Aviv, Israel

M. Hartman, Dept. of Cell Research and Immunology, Tel Aviv University, Ramat Aviv, Tel Aviv 69978, Israel

G. Hortobagyi, Dept. of Medical Oncology, The University of Texas M.D. Anderson Cancer Center, 1515 Holcombe Blvd., Houston, TX 77030

T. Irimura, Dept. of Chemical Toxicology and Immunochemistry, The University of Tokyo, Tokyo 113, Japan

S. Kelley, Bristol-Myers Squibb Company, Wallingford, Connecticut 06492

I. Keydar, Dept. of Cell Research and Immunology, Tel Aviv University, Ramat Aviv, Tel Aviv 69978, Israel

M.B. Khazaeli, Comprehensive Cancer Center, University of Alabama at Birmingham, Birmingham, Alabama 35294

D.J. King, Oncology Biology, Celltech Research Division, 216 Bath Road, Slough, Berks., U.K. SL1 4EN

R. Kiwan, Cancer Research Fund of Contra Costa, 2055 N. Broadway, Walnut Creek, CA 94596

R. Koganty, Immunotherapeutics Div., Biomira Inc., 2011 - 94 Street, Edmonton, Alberta, Canada T6N 1H1

H. Kohler, Lucille Markey Cancer Center, University of Kentucky College of Medicine, Lexington, KY 40536

B. Korczak, Samuel Lunenfeld Research Institute, Mount Sinai Hospital, 600 University Ave., Toronto, Ontario, Canada M5G 1X5 and Allelix Inc., Goreway Drive, Mississauga, Ontario

E.L. Kramer, New York University Medical Center/Bellevue Hospital Center, 560 First Avenue, New York, NY 10016

K. Krauer, The Austin Research Institute, The Austin Hospital, Studley Road, Heidelberg VIC 3084, Australia

L. Kroger, Section of Radiodiagnosis and Therapy, University of California at Davis, Sacramento, CA

A.D.G. Lawson, Oncology Biology, Celltech Research Division, 216 Bath Road, Slough, Berks., U.K. SL1 4EN

G.D. Lewis, Dept. of Cell Biology, Genentech, Inc., 460 Point San Bruno Blvd., So. San Francisco, CA 94080

L. Liebes, New York University Medical Center/Bellevue Hospital Center, 560 First Avenue, New York, NY 10016

A.F. LoBuglio, Comprehensive Cancer Center, University of Alabama at Birmingham, Birmingham, Alabama 35294

B.M. Longenecker, Immunotherapeutics Div., Biomira Inc., 2011-94 Street, Edmonton, Alberta, Canada T6N 1H1, Dept. of Immunology, University of Alberta, Alberta, Canada T6N 2H7, and Cross Cancer Institute, 11560 University Avenue, Alberta, Canada T6G 1Z2

A. Lyons, Oncology Biology, Celltech Research Division, 216 Bath Road, Slough, Berks., U.K. SL1 4EN

G.D. MacLean, Dept. of Medicine, University of Alberta, Edmonton, Alberta, Canada T6N 2R7, and Cross Cancer Institute, 11560 University Avenue, Alberta, Canada T6G1Z2

I.F.C. McKenzie, The Austin Research Institute, The Austin Hospital, Studley Road, Heidelberg VIC 3084, Australia

A. Mountain, Oncology Biology, Celltech Research Division, 216 Bath Road, Slough, Berks., U.K. SL1 4EN

E. Mrozek, Molecular Immunology, Roswell Park Cancer Institute, Buffalo, NY

S. Mukerjee, Molecular Immunology, Roswell Park Cancer Institute, Buffalo, NY

J.L. Murray, Dept. of Clinical Immunology and Biological Therapy, The University of Texas M.D. Anderson Cancer Center, 1515 Holcombe Blvd., Houston, TX 77030

M.E. Noz, New York University Medical Center/Bellevue Hospital Center, 560 First Avenue, New York, NY 10016

L.F. O'Grady, Dept. of Internal Medicine, University of California Davis Medical Center, Sacramento, CA

R.J. Owens, Inflammation Biology, Celltech Research Division, 216 Bath Road, Slough, Berks., U.K. SL1 4EN

L. Ozzello, College of Physicians and Surgeons, Columbia University, New York, NY 10032

E.A. Padlan, Laboratory of Molecular Biology, National Institute of Diabetes and Digestive and Kidney Diseases, National Institutes of Health, Bethesda, MD 20892

J.A. Peterson, Cancer Research Fund of Contra Costa, 2055 N. Broadway, Walnut Creek, CA 94596

G.A. Pietersz, The Austin Research Institute, The Austin Hospital, Studley Road, Heidelberg VIC 3084, Australia

J. Prenzoska, The Austin Research Institute, The Austin Hospital, Studley Road, Heidelberg VIC 3084, Australia

M. Raber, Dept. of Medical Oncology, The University of Texas M.D. Anderson Cancer Center, 1515 Holcombe Blvd., Houston, TX 77030

M. Reddish, Immunotherapeutics Div., Biomira Inc., 2011 - 94 Street, Edmonton, Alberta, Canada T6N 1H1

M. Refaat Shalaby, Dept. of Medicinal and Analytical Chemistry, Genentech, Inc., 460 Point San Bruno Blvd., So. San Francisco, CA 94080

C.M. Richman, Dept. of Internal Medicine, University of California Davis Medical Center, Sacramento, CA

M.L. Rodrigues, Dept. of Protein Engineering, Genentech, Inc., 460 Point San Bruno Blvd., So. San Francisco, CA 94080

M.R. Rolfe, Oncology Biology, Celltech Research Division, 216 Bath Road, Slough, Berks., U.K. SL1 4EN

D. Sagiv, Dept. of Cell Research and Immunology, Tel Aviv University, Ramat Aviv, Tel Aviv 69978, Israel

M.K. Schwartz, Dept. of Clinical Chemistry, Memorial Sloan Kettering Cancer Center, New York, NY 10021

M. Sehdev, Oncology Biology, Celltech Research Division, 216 Bath Road, Slough, Berks., U.K. SL1 4EN

N.I. Smorodinsky, Dept. of Cell Research and Immunology, George S. Wise Faculty of Life Sciences, Tel Aviv University, Tel Aviv 69978, Israel

M. Tepper, Bristol-Myers Squibb Company, Wallingford, Connecticut 06492

J. Trapani, The Austin Research Institute, The Austin Hospital, Studley Road, Heidelberg VIC 3084, Australia

D.H. Wreschner, Dept. of Cell Research and Immunology, Tel Aviv University, Ramat Aviv, Tel Aviv 69978, Israel

P.X. Xing, The Austin Research Institute, The Austin Hospital, Studley Road, Heidelberg VIC 3084, Australia

R. Yarden, Dept. of Cell Research and Immunology, George S. Wise Faculty of Life Sciences, Tel Aviv University, Tel Aviv 69978, Israel

G.T. Yarranton, Oncology Biology, Celltech Research Division, 216 Bath Road, Slough, Berks., U.K. SL1 4EN

S. Zrihan-Licht, Dept. of Cell Research and Immunology, Tel Aviv University,
Ramat Aviv, Tel Aviv 69978, Israel

# INDEX

The manufacturer's authorised representative in the EU is Springer
Nature Customer Service Centre GmbH, Europaplatz 3, 69115 Heidelberg,
Germany. If you have any concerns regarding our products, please
contact ProductSafety@springernature.com

Printed and bound by CPI Group (UK) Ltd, Croydon, CR0 4YY
23/04/2026
02095607-0012